Modeling and Simulation in Science, Engineering, & Technology

A Survey of Models for Tumor-Immune System Dynamics

John A. Adam
Nicola Bellomo
Editors

Birkhäuser
Boston • Basel • Berlin

John A. Adam
Department of Mathematics
Old Dominion University
Norfolk, Virginia 23529-0077
USA

Nicola Bellomo
Dipartimento di Matematica
Politecnico di Torino
10129 Torino
Italy

Library of Congress Cataloging-in-Publication Data

Adam, John A.
A survey of models for tumor immune systems dynamics / John Anthony Adam, Nicola Bellomo.
p. cm. -- (Modelling and simulation in science, engineering, and technology)
Includes bibliographical references.
ISBN 0-8176-3901-2 ISBN 3-7643-3901-2
1. Tumors--Immunological aspects--Computer simulation. 2. Tumors--Immunological aspects--Mathematical models. I. Bellomo, N.
II. Title. III. Series.
QR188.6.A33 1996
616.99'2079--dc20 96-38754
CIP

Printed on acid-free paper

Birkhäuser

ISBN 0-8176-3901-2
ISBN 3-7643-3901-2
Camera-ready text prepared by the Author in TEX.
Printed and bound by Maple-Vail, York, PA.
Printed in the U.S.A.

9 8 7 6 5 4 3 2 1

CONTENTS

Preface xi

Chapter 1. A Brief History of Immunologic Thinking: Is it Time for Yin and Yang? 1

1.1 Koch's Postulates 2

1.2 Aristotle's Laws of Logical Argument 4

1.3 Antigens and T-Cell Responses 5

1.4 Thinking About the Immune System 8

1.5 Fuzzy T-Cell Model 10

1.6 Acknowledgment 13

Chapter 2. General Aspects of Modeling Tumor Growth and Immune Response 15

2.1 Introduction 15

2.2 What is a Mathematical Model? 17

2.2.1 Why are mathematical models useful? . . 17

2.2.2 Limitations of mathematical models . . . 17

2.2.3 Other considerations 18

2.3 Introduction to Deterministic Tumor (or Spheroid) Growth Models 21

2.3.1 Basic models: Description 21

2.3.2 Basic diffusion models: Mathematical aspects 26

2.3.3 Diffusion of growth inhibitor 29

2.3.4 Time-evolutionary diffusion models . . . 34

2.4 A Predator-Prey Approach 48

2.5 A Model of Tumor Cell/Immune System Interaction 54

2.6 Models, Metaphors and Similes: Some Alternative Paradigms . . . 62

2.6.1 The tunneling phenomenon . . . 63

2.6.2 Some speculation . . . 64

2.7 References . . . 66

2.8 Appendices . . . 75

2.8.1 Appendix I – Comments on catastrophe theory . . . 75

2.8.2 Appendix II – Solution existence, uniqueness, stability and bifurcation and the inverse problem . . . 82

Chapter 3. Mathematical Modeling of Tumor Growth Kinetics . . . 89

3.1 Introduction . . . 90

3.2 Tumor Growth as a Dynamical System . . . 92

3.2.1 Construction of growth rate functions . . . 93

3.3 The Gompertz Model . . . 97

3.3.1 Gompertz model as a simple dynamical system . . . 98

3.3.2 Gompertz model as an S-system . . . 99

3.3.3 Gompertz model and quiescence . . . 100

3.3.4 Gompertz model and cell kinetics . . . 101

3.3.5 Gompertz model and entropy . . . 103

3.3.6 Gompertz model and tumor heterogeneity 105

3.3.7 Other explanations and analyses of Gompertz model . . . 107

3.4 The Logistic Model . . . 107

3.5 Models of von Bertalanffy . . . 109

3.6 Tumor Growth Modeled by Specific Mechanisms . . . 111

3.6.1 Competition among cell populations . . . 111

3.6.2 Cell cycle kinetics and regulation by growth factors . . . 113

3.6.3 Positive feedback mechanisms in tumors . 117

3.7 Mathematical Models and Measured Growth Curves 122

3.7.1 Growth data and Gompertz model . . . 122

3.7.2 Comparative studies of deterministic tumor growth models 123

3.8 Concluding Outlooks 126

3.9 Acknowledgment 127

3.10 References 128

Chapter 4. Tumor Immune System Interactions: The Kinetic Cellular Theory 135

4.1 Introduction 136

4.2 A Concise Guide to the Literature 137

4.3 Guidelines: From Observation to Simulation . . 140

4.4 Cell Population and Activity 142

4.5 Modeling Cell Interactions 145

4.6 Evolution Kinetic Equations 148

4.7 Experimental Activity 154

4.7.1 Transition to neoplastic behavior and tumor proliferation 154

4.7.2 Preimmunization and recognition of antigens 156

4.7.3 Cytokine genes 158

4.8 Simulation and Validation Problems 159

4.8.1 Simulation methods 160

4.8.2 Some identification and validation problems 161

4.8.3 Discrete models 175

4.9 Remarks Addressed to Applied Mathematicians 176

4.10 Perspectives 178

4.11 References 180

Chapter 5. From Mutation to Metastasis: The Mathematical Modelling of the Stages of Tumour Development 187

5.1 Introduction 188

5.2 Avascular Tumour Growth: The Multicell Spheroid Model 190

5.2.1 Results 195

5.3 Tumour Angiogenesis. Capillary Sprout Formation and Growth 200

5.3.1 Model improvements and extension . . . 211

5.3.2 Numerical simulations 212

5.4 Vascular Tumour Growth 219

5.4.1 Results 223

5.5 Discussion and Conclusions 226

5.6 References 229

Chapter 6. Basic Models of Tumor-Immune System Interactions Identification, Analysis and Predictions . 237

6.1 Introduction 238

6.2 Kinetics Models of Cellular Cytotoxic Reactions at the Effector Stage of Immune Response . . 241

6.2.1 Solutions of the model at quasi-stationary approximation 244

6.2.2 Comparison of the minimal model with experimental data 245

6.3 Regulatory Cells at the Effector Stage of the Cellular Immune Response 257

6.4 Modeling of the Recognition Mechanisms of Tumor Cells by NK-like Cells 261

6.5 Switch of Cytolytic Mechanisms: Effector Cells, Target Cells and Bispecific Regulating Molecules 270

6.5.1 Kinetics of the multiple cytotoxic reactions 271

6.5.2 General model 273
6.5.3 Kinetics of ADCC/LDCC reactions . . . 275
6.5.4 One effector cell and two molecular mechanisms recognition 277
6.5.5 Conclusion 279
6.6 Propagation and Interaction of Tumor Specific Macromolecules in Multicellular Tumors . . . 279
6.7 Conclusion 284
6.8 Acknowledgment 285
6.9 References 285

Chapter 7. Tumor Heterogeneity and Growth Control 295
7.1 Introduction 296
7.2 The Goal 296
7.3 The Plan 297
7.4 The Foundation and Tools 298
7.4.1 Distributional heterogeneity and models of the cell cycle 298
7.4.2 Epigenetic heterogeneity and environmental factors in the development of a heterogeneous milieu 300
7.4.3 Intrinsic heterogeneity and subpopulation emergence 302
7.4.4 Intrinsic heterogeneity and interacting populations 304
7.4.5 Our models of tumor growth 307
7.5 The Structure 310
7.5.1 Paradigm #1: Tumor dormancy 310
7.5.2 Paradigm #2: Interlocking growth control 315
7.5.3 Paradigm #3: Concomitant resistance . . 320
7.6 Conclusions 325
7.7 References 326

Chapter 8. Biological Glossary 335

Editors' Acknowledgment

I gratefully acknowledge the patience and writing help of Gayle Tarkelson and Barbara Jeffrey, without whom my (J.A.) chapter bound not have been completed, and the mechanics of co-editing this book would have been very complex! I would also like to thank my friend and colleague, Dr. John Tweed, for his constant encouragement, and who, as Chair of the Department, provided a working environment that was conducive to the many activities associated with the completion of this project.

Finally, I would like to thank my wife Susan, for her love and companionship over the years, and who was willing to leave the country and continent and settle on the other side of Atlantic Ocean. To her I dedicate my contribution to this book.

John Adam

This book is dedicated to my wife Fiorella and to my son Piero.

Nicola Bellomo

PREFACE

Mathematical Modeling and Immunology

An enormous amount of human effort and economic resources has been directed in this century to the fight against cancer. The purpose, of course, has been to find strategies to overcome this hard, challenging and seemingly endless struggle. We can readily imagine that even greater efforts will be required in the next century. The hope is that ultimately humanity will be successful; success will have been achieved when it is possible to activate and control the immune system in its competition against neoplastic cells.

Dealing with the above-mentioned problem requires the fullest possible cooperation among scientists working in different fields: biology, immunology, medicine, physics and, we believe, mathematics. Certainly, biologists and immunologists will make the greatest contribution to the research. However, it is now increasingly recognized that mathematics and computer science may well able to make major contributions to such problems. We cannot expect mathematicians alone to solve fundamental problems in immunology and (in particular) cancer research, but valuable support, however modest, can be provided by mathematicians to the research aspirations of biologists and immunologists working in this field.

The interplay between mathematics and the natural sciences occurs in the arena of modeling complex systems and computer-aided simulations of analytic or numerical models. A mathematical model therefore finds its location midway between phenomenological observation and physical reality. It can be regarded as an attempt to provide a description of that reality by means of mathematical constructs and/or computational algorithms. It is not claimed that a model may precisely simulate physical reality, but that it may in some sense be a good approximation.

Ideally, then, mathematical models contribute to an understanding of the real system which is being modeled. Such simulation helps us to look at reality more deeply and with heightened understanding, but in many case, however accurate the observations and however sophisticated the experimental devices used for measurements may be, the system is still too complex to be deeply understood. A mathematical model may decompose the system into relatively simple elements and attempt to reproduce some particular behaviors of those elements. Eventually, it may contribute to a substantial understanding at least of some selected aspects of such a system.

Simulation provides the capability of visualizing the above-mentioned behaviors. This can be of considerable support to experimental research by reducing the cost of expensive experiments and shortening the investigation times. Thus the cost-effectiveness of collaboration between mathematicians and immunologists may be very high, especially in view of the potential social impact success would bring.

Ideally we anticipate that a physico-mathematical theory will eventually be available to describe the dynamics of the immune system and its competition with tumor cells. We are not close to this objective. It seems that it may be necessary to develop new mathematics (or at least, utilize other existing mathematical approaches) and design architectures in computer devices for such a purpose. Obviously it is necessary to make a serious commitment to this ultimate goal in order to promote high quality research. This collection of surveys was designed with the aim of addressing the above-mentioned objective. Although the final result is extremely distant, the surveys represent, it is to be hoped, a small but valuable step towards the desired outcome.

This book reports some of the current research modeling the interactions between tumor cells and the immune system. We hope that a synergistic collaboration between applied mathematicians and immunologists will become recognized by the broader scientific community. As a result of editing this book, we have become convinced that such collaborations are already developing.

The contents should also be of interest to applied mathematicians not currently in this field, who may nonetheless be stimulated by some of the new and challenging problems posed within the book. These problems often relate to qualitative analysis of initial and initial-boundary value problems associated with the models described in the book, as well as relating to the development of computational methods appropriate for quantitative analysis and simulation. Some of these problems are on the frontiers of applied mathematics.

Contents

The contents are organized into eight chapters. The first two chapters also play the role of introduction. The first is the viewpoint of the immunologists; the second from that of an applied mathematician. The chapters that follow develop more specific technical features, which are briefly described below. The final chapter is a glossary which collects terms in the field of immunology and biology that have been used throughout the book. Its purpose is to alleviate the sometimes difficult dialogue between applied mathematicians and immunologists.

The first chapter by Curti and Longo is an introduction to the topics under discussion from the viewpoint of immunologists. This chapter concisely summarizes the historical background of the general philosophical framework in immunology. It subsequently addresses the description of current research activity in molecular biology and of its relationship with cancer research. It is noted that despite the great expansion and advances in this field, the level of success in devising effective therapy against cancer has been modest at best. The pertinent question to be asked is: why has such knowledge not been translated into more effective methods of cancer treatment?

The Authors, in developing an answer to the above question, start a dialogue with mathematicians and suggest examination of the interplay between cellular immune system and T-cell by examining fuzzy T-cell models. Immunologists who may not be well-acquainted with the formalized structures of mathematics nevertheless have great insight: they suggest that the governing mechanisms are developed at a cellular level with non-deterministic interactions. Such insight can also help indicate where to look for the most interesting (i.e. fundamental) interactions.

The dialogue between immunologists and mathematicians is not an easy one. The two languages are well separated. However in this chapter mathematicians are challenged by two immunologists to a demanding but fascinating collaborative effort. As noted above, mathematicians are beginning to understand that new paths (and perhaps new mathematics) are (is) necessary to meet the challenge. Each step of the way must be verified by immunologists. Some replies by mathematicians are already contained in this book, in that several of the chapters refer directly or indirectly to the content of this first essay.

The second chapter by Adam can be regarded as a link between the approach which is appropriate for biologists and the procedures developed in the field by mathematicians. This chapter is about mathematical modeling and is a review of many of the models proposed in the literature, particularly those which are based on diffusion processes in the spheroid or pre-vascular nodular state. The governing equations are closely related to those of classical mathematical physics (and as such this chapter is a suitable precursor for chapter 5 by Chaplain), e.g. the diffusion equation, Poisson's equation, reaction-diffusion equations, etc. The chapter commences with a summary of the philosophy and methodology of mathematical modeling, followed by a brief description of the observational features of prevascular spheroid growth that are relevant to deterministic, continuum-type models. The mathematical aspects of basic growth and diffusion models are set in a somewhat historical context, and, not surprisingly therefore, utilize increasingly sophisticated mathematics (though of course a simple model may well be more valuable at times than a more complicated one!). The process of modeling is subsequently illustrated by means of both a predator-prey paradigm (for lymphocyte/tumor cell dynamics) and a one-dimensional reaction-diffusion equation (illustrating other aspects of tumor cell/immune system interaction). The chapter concludes with a somewhat speculative section on possible alternative levels of description, i.e. other windows through which to view cancer/immune response phenomena: catastrophe theory and (non-quantized) scattering or tunneling theory. Two appendices (one describing aspects of catastrophe theory) are provided.

The third chapter by Bajzer, Huzak and Vuk-Pavlović provides a coherent and integrated survey of mathematical models, wherein the growing tumor is regarded as a deterministic dynamical system represented by ordinary differential equations.

They first examine general features of a single first-order autonomous equation, discuss the construction of growth rate functions, and then analyze in considerable detail the mathematical structure and biological implications of the Gompertz growth law. The logistic and von Bertalanffy models are also briefly examined. Different aspects of tumor growth kinetics are reviewed: competition among cell populations, cell cycle kinetics and regulation by growth factors and positive feedback mechanisms in tumors.

The authors also point out that, despite the many mathematical models proposed in the literature to describe and predict various aspects of tumor growth, only the Gompertz model has been extensively tested against measured tumor growth data. A summary of such work to date is provided, along with guidelines on direction of future studies.

The fourth chapter by Bellomo, Preziosi and Forni is a survey of the the so-called *cellular kinetic theory*. This theory is based on methods, typical of nonequilibrium statistical mechanics, which describe interactions and their evolution at the cellular level. This class of models deals with several populations of interacting cells belonging to degenerate neoplastic cells, the environment and the immune system.

The activity of a cell is regulated by genes contained on its nucleus. These are activated or suppressed by signals from their environment received by selective receptors expressed on the cell surface and transduced to the nucleus. In extreme cases, particular signals can induced a cell to (i) reproduce itself in the form of a clone of identical descendants (clonal expansion) or (ii) die and disappear virtually without trace (apoptosis or programmed cell death).

The cellular kinetic theory describes the evolution of the statistical distribution of cell populations due to cellular interactions that are governed by such signals. This theory is developed for the early stage of the tumor, when neoplastic cells have not yet condensed or are still at the stage of small clusters.

The contents of this chapter can be regarded as an attempt to develop a physico-mathematical theory in a similar vein to the approach of

Chapter 5, the differences being due essentially to scale. Chapter 4 applies to the cellular regime whereas Chapter 5 is formulated in the framework of continuum theory.

The fifth chapter by Chaplain is a review of modeling growth of solid tumors by means of partial differential equations of mathematical physics (see also Chapter 2), generally reaction diffusion and related equations. The models describe several interesting features that are typical of such physical systems, e.g. moving boundaries, surface interactions, energy distribution, stability/instability etc.

In more detail the development of solid tumors occurs typically in two stages: the avascular growth phase and the vascular growth phase. During the former phase, the tumor remains in a diffusion-limited, dormant state with the geometry being that of a spheroid (again, this relates to material in Chapter 2). During the latter phase, more sophisticated surface phenomena occur. Tumors may secrete diffusible substances (called tumor angiogenesis factors) into the surrounding tissues. Endothelial cells respond to this chemotactic stimulus in an ordered sequence of events. Capillary sprouts are formed which migrate towards the tumor, eventually penetrate it and vascular growth takes place. In this stage, or shortly thereafter, invasion and metastasis may occur.

The models reviewed in this chapter can be regarded as developments of models of classical mathematical physics to describe the complex events outlined above. It is worthy of mention that the models are able to describe, and at macroscopic level, explain several characteristic features of tumor growth and development. They are closely tied to observational data.

The structural difference between the contents of Chapter 4 and Chapter 5 is analogous to that which in mechanics can be observed between molecular kinetic theory and continuum theory. The exact nature of the link between the two theories is still an open problem. As we have already noted, an important contribution to the development of kinetic cellular theories is the analysis of cellular interactions. Again, the contribution is of similar type to the one provided by molecular physics to nonequilibrium statistical mechanics. Some aspects of this analysis are developed in Chapter 6.

The sixth chapter by Kuznetsov reports the relevant research developed by a cadre of Russian scientists.

The analysis proceeds by modeling the phenomena in terms of ordinary differential equations in the framework of population dynamics models. This survey illustrates how the parameters of the models can be related to physical interpretation of the phenomena and the experimental activity.

Chapter 7 by Michelson and Leith deals with tumor heterogeneity and growth control. They define four types of heterogeneity that may occur *in vivo*, and the mathematical tools that have been developed to describe them. In the process they address the importance of stochastic models in describing cellular population growth (e.g. consistent with the observed asynchronous growth of such populations). They describe models of tumor growth based on the equations for species competition, but including terms describing sub-population emergence. The authors then apply the model to three different tumor growth phenomena: dormancy, interlocking growth control, and concomitant resistance. In each case they summarize the model by stating (i) what we know; (ii) what we think we know; (iii) what we wish we know; and in the light of (i)-(iii), (iv) a description of the appropriate experiments and their analyses.

The eighth chapter by Federica Cavallo and Katia Boggio is a glossary of scientific terms in biology and immunology addressed to applied mathematicians. We have already mentioned that the collaboration of mathematicians with scientists working in medical and immunological sciences may be of great value, and may indeed be necessary, however difficult this dialogue appears to be. This simple and concise guide towards the creation of a common language is a first step to overcome these difficulties.

Closure

The Editors of this volume have made a sincere effort to present to the scientific community some aspects of the "state of the art" in the field. Completeness is not claimed. Perhaps it cannot ever be realistically claimed in a field which is constantly developing and open to new ideas. On the other hand, we believe that this is an appropriate time to collect ideas and research reports in order to offer them both to scientists and mathematicians who will, it is to be hoped, continue this "battle" with renewed efforts.

John Adam and Nicola Bellomo

1

A Brief History of Immunologic Thinking: Is it Time for Yin and Yang?

B.D. CURTI

National Cancer Institute-Frederick
Cancer Research and Development Center
Clinical Research Branch, Division of Clinical Sciences
Frederick, MD, USA

AND
D.L. LONGO

National Institute on Aging
National Institutes of Health
Baltimore, MD, USA

ABSTRACT. Our understanding of tumor biology and the immune system has expanded greatly in the last decade. This explosion of knowledge can be attributed to advances in molecular biology. Despite these advances, our success in devising effective therapy against cancer has been modest at best. Why hasn't this new knowledge translated into more effective cancer treatment? This chapter discusses the limitations of applying traditional Aristotelian logic to complex biological systems. Alternative approaches for solving problems in immunology and cancer research, such as "fuzzy logic" are described.

1.1 Koch's Postulates

There has been an explosion of information about the immune system in the last two decades. Most of these new facts have been discovered by applying molecular and cell biology techniques. This technology has been a transforming event in biological sciences, and particularly in immunology. Classical immunologists described many facets of cellular and humoral immunity, and its power to destroy foreign tissues, organisms, or even tumors. However, the reasons for these powers were ill-defined, and deduced indirectly. Subjective descriptions of immunologic events using a qualitative scale were the only means of characterizing immune activity. These characterizations were usually based on challenging the immune system with a complex stimulus (e.g., heat-treated bacteria) and measuring a complicated response (e.g., resistance to future infections) on a scale from 1+ to 4+. Despite these crude methods, successful vaccines were developed against a range of pathogens including small pox, anthrax, diphtheria, and rabies.

KOCH's POSTULATES

1) The organism is regularly found in the lesions of the disease.
2) The organism can be isolated in pure cultures on artificial media.
3) Inoculation of this culture produces a similar disease in experimental animals.
4) The organism can be recovered in the lesions of the inoculated animals.

Jenner, Pasteur, and Koch made these advances with less knowledge about the mechanics of the immune system than many individuals today have about the Internet. The intellectual foundation for many of these discoveries are Koch's Postulates, which are still used today to solve problems in clinical medicine and all basic biologic sciences. Koch established the ground-rules for biologic discovery. They are as important to biology as Euclid's Postulates are to geometry. By using Koch's framework to interpret the results of our more sophisticated experiments today, we can routinely identify different immune cell types and behaviors, specific antibodies, antigens, signaling proteins, cell surface receptors, cytokines, growth factors, and the genes and regulatory proteins that control them.

Paradoxically, many recent insights about the immune system have come from the study of AIDS, a disease that destroys immune function.

This new knowledge suggests that we are entering an age of enlightenment about the immune system that will easily translate into treatment advances in cancer, AIDS, infectious diseases, and autoimmune processes. We should be making impressive advances in immune-based treatments, since our understanding of normal immune function and pathophysiology has increased exponentially. Although the complexity of immunotherapy regimens in cancer has also increased exponentially, the increase in efficacy of these treatments is changing in a linear fashion. It is as yet unclear if the slope of the line that describes treatment efficacy is positive or negative. One could even suggest that chance, and not reason, links basic knowledge in biology, and progress in clinical medicine, at least as it applies to cancer treatment. The vast majority of agents and regimens in use today were not the product of rational design; they were discovered empirically or even accidentally. This observation is particularly true of cancer therapy, and is magnified with immunotherapy regimens. When progress does occur, a rationale is chosen post hoc. For trials that fail or generate unexpected toxicities, it is distinctly unusual to find supported explanations for why they failed. Despite the apparent failure of reason in the design of successful cancer treatments, there have been some remarkable successes, just as in the development of early vaccines for infectious diseases. Examples include chemotherapy for Hodgkin's and non-Hodgkin's lymphoma, testicular cancer, and some leukemias. Intermittent reinforcement is even more prevalent in cancer immunotherapy, where interleukin-2 and a variety of other agents produce occasional dramatic and durable responses in solid tumors refractory to chemotherapy and radiation therapy. However, the journals are literally packed with clinical trials based upon a clear scientifically justified rationale, sometimes even an elegant one, that simply did not work. And we do not know why.

Why have huge increases in basic knowledge not translated into clinical success? Even simple prokaryotic organisms are complicated; perhaps we need even more basic knowledge about normal human molecular physiology and the changes that occur in cancer to design effective treatments. Although several million compounds have been screened for anticancer activity, only a few dozen have proved clinically useful. It is possible that we have sufficient knowledge to design successful chemo- or immunotherapy regimens, but we lack good medications. Certainly there is no shortage of clever hypotheses about how to use new knowledge or new agents to treat cancer and other medical conditions. Perhaps the occasional victories in cancer treatment are counter-productive, because they serve as a reason for clinical researchers to persist in thinking in the same ways about disease, and about the agents we have at our disposal. If arriving at an effective treatment by one approach was successful, why not employ the same thought process as we gain new (and presumably more perfect) knowledge about cancer biology, treatment agents, and the immune system? To decide if our clinical thinking is sound, let us examine how basic scientific facts are assembled by researchers and applied by clinicians to design new cancer treatments.

1.2 Aristotle's Laws of Logical Argument

Virtually all medical thinking is derived using variations of Koch's Postulates, which are a biologic application of Aristotelian logic, and are descended from the scientific method described by Galileo. Aristotle's Organum first laid out the framework for logical argument.

ARISTOTLE'S LAWS OF LOGICAL ARGUMENT

1) The law of identity (If A is true, then A is true)
2) The law of contradiction (A cannot be both true and false)
3) The law of the excluded middle (A is either true or false)

This framework can be distilled into a sequence of three propositions (two premises and a conclusion), which together compose a syllogism (i.e., if A implies B, and B implies C, then A implies C). In addition, there are three basic laws of Aristotelian logic: the law of identity (If A is true, then A is true); the law of contradiction (A cannot be both true and false); and the law of the excluded middle (A is either true or false). In basic medical science, biologic events are dissected in a similar fashion. We'll use a simple example from basic cellular immunology to illustrate a "biologic proof". This proof will take us through the medical thought process that is commonly used to develop both chemotherapy and immunotherapy regimens for cancer. The elements of the proof are as follows: If a T-cell receptor encounters an antigen specific for that receptor, then a signal is sent from the receptor to the nucleus. This signal will cause T-cell activation. Therefore an appropriate receptor-antigen encounter causes T-cell activation. There are of course many additional steps and conditions involved in the activation of a T cell after encountering an antigen, but we won't consider any of these complexities for now. Let's now examine how each of these biologic propositions comes together to form a syllogism. We are presuming that each statement in this causal chain is axiomatic. Indeed, each statement is accepted as a biologic fact or ground rule (we will later examine how each statement became an axiom). The proposition "A" corresponds to the T-cell receptor encountering an appropriate antigen. "B" is the signaling event between the receptor-antigen complex and the nucleus. "C" is the activation of the T cell. Selected examples of how events in this causal chain comply with Aristotle's Laws are as follows: A particular T-cell receptor always interacts with one and only one antigen (If A is true, then A is true). The T-cell receptor cannot simultaneously interact with its specific antigen and some other antigen [A cannot be both true and false (in this case a "false receptor" would be a T-cell receptor for another antigen)]. Similarly, the T-cell receptor either encounters its antigen and sends a signal, or it encounters the wrong antigen and does nothing (A is either true or false). According to this model, a T-cell receptor does not send a 50% signal under any circumstances.

1.3 Antigens and T-Cell Responses

Why is each statement in our biologic proof axiomatic? Each proposition was derived using a variant of Koch's Postulates (KP), and is therefore "proven". Instead of organisms and diseases, which were the causes and effects of interest to Koch, we shall refer to antigens and T-cell responses. We'll take an example from recent work in cancer immunology performed by Dr. Steven Rosenberg's lab at the National Cancer Institute. This work has translated into a number of clinical protocols. MART-1 is a peptide antigen regularly found in melanoma deposits, along with specific T cells that react with MART-1 (KP#1). MART-1 can be isolated from melanoma cell lines (KP#2). Inoculation (vaccination) with MART-1 in an appropriate animal model can expand T cells that react with MART-1, but other proteins will not cause the same expansion of specific T cells (KP#3). MART-1 can be isolated from tumor nodules arising after inoculation of MART-1-expressing cell lines into suitable animals (KP#4). Basic scientists usually make biologic proofs more stringent by demonstrating that removing or blocking the protein or gene of interest will abrogate the expected effect. In this example, antibodies to MART-1 should abrogate T-cell responses to MART-1, and indeed they do. A large number of biologic axioms have been accumulated by the process described above. These axioms are then strung together to describe larger chunks of biologic behavior. Clinical researchers design treatment regimens around axioms that are proven or suspected to be involved in a particular disease. In cancer research, new drugs, drug combinations, or manipulations of the immune system seek to correct or delete the biologic axioms corrupted by the cancer (surgeons provide a trivial but sometimes highly effective solution by removing all visible manifestations of the cancer).

It would seem that designing an effective treatment is easy, once valid biologic axioms and syllogisms are known. To continue with the example described above, MART-1 and other antigen-specific cancer vaccines have been given to appropriately selected patients. The expected result was that MART-1-specific T cells should activate and attack tumor cells bearing the MART-1 antigen. Although clinical trials based on such specific mechanisms are still early in their evolution, the results thus far are extremely disappointing. What went wrong? One possible answer (although there are many other alternative answers) is suggested by our work together with our colleague, Dr. Augusto Ochoa, describing defects in the T-cell receptor and signaling pathways in cancer patients. We found that the zeta chain, a normal component of CD3 (a multimeric protein found in association with the T-cell receptor complex), was absent or diminished in peripheral blood T cells of approximately 50% of cancer patients. In addition, T cells infiltrating tumor masses show these defects more commonly. Furthermore, melanoma patients who had no zeta expression in their peripheral blood T cells had a significantly shorter overall survival than melanoma patients who had normal zeta expression. The zeta chain is the component of the T-cell receptor complex that generates the signal to the nucleus that activates the T cell. So if there is no zeta chain in a significant proportion of cancer patients, then no activation signal can be generated if our proof is otherwise correct. Any cancer treatment based on the previously described T-cell syllogism falls apart when the zeta chain is absent. One can argue that our syllogism broke down because of a less than perfect knowledge of T-cell behavior in cancer. The answer is to fix the zeta chain.

Did this system break down from a lack of knowledge, or some other problem? As we probe more deeply into the molecular machinery of normal cells, organs, and tumors there seems to be no limit to the number of physiologic pathways, signaling molecules, genes, and regulatory elements that play important roles. The number of biologic pathways and components may be vast, but not infinite, since even cancer cells have a finite number of constituent molecules. Certainly, our knowledge is less than complete. We do not know how many interleukins, inflammatory mediators, chemokines, or interferons the immune system produces. Interleukin-132 (expected discovery by the year 2046) may be the most potent anti-cancer cytokine. Many of our biologic syllogisms suffer from our intellectual hubris. We know many more isolated facts than we did even a few years ago, but we are too willing to fill in gaps in our knowledge with results from necessarily simplistic in vitro or animal models.

We try to deduce things about cancer from the fragments of information that we have about it. Of course, Sherlock Holmes was the master of deduction. At the beginning of "The Sign of Four", Watson hands Holmes a pocket watch he has recently come to own and asks him to tell him about its owner. After careful inspection, Holmes states that the watch belonged to Watson's elder brother, who inherited it from his father. The brother was a man of untidy habits who was left with good prospects, but he squandered his resources, lived for a considerable time in poverty punctuated by intermittent intervals of prosperity. He finally took to drinking heavily and died. The account was accurate in every detail. How did he know all this? The watch had the initials HW on the back and was an old watch. Because jewelry generally passes to the eldest son, he assumed it was John Watson's father's watch originally that became his older brother's watch. The lower part of the watch case was scratched and dented suggesting that the watch was kept in the same pocket with other metal objects such as keys and coins, clearly the action of a careless man of untidy habits. If he had inherited such an expensive watch, it was likely he had inherited other wealth. It must have been squandered away because there were numbers etched into the case by pawnbrokers who had provided cash in its exchange. There were four sets of numbers suggesting that the watch had been pawned and redeemed several times, thus, the intermittent financial solvency of the owner is inferred. Finally, the inner plate contained the keyhole which displayed thousands of scratches all around the hole where the key had slipped. It was customary to wind the watch at night before bedtime and the scratches reveal the unsteady hand of a drunkard. Elementary. Holmes accurately perceives all that he can objectively, uses a rather focused comprehensive body of knowledge that he has mastered, and makes some lucky guesses.

Now let's look at an example from another well-known deductive logician, Winnie-the-Pooh. Winnie desires some honey and knows there is a bee hive high in a particular tree. He thinks very hard about the problem and decides that he will disguise himself as a rain cloud by covering himself with dark mud and he will float up to the hive with a blue balloon that looks like the sky. However, it is an otherwise sunny day. As he implements the plan, it is quite clear that the bees are not fooled by his disguise, so he gets Christopher Robin to march around underneath the tree with an open umbrella saying things like "It looks like rain". His plan fails and he gets no honey. His interpretation of his failure is that the bees were the wrong sort of bees.

The path from effects to causes is an obscure one for mere mortals. Three things are required: the power of observation, the power of deduction, and a comprehensive knowledge of the nature of things. According to Sherlock Holmes, all of life is a great chain, the nature of which is known whenever we are shown a single link of it. From a drop of water, one could infer the possibility of an ocean or a waterfall without having seen or heard of them. Unfortunately, for those of us trying to understand human cancer and the host response to it, such insights are not generally present. We are capable of making observations and deductions based on those observations, but we have nowhere near enough knowledge of the nature of things to intuit from our observations how to intervene to alter the course. We resemble Winnie-the-Pooh to a much greater extent than we do Sherlock Holmes.

1.4 Thinking About the Immune System

There is no general comprehension of the biological world. There is nothing remotely approaching a unified field theory that ties together the current extent of molecular knowledge in cellular biology, immunology, and cancer. Of course, there are some scientific observations that are simplifying and clarifying. From the structure of DNA, its replication became more readily understandable. The complexity of the class I Major Histocompatibility Complex antigens became immeasurably clarified by the insight by Donald Shreffler that the myriad of epitopes recognized by a bewildering panoply of antisera were identifying two different gene products at different loci. By contrast, we seem currently to be at a stage where each new discovery, rather than simplifying, adds complexity to our image of how things work. Sir Francis Bacon in the 1620's observed this problem in Western science based on Aristotelian thinking. The quote from the Novum Organum eloquently expresses these sentiments. Hard work, modesty, patience, and a large supply of graduate students would only be a partial solution to this knowledge gap.

> *The human understanding from its peculiar nature, easily supposes a greater degree of order and equality in things than it really finds; and although many things in nature be sui generis and most irregular, will yet invent parallels and conjugates and relatives, where no such thing is.*
>
> Sir Francis Bacon, *Novum Organum*

There is deeper problem in our thinking about biologic processes, and particularly about the immune system. Virtually all immunologically important molecules (cytokines, chemokines, growth factors, and interferons) have a very wide range of biologic effects.

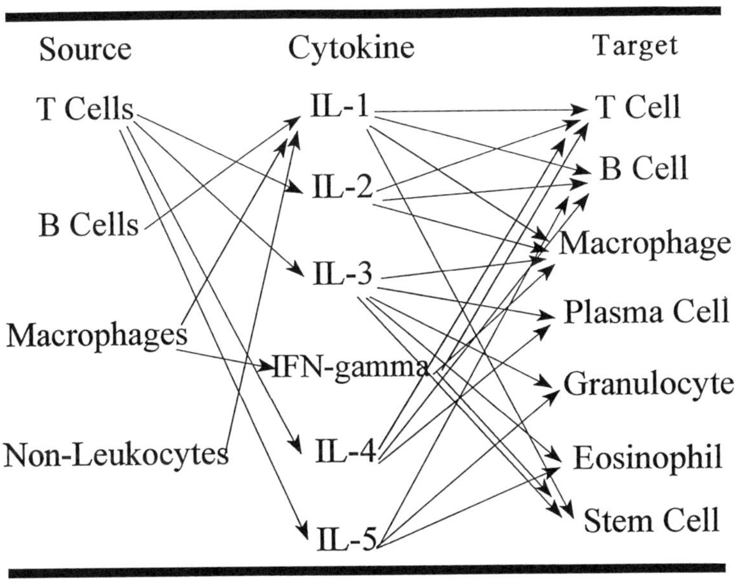

Figure 1.1 — Partial listing of overlapping properties for cytokines in the immune system.

As illustrated in the accompanying figure, the activity of one cytokine almost universally overlaps other cytokines, influences the behavior of many cell types, and can be stimulatory or inhibitory depending on the circumstances. These contradictory axioms can all be proven independent of each other and are consistent in simple systems, but when juxtaposed create mayhem. For instance, sometimes an antigen can stimulate a T cell, other times the same signal is inhibitory, or can even result in cell death. T cells can be resting, a little activated, or fully activated. Sometimes only humoral immunity is promoted (Th2 behavior), while at other times T cells will predominantly stimulate cellular immunity (Th1 behavior). A T-cell receptor can be activated not only by one specific antigen, but other antigens that are similar, or by superantigens that activate entire families of T cells. Superantigens bind to a portion of the T-cell receptor outside the normal antigen-binding groove, and thus can activate multiple clones of T cells. The "amount" of yin and yang displayed not only in the immune system, but in all biologic systems, violates the laws of Western logic. Our current notions of identity, contradiction, and the excluded middle and how we apply them are not consonant with biologic reality. It appears that Aristotle was not consulted in the design of the immune system. Unfortunately, in our devotion to Aristotle, we select those axioms that support the particular biologic proof we wish to create and ignore the inconsistencies that might refute our proof. It should be no surprise that predicting the success of clinical trials based on such selective logic requires the services of a crystal ball.

If Aristotle can't help us to do clinical cancer research and immunology, then who can? Certainly the tools of applied mathematics and statistics are useful. This book is devoted to modeling ideas that describe tumor growth kinetics, patterns of angiogenesis and tumor growth, and how the immune system interacts with tumors. This approach will allow basic scientists and clinicians to view tumors and the immune system as dynamic entities. It is reasonable to propose that treatment hypotheses will be tested in computer models that are perhaps better approximations of reality than current animal or in vitro models. Unfortunately, very few clinical or basic scientists have even rudimentary "literacy" skills in mathematics and statistics. It will be a challenge to overcome this gap in our training and bring these valuable modeling tools to the clinic and lab.

1.5 Fuzzy T-Cell Model

Another possible answer to the shortcomings of Aristotle comes from the relatively new science of "fuzzy logic". This field traces its formal origins to the philosopher Max Black, who published a paper in 1937 entitled: "Vagueness: An Exercise in Fuzzy Analysis". More recently, Bart Kosko has popularized these ideas in a book called Fuzzy Thinking. The term fuzzy logic is unfortunate because it connotes an imprecision that is antithetical to Western scientific thought, although quite in keeping with Eastern philosophical traditions. The rules that govern fuzzy logic are just as formal as the laws in Aristotle's Organum. Indeed, these fuzzy rules could be called "Buddha's Organum". Fuzzy logic applications have proven their utility in a variety of engineering problems ranging from designing a "smart" washing machine to running the Tokyo subway system. What makes fuzzy logic a more powerful tool than Aristotelian logic for biological problems? The answer lies in the ability of fuzzy logic to deal with shades of gray.

A T cell can be a little activated, moderately activated or fully activated in a fuzzy system. As we saw above, this situation is poorly handled by an Aristotelian approach. To illustrate the power of this new thinking tool, let us construct a fuzzy T-cell model.

FUZZY T-CELL MODEL
1) If the IFN-γ core promoter (CP) is hypomethylated, then T-cell behavior will be predominantly Th1.
2) If the CP is partially methylated, then T cells have both Th1 and Th2.
3) If the CP is highly methylated, then T cells will be predominantly Th2.

Fuzzy models approximate reality with a series of if-then rules. More rules can be written as more facts are known about a system. The rules are stated in words, but they can be translated into numbers. As shown in the model above, if-then clauses relate a measured lab test (the status of the interferon-γ core promotor protein) to different T-cell behaviors. One way to measure T-cell behavior is by assessing cytokine output. Th1 cells make IL-2 and interferon-γ. Th2 cells make predominantly IL-4, IL-5 and IL-10. Although this model is extremely simple, it is also relevant to cancer immunology. Th1 behavior is thought to be much more important in the immune response against tumors. The balance of Th1 and Th2 behavior can be assessed by measuring the methylation state of the interferon-γ core promoter binding protein. In preliminary clinical work, patients with renal carcinoma whose T cells were predominantly Th1 in phenotype had substantially higher response rates to treatment than patients who were Th2. This story also has ties to the zeta chain and signal transduction anomalies described above, but that is the subject of another model. How are these if-then clauses helpful? As shown in the accompanying figure, each "if" and "then" statement from the model is defined by a triangular range. Overlapping ranges describe a "patch" of immunologic behavior. If specific cytokine and CP methylation data are available, then a prediction can be made about the behavior of an individual patient's immune system. There are areas where Th1 and Th2 behavior overlap in this model. The less that is known about a system, the larger the areas of overlap have to be. The salient feature of this model is that a T cell doesn't have to be either fully activated, or completely inactive. The fuzzy middle is not excluded. These shades of gray provide a much better approximation of immunologic reality than does the Aristotelian model. Of course much more validation is needed before this particular model is clinically useful. Fuzzy systems can be built that teach themselves new rules. This feature is particularly attractive for describing normally homeostatic systems that have gone awry.

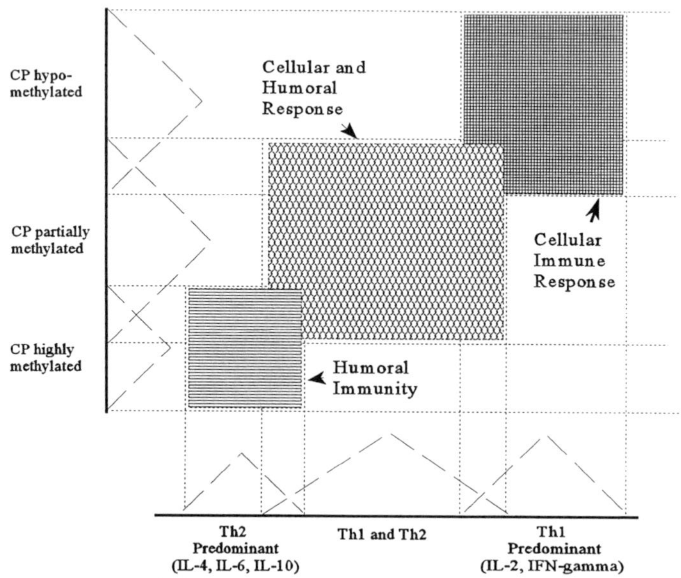

Figure 1.2 — Fuzzy model for Th1 and Th2 behavior in T cells.

We have found that even in disease states, human physiology is tightly regulated. When we push the system, it pushes back. When we strive to activate components of the immune response, we find negative regulatory pathways acting to dampen them. In order to model a remarkably complex system, fuzzy systems capable of learning new things may be valuable. Such learning systems have great potential in clinical research, and may supplant the need for crystal ball gazing in predicting medical outcomes in clinical trials.

The tools of molecular and cell biology have revealed a marvelous and daunting complexity inherent to biologic systems. As we probe the mysteries of the cell, more is found. We don't even have an appreciation of the limits of what we may find in normal cellular physiology and the abnormal behaviors of tumors. Although molecular and cell biology have allowed us to amplify our senses, they have not amplified our intellects to deal with this complexity. Our old methods of analysis hinder a useful comprehension of the immune system and how tumors interact with it. New intellectual tools are needed to expand our medical consciousness so that new clinical designs will reflect the non-Aristotelian reality of complex biological systems. The models described in this book are a positive step in the evolution of our thinking about the immune system and tumor biology.

1.6 Acknowledgment

The authors would like to thank Dr. Gregory Alvord for his critical reading of the chapter and many useful suggestions. Also, we are grateful for the help provided by Terry Jones in preparing the manuscript.

2

General Aspects of Modeling Tumor Growth and Immune Response

JOHN A. ADAM

Old Dominion University
Department of Mathematics and Statistics
Norfolk, VA, USA

ABSTRACT. This chapter opens with a summary of the philosophy and methodology of mathematical modeling (Sections 2.1 and 2.2). In Section 2.3 a survey of deterministic diffusion models of spheroid growth is provided. Section 2.4 addresses a particular type of model, based on a predator-prey description of the immune response to cancer illustrating the modeling process in some detail. This is followed in Section 2.5 by a spatially-dependent approach to the immune response in a one-dimensional system. Section 2.6 is more speculative in nature: the suggestion is made that the concepts of "tunneling" (as used in quantum mechanics) and "catastrophe" may be applicable to both the development of cancer and the effectiveness of the immune response. Two appendices follow on (i) catastrophe theory and (ii) certain mathematical properties of solutions to diffusion equations.

2.1 Introduction

Throughout this chapter, examples are chosen to illustrate some of the basic principles of mathematical modeling. Many of these are taken from the literature in the stated field. While to some extent they reflect the author's interest in this field, the examples are also chosen because, to one degree or another, they represent formative work or contain significant results that have provided the basis for a better understanding of the processes involved. In a "meta-modeling" sense, it is interesting to note how punctuated the evolutionary track of such models has been!

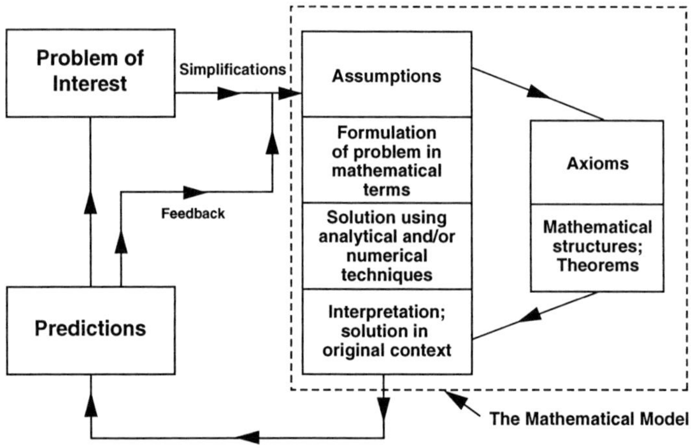

Figure 2.1 — Schematic representation of the basic stages of the mathematical modelling process, and their inter-relationships.

Much of mathematics is concerned with the derivation of hidden implications of systems of axioms: in "applied mathematics" these axioms are deemed to have been "distilled" from the original context of the subject of interest (e.g. Newton's laws of motion in classical mechanics). Mathematical modeling (which we discuss in detail below) has a characteristic philosophy and methodology (see the flow chart in Figure 2.1), which is to be contrasted with an empirical approach of inferring mechanisms from a finite (perhaps small) set of observations. While both approaches are prone to error, mathematical models operate in the opposite direction by postulating mechanisms and using mathematics to examine the consequences of those postulates (for a discussion of this in the context of immunology using the notion of rugged landscapes, see [PEa]). Related to these ideas is the question; given a general process (such as neoplasia), are there any general principles or universal features inherent in the process which may be subject to some level of mathematical analysis? With these comments in mind, we ask the following question:

2.2 What is a Mathematical Model?

Following [BDa], one definition might be: a mathematical model is an abstract, simplified mathematical construction related to part of the "real world" and created for a specific purpose. That is, it is designed to mimic reality by using the language of mathematics. (For the sake of completeness, we include computer simulations as part of the modeling process, though that will not be addressed in this chapter).

2.2.1 Why are mathematical models useful?

a) If we formulate our ideas precisely we are less likely to let implicit assumptions slip by us unnoticed.

b) We have at our disposal a concise language which encourages manipulation.

c) We have a large number of potentially useful theorems available.

d) Computational resources are generally available for carrying out calculations. More specifically, mathematical models can be used to:

   i) help confirm or reject hypotheses about complex systems;

   ii) reveal contradictions or incompleteness of data and/or hypotheses;

   iii) predict system performance under untested or presently untestable conditions;

   iv) predict and supply information on the values of experimentally inaccessible variables;

   v) mathematical models may suggest the existence of new phenomena. Indeed, in some respects it is the predictive capability of a model that is its most important feature (certainly for the scientist).

2.2.2 Limitations of mathematical models

a) The mathematically-accessible features of the model may be suboptimal.

b) Incorrect models may well fit limited data, leading to erroneous conclusions.

c) Simple models are easy to manage, but complicated models are often needed! There is a trade-off here. Models of the "back of the envelope" variety can be of great use, and may be more cost-effective than more sophisticated models. However, theory is useful for drawing general conclusions from simple models, and computers are useful for drawing specific conclusions from more complex models. Related to this point is:

d) Realistic simulations often require a large number of parameters (the values of which may be difficult to obtain). The resulting "parameter space" may be too large to draw meaningful conclusions for anything but lower-dimensional models (e.g. by "turning off" one or more parameters).

Thankfully for mathematicians (and others!) however, the advantages of modeling usually outweigh the disadvantages in the hands of a skilled practitioner of the art (yes, ART). Modeling can help us avoid, or reduce the need for costly, undesirable or impossible experiments with the real world. (Even scaled-down test models can be expensive). Examples are weather forecasting (there are some inherent limitations here quite apart from the modeling aspects we consider), space flight planning, germ warfare, nuclear reactor accidents, or even inferring how large a meteor was needed to eliminate the dinosaur population some 65 million years ago!

In mathematics we deal with abstract ideas and relationships between them; ideas like the concept of points, lines and planes. They may represent features of the real world such as a dot on a page, a line drawn on a page, or the page itself. Predictions based on the theory may lead to interesting results in the real world, and conversely, situations in the real world may suggest the development of mathematical ideas. This "two-way-ness" is very important; it does not necessarily always exist, but it has prompted the following comment by a physicist: "Ask not what physics can do for biology, but what biology can do for physics!" [STa]. We might well seek to replace the word "physics" by the phrase "mathematical modeling" in the present context!

2.2.3 Other considerations

As far as a mathematical model is concerned, the "world" can be divided into three components [BDa]:

i) Things whose effects are neglected.

ii) Things that affect the model but whose behavior the model is not designed to study. These are called independent (or exogenous variables).

iii) Things the model is designed to study (the dependent or endogenous variables).

This classification is important because it is implicit in every model we make, even if we are not aware of it! The model will be useless if we neglect the wrong things. If too much is included, the model will be too complex and confusing. Different models of the same situation, with different simplifying assumptions, can provide useful complementary insights and levels of description. However, "It is not possible to maximize simultaneously generality, realism, and precision" [LVa]; for example, in the social sciences one is often content with a statement that under certain circumstances, something will increase. Precision has been sacrificed for realism (hopefully) and generality. On the other hand, computer simulation models usually sacrifice generality for precision and realism.

Definitions of variables and their inter-relationships form the model (summarized in greater detail in the following scheme), i.e. if the assumptions are true, the conclusions must also be true. A false prediction implies the model is wrong in some respect.

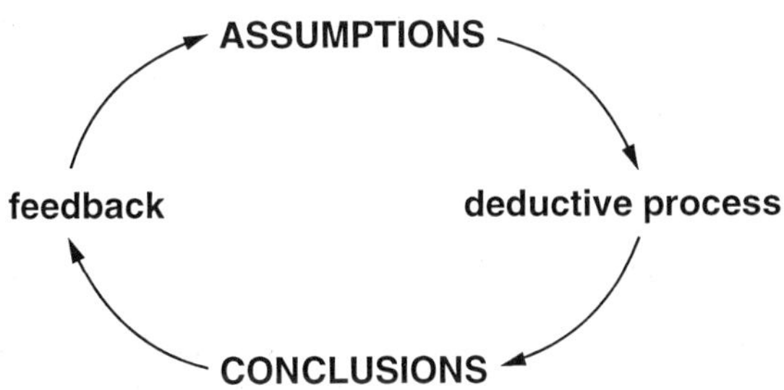

However, things are not generally as clear-cut as this; since the model is only an approximation, the conclusions drawn from it are in some sense, only approximate. Some models may be very sensitive to the assumptions built into them; other may be less so (that is, more robust).

The models provide **descriptions** of the situation, rather than **explanations**: two different models may have the same predictions but provide different descriptions (e.g. a symphony can be described in terms of physics or musical language).

Finally, it should be remembered that we are finite, limited, often biased human beings. The more open-minded, communicative and creative we can be, the better our model is likely to be. The onus is **us** to explain **our** model to the users (biologists, sociologists, etc.), not to leave **them** struggling to draw **their own** conclusions from **our** mathematics. In summary, the following abbreviated points can be made:

- Mathematical Model:
  The formulation in mathematical terms of the assumptions and their consequences believed to underlie a particular "real world" problem.
- The Aim of Mathematical Modeling:
  The practical application of mathematical models to help unravel the underlying mechanisms involved in biological (or other) processes.

- Pitfalls:
  Indiscriminate, naive or uninformed use of models.
- Models can:
  i) Provide insight into the nature of the problem.
  ii) Be useful in interpreting data.
  iii) Stimulate experiments.
- There is not necessarily a "right" model; producing results which are consistent with observations is only a first step and does not imply that the model is the only one that applies, or even that it is "correct".
- Mathematical descriptions are not explanations, and can never on their own provide a complete solution to the biological problem — there often may be complementary levels of description within the scientific paradigm.
- Collaboration with biologists is needed for realism and help in modifying the model mechanisms to reflect the biology more accurately.
- The biologists need to appreciate what mathematics (and its practitioners) can and cannot do! The mathematician needs to do the educating here! Good communication is necessary!
- The Art of Good Modeling relies on
  1) A sound understanding and appreciation of the biological problem.
  2) A realistic mathematical representation of the important biological phenomena.
  3) Finding useful solutions, preferably quantitative ones.
  4) A biological interpretation of the mathematical results (insights, predictions, etc.).
- The mathematics is dictated by the biology and not, in general, vice versa. Sometimes the mathematics used can be very simple. The usefulness of a mathematical model should not be judged by the sophistication of the mathematics, but by different (and no less demanding) criteria.
- While the techniques of statistical analysis may well be used in portraying and interpreting data, the term "Mathematical Model" here refers to deterministic (i.e. causal) models as opposed to probabilistic or statistical ones, though much of the above applies to these types of mathematical model also.

2.3 Introduction to Deterministic Tumor (or Spheroid) Growth Models

2.3.1 Basic models: Description

Within the last several decades a number of deterministic mathematical models of tumor growth by diffusion have been developed in the literature (e.g. Burton [BNa], Deakin [DEa], Greenspan [GRa–c], McElwain and Ponzo [MCa], King, Schultz and Gatenby [KIa]). Many of these models can be regarded as highly simplified but complementary levels of description for one aspect of a complex biological phenomenon: the growth and stability of tissue. The main objective of most of these models has been to describe in a qualitative fashion, the early (prevascular) stages of growth and stability of tissue, principally that of tumor tissue, under various simplifying assumptions. If the results so obtained can be compared and contrasted with the observations of tissue growth in vitro, then it may be possible to identify which simplifications are appropriate, and which are not, and subsequently to develop more sophisticated models. The principal advantage of those developed so far has been their mathematical simplicity, which has allowed the basic physics of diffusion processes in biological tissue to remain unobscured. Thus, in many cases, one-dimensional models have been studied, and the solutions have afforded considerable insight into the nature of the growth processes in more realistic geometries. In this section several basic models are discussed and the mathematical details are addressed in Section 2.3.2.

Perhaps the simplest and most schematic of these models has been that by Glass [GLa]. The basic mechanism in this model is that of tissue size regulation via negative feedback from the tissue itself (there is evidence that control of cellular replication in some mammalian tissue is at least partially determined by such a mechanism (Bullough, [BUa]). The agents of negative feedback ("chalones", or in more recent nomenclature, growth inhibitors) are tissue-specific, mitotic inhibitors produced by tissue, and it has been suggested that a breakdown in the normal functioning of the chalone mechanism may be responsible for limitless tissue growth in at least some types of cancer. Strong supporting evidence for this hypothesis comes from a study of the pattern of tumor growth (Bullough and Deol, [BUb]).

Glass's model [GLa] provides a limiting size for stable tissue growth, without describing the time-evolution of the tissue prior to that limiting state. He solves the one-dimensional diffusion equation in terms of a dimensionless number, n, which is defined by biological parameters describing the system. Shymko and Glass [SHa] carried over these ideas in considerable detail to take account of a more realistic spherical geometry obtaining agreement with results from tissue culture experiments of Folkman and Hochberg [FOd] (also see details in Folkman and Greenspan [FOb]). This was further developed for non-uniform production of inhibitor in [ADa–d].

Burton [BNa] studied the spatial distribution of oxygen and other nutrients diffusing in tissue, and later Greenspan [GRa,b] developed detailed models in which the effects of both inhibitor and nutrient were considered. In the latter paper, Greenspan examined a one-dimensional column of tissue and its subsequent self-regulating development, whereas in the former a spherically symmetric three-dimensional counterpart to this model was developed. That paper sets out with great clarity the basic assumptions that are built into such deterministic models. Both Burton and Greenspan assumed that the oxygen consumption for living cells was independent of the oxygen concentration in the living tissue (noting that a necrotic core is usually present in these models). Deakin [DEa] used a consumption rate which was a piecewise linear function of the nutrient concentration. This can lead to growth inhibition also, and considerable deviation in the limiting size of prevascular tumors compared with that obtained in uniform-nutrient consumption models, as McElwain and Ponzo [MCa] have shown. In Greenspan [GRa,b], the governing differential equation for the outer tumor radius (or length, in one dimension) is derived, and solved, subject to the appropriate relationships between the nutrient or inhibitor concentrations and various inner radii (for example the radius of the necrotic core). These relationships are obtained by solving the diffusion equation for the nutrient or inhibitor concentration. The models are examples of moving-boundary value problems and can be adapted to take account of types of volume loss mechanisms other than necrosis (McElwain and Morris, [MCb]).

It also seems desirable to examine the effect of a spatially-dependent inhibitor production rate to see how sensitive the models are to the source distribution. The idealized tumors in these more complex systems in general develop a three (or possibly four) level structure: an outer layer or shell of normally proliferating cells overlaying a region of living cells of very low mitotic index, which in turn overlay a necrotic core. In these models the necrotic core exists because cells are assumed to die if the nutrient concentration falls below a certain threshold value. The following question can be asked: what is the source of the growth inhibition for cells in the viable middle region? In Greenspan's papers the inhibitor was assumed to be produced (i) by necrotic debris freely diffusing out from the tumor core, or (ii) by the metabolic processes associated with the outer growing cells. By comparing these models with the results of Sutherland, McCredie and Inch [SUa], Greenspan tentatively identified the source of the inhibitor as the necrotic debris. McElwain and Ponzo [MCa] considered a third possibility, namely that nutrient depletion combined with a concentration-dependent cell proliferation rate was the sole inhibitory mechanism. Non-uniform production rates of inhibitor have been examined in [ADa–d], [MAb], [SWb] with more recent work by Chaplain and co-workers [CHa–f] discussed in Section 2.3.2. Of course, the advantage of all these models is that by being limited to one particular inhibitory mechanism, convenient comparisions can be made, in principle, with observations. In practice, a combination of these and possibly other mechanisms may be responsible for growth retardation in the prevascular stage of growth.

Realistic models of spheroid growth by diffusion should incorporate, ideally, at least some of the following processes or constraints:

a) Non-uniform inhibitor production;
b) Non-uniform consumption rate of nutrients, and associated non-uniform cell proliferation;
c) Continuous, as opposed to discontinuous mitotic rate as a function of growth inhibitor concentration;
d) Geometric constraints;
e) Central necrosis (though this does not always occur).

These five areas are not necessarily mutually exclusive, and initially they are not all necessarily appropriate in one model, for it is useful to be able to compare the success or failure of limited models in accounting for experimentally observed results. Ultimately, it would be advantageous to have a model that incorporated all of a)-e) above (and any other features deemed appropriate). Then various features could be "turned" on or off as necessary to compare with the known results, but the parameter space for such a model would be of (relatively) large dimension. The beauty of many existing models is their analytic simplicity; however, three-dimensional spherical structures are of obvious and particular interest both from a mathematical and an experimental viewpoint. Mathematically, the radial dependence induced by spherical symmetry introduces considerable simplifications in the analysis while retaining the basic physics and appropriate geometric features. Experimentally, the spherical geometry is mimicked closely in the growth of **multicellular spheroids** in the laboratory (Sutherland and Durand, [SUc]). Multicellular spheroids are spherical avascular structures which can be cultured in-vitro under well-defined supply conditions and which make it possible to model the microenvironments of cells in-vitro. In contrast to conventional monolayer cultures, spheroids exhibit (i) a three-dimensional array of intercellular junctions, (ii) an extracellular matrix similar to that found in tissues in vivo and (iii) a diffusion-limited supply of nutrients and removal of metabolic wastes.

By growing multicellular (or multicell) spheroids, so-called "microenvironmental" conditions can be created for the cancer similar to those the cells are exposed to in solid tumors (Sutherland, [SUd]). Since oxygen has been considered a major and decisive factor in the control of cellular metabolism, viability, and development of necrosis both in solid tumor and in spheroids, a number of studies have been undertaken to assess oxygen levels in experimental tumors (a review can be found in Vaupel, [VAa]) and in the tumor spheroids (Müller–Klieser and Sutherland, [MKa,b]). Recent work by Müller–Klieser and Sutherland, [MKc] indicates that spheroids may represent a valuable model to provide evidence for the way oxygen-tension histograms are influenced by the density of capillaries and by the cellular oxygen consumption. A detailed model of spheroids is presented by [CAa]. (See also [BJa,b]).

In view of this, multicell spheroids represent an in-vitro tumor model, insofar as conditions for the tumor cells can be generated similar to those of cancer cells located between nutritive vessels in solid tumors, (and being supplied by diffusion of substrates from tumor capillaries). Restrictions in blood supply, which may occur in solid tumors with increasing tumor weight (Vaupel, [VAa]) can lead to a decrease of the concentration of nutrients, such as oxygen in the tumor capillaries (Vaupel et al., [VAb,c]). This situation can be stimulated in laboratory-grown spheroids by lowering the oxygen content in the growth medium.

The information obtained from spheroid models provides a base from which to undertake detailed studies (which are not possible in experimental tumors) of controlled manipulation of spheroid microenvironments. The interrelationships between nutrient supply, cellular microenvironment, cellular proliferation and metabolism, development of necrosis, and resistance of cells to therapy can be studied quantitatively in spheroids [FKa], [FRa,b].

Multicellular tumor spheroids in summary, therefore, represent a useful in-vitro model for studying the impact of tumor microenvironments on cellular proliferation and on the resistance to certain therapeutic techniques (e.g. ionizing radiation (Sutherland and Durand, [SUb])). Cellular heterogeneity in spheroids may be similar on a microenvironmental level to conditions in solid tumors, and since the former can be investigated systematically, these studies may be of great practical importance, since heterogeneous cell populations are a major problem in tumor therapy [SUc].

Nevertheless, it is clear that the models of **prevascular** growth are somewhat limited, despite the considerable interest in them. Following this phase of growth, vascularization takes place, leading of course, to a vascular phase of growth. Existing models of prevascular growth are valid up to the "dormant" phase of avascular nodules (1–2 mm in diameter), which may last for several months. Near this dormant state, the concentration of tumor angiogenesis factor (TAF) rises (McElwain, Callcott and Morris, [MCc]). (The word "angiogenesis" means formation of new blood vessels. Blood vessel growth is most active in the developing embryo and normally very inactive in adults, except in special circumstances such as during wound healing, placenta formation and tumor growth). This factor promotes the growth of capillary sprouts which grow toward and eventually penetrate the tumor.

After vascularization, the tumor no longer has to depend solely on diffusion processes for nutrient, oxygen and waste transport and thus is no longer confined to a dormant state and rapid growth ensues. However, this exponential growth is not maintained indefinitely. When the diameter of the tumor reaches 1–3 cm (Folkman, [FOa]), the growth rate again slows down, and the growth curve appears to be well described by a Gompertzian rather than an exponential curve. This description has been shown to be excellent for a wide variety of mouse, rat and rabbit tumors by Laird [LAa]. Nearly all of the tumors studied showed the slow-down in growth as the tumor became larger and some appeared to be approaching a steady state asymptotically.

Several ideas have been proposed to explain the overall deceleration of the vascular stage. Tannock [TAa] observed that in a mouse mammary tumor, the capillary endothelial cells turnover time was longer than that of the tumor cells. This means that the distance between capillaries increases as the tumor grows and the proliferation rate far from the capillaries decreases, giving rise to an overall decrease in the growth rate of the tumor as a whole.

Another observation is that when a tumor is about 1–3 cm in diameter, vascular obstruction occurs (Goldacre and Sylven, [GOa]). This confines flow to the outer periphery of the tumor and may rise to the formation of large regions of necrosis (Folkman, [FOa]). Folkman also put forward the idea that there may be a critical depth within most tumors beyond which there is no blood flow due to external pressures.

Very little theoretical work has been done in this area. McElwain, Callcott and Morris [MCc] have assumed that, in the vascular phase, compression of the blood vessels in the tumor interior causes the decline of rapid early growth referred to above. In this model, the tumor develops into an avascular nodule surrounded by a shell of vascularized tumor tissue. Eventually, a four-layer structure occurs, with an outer peripheral layer in which the vascularized tissue behaves normally; below this there is a region in which the blood vessels are collapsed and transport is by diffusion. In the region below this, the proliferation rate is reduced due to lack of nutrient, or build-up of mitotic inhibitor (or both, as was suggested above for the prevascular models). Finally, there is a core of necrotic material. It is clear that such models are natural generalizations of the prevascular models already discussed, and a greater degree of generality for such models may be very useful for models of vascular compression. Indeed, it has been suggested that such models may well be of relevance to the study of cell migration in tumors as a result of pressure gradients within the tissue. It is of great interest, therefore to try to adapt the prevascular models to compare with experimental data for the more "dangerous" phase of tumor growth, namely the vascular phase (we refer to tumors with this structure as partially solid tumors).

While many of these deterministic models were developed in the 1970's, there has been renewed interest very recently in tumor angiogenesis (Folkman and Klagsbrun, [FOc]) and necrosis (Old, [OLa]) following the isolation over the past three or four years of several proteins that stimulate angiogenesis-angiogenin, fibroblast growth factors (acidic and basic), and transforming growth factors α and β [MAa]. The latter factor apparently attracts macrophages-cells frequently found in tumors.

Diffusion models can also be used in studies of drug transport in solid tumors, with particular reference to chemotherapy. Realistic models need to take account of the existence of necrosis and non-uniform blood flow (King, Schultz and Gatenby, [KIa]), so a quantitative understanding of detailed mass-transport in tumors will obviously be of service in attempting to improve chemotherapy and other methods of cancer treatment [JAa,b]. Models may, for example, predict oxygen or drug profiles that could allow manipulation to optimize the therapeutic effect (Swan, [SWa]). King, Schultz and Gatenby [KIa] have demonstrated that multi-region models can often accurately reproduce clinical measurements, and may therefore serve as predictors for establishing new oxygen levels within a tumor that result from increasing systemic oxygen through the intake of pure oxygen under atmospheric or hyperbaric conditions. (They point out, furthermore, that solutions to the time-dependent version of the model(s) may provide an estimate of the time period required to adequately oxygenate tumors before therapy ensues).

In the light of these qualitative comments we now turn to the mathematical aspects of these models.

2.3.2 Basic diffusion models: Mathematical aspects

The simplest empirical model for population growth is Malthusian, in which the rate of change of population is proportional to the population itself:

$$\frac{dN}{dt} = kN\,, \qquad k > 0\,. \tag{2.1}$$

Clearly, this is less than satisfactory for any system with limited resources or "self-competition," so a simple modification to allow for population saturation yields the logistic differential equation (with carrying capacity θ)

$$\frac{dN}{dt} = kN\left(1 - \frac{N}{\theta}\right). \tag{2.2}$$

However, the function $N(t)$, which is a solution of this equation, possesses a symmetry about the point of inflection which renders it less useful for curve fitting than a more general profile would be. A family of empirical curves of growth that saturates either more slowly or more rapidly than the solution of (2.2) can be derived from a generalization of the Verhulst equation, namely

$$\frac{dN}{dt} = \frac{k}{\alpha} N \left(1 - \left(\frac{N}{\theta}\right)^{\alpha}\right), \tag{2.3}$$

which reduces to (2.2) when $\alpha = 1$. It also has the advantage that in the limit $\alpha \to 0^+$, the equation reduces to the Gompertz equation:

$$\frac{dN}{dt} = -kN \ln \frac{N}{\theta} \cdot \tag{2.4}$$

By making the transformation $v = \ln(N/\theta)$ it may be shown that the solution of Eq. (2.3) is

$$N(t) = \theta \left(\frac{N_0^{\alpha}}{N_0^{\alpha}(1 - e^{-kt}) + \theta^{\alpha} e^{-kt}}\right)^{\frac{1}{\alpha}}, \tag{2.5}$$

where $N_0 = N(0)$. This result contains the logistic solution (when $\alpha = 1$)

$$N(t) = \frac{\theta N_0}{N_0 + (\theta - N_0)e^{-kt}} \tag{2.6}$$

and the Gompertzian solution (as $\alpha \to 0^+$)

$$N(t) = \theta \exp(-Ae^{-kt}), \tag{2.7}$$

where

$$A = \ln \frac{\theta}{N_0} \cdot$$

Other models have been developed by Marusic and co-workers [MRa–d] and in [VYa] (see the chapter by Bajzer). Many prevascular diffusion models of tumor growth predict growth curves which are qualitatively similar to the above saturated-growth curves, but a major advantage of these models is that the governing differential (or integro-differential) equations of growth are based on plausible physical assumptions. Thus any comparison of model-generated curves of growth with experimental data can, at least in principle, provide some information on the appropriate parameter ranges necessary for consistency with the data. As pointed out by Wheldon [WHa], the value of modeling to a science will depend on the extent to which that science incorporates defined assumptions which lend themselves to quantitative expression. This is the basis of the model by Greenspan [GRa] which gives the outer radius (and various inner radii, e.g. the radius of the necrotic core) as a function of time. The first mathematical model we review, however, is that by Burton [BNa].

Burton was the first to introduce diffusion into a model of spheroid growth, taking the model out of the realm of pure phenomenology into a more biologically-driven environment. Interestingly, by considering a diffusion problem alone Burton was able to glean important information about the relative thickness of the viable layer (the outer rim of proliferating cells) without utilizing an evolution equation for the outer tumor radius. The main features of models are easily summarized: assumptions include spherical symmetry and diffusive equilibrium. The oxygen consumption rate per unit volume of non-necrotic tissue is assumed to be constant, so if $X(r)$ is the oxygen concentration distribution in appropriate units, it satisfies the equation

$$\frac{d}{dr}\left(r^2\frac{dX}{dr}\right) = \frac{m}{D}r^2 = Kr^2 , \tag{2.8}$$

where the constant K is the ratio of the consumption rate m and the constant diffusion coefficient D for oxygen (or whatever other nutrient is deemed appropriate). The necrotic core is defined by $0 \leq r \leq R_N$, with a zero flux boundary condition at R_N, where $X = X_c$ (a critical oxygen concentration below which cells are assumed to die). Further, at the outer surface of the spheroid ($r = R_0$) the oxygen concentration is maintained at a constant value X_m. Under these circumstances the following relationship between these quantities is readily established:

$$X_m - X_c = \frac{1}{3}K\left(\frac{1}{2}R_0^2 + \frac{1}{R_0}R_n^3 - \frac{3}{2}R_n^2\right) . \tag{2.9}$$

As is frequently the case in modeling, a dimensionless or relative measure of such relationships is of great value. To this end, Burton introduces a critical radius R_c which is the value of R_c when necrosis first occurs, i.e. when $X(0) = X_c$. Thus when $R_0 \geq R_c$, $R_n \geq 0$, the equalities corresponding. This implies

$$X_m - X_c = \frac{KR_c^2}{6}$$

whence from (2.9) in terms of the relative radii $p = R_0/R_c$ and $p_n = R_n/R_c$

$$p^2 - 1 = p_n^2\left(3 - \frac{2p_n}{p}\right) . \tag{2.10}$$

This is an exact cubic relationship for the model as stated; there is no limit in principle to the size of the spheroid (clearly a deficiency of the model!), but even here a useful result can be found for the relative size of the viable layer $(p - p_n)$. If p is large compared with 1, then $p/p_n = \alpha$ satisfies the approximate result

$$\alpha^3 - 3\alpha + 2 = 0\,,$$

which has a double positive root $\alpha = 1$ (the other root being $\alpha = -2$). Hence as p becomes unbounded the quantity α approaches unity (from above) and $p - p_n$ approaches a limiting value, T. To see this, substitute for p_n in Eq. (2.10) to obtain

$$p^{-2} = 3(Tp^{-1})^2 - 2(Tp^{-1})^3\,. \tag{2.11}$$

If Tp^{-1} is small compared with 1, so that the cubic term can be neglected it follows that $T \approx (3)^{-\frac{1}{2}} \approx 0.58$. Recalling that $T = (R_0 - R_n)/R_c$ we interpret this to mean that within the confines of this two-layer model, the viable layer approaches a constant thickness, equal to 58% of the critical tumor radius R_c.

There are several other aspects of Burton's paper that are of considerable interest. Equation (2.10) in particular is shown to give a good empirical fit to a Gompertzian relation over at least a hundred-fold range of tumor volume, predicting a value of the Gompertzian parameter θ (in our notation) in Eq. (2.7) close to the experimental value discussed by Laird [LAa].

2.3.3 Diffusion of growth inhibitor

In 1973, Glass [GLa] published a one-dimensional model of growth-inhibitor production by tissue; that model has proven to be seminal because of its simplicity and its usefulness. For completeness, the symmetric two- and three-dimensional versions will be given here also, but it should be noted that in another fundamental paper, with more biologically realistic boundary conditions, Shymko and Glass [SHa] dealt fully with the corresponding three-dimensional problem.

Consider a "slab" of slowly growing tissue of width L, centered on the origin, producing growth-inhibitor at a rate P (molecules/unit volume/second) which is depleted or decays at a rate λ. This central tissue is embedded in an infinite expanse of non-active tissue. For simplicity, the diffusion coefficient D for the inhibitor is assumed to be constant everywhere. A fundamental assumption made is that of diffusive equilibrium: the timescale for significant tissue growth is considered large compared with the timescale for readjustment of the inhibitor concentration profile due to such growth: the system is essentially in a steady state. This is a reasonable assumption for central tissue sizes not in excess of, say, 1 mm, for which the typical diffusion time (for oxygen) is of order 10 minutes [EDa].

The most simple boundary conditions of interest to us here are that the concentration of growth inhibitor C (in units of molecules/unit volume) should be smoothly varying across

$$x = \pm \frac{1}{2} L ,$$

with the obvious symmetry condition that $C'(0) = 0$, where the prime denotes first order ordinary derivative. More precisely, the governing mathematical description can be described by an ordinary differential equation (rather than by a partial differential equation, in view of diffusive equilibrium) as follows:

$$D \frac{d^2 C}{dx^2} - \lambda C = -PS(x) , \qquad (2.12)$$

where the source term

$$S(x) = \begin{cases} 1 & |x| \leq \frac{1}{2} L \\ 0 & |x| > \frac{1}{2} L \end{cases}$$

subject to the conditions $C'(0) = 0$, $C(\pm\frac{1}{2}L)$ and $C'(\pm\frac{1}{2}L)$ continuous, and $C(x)$ bounded as $|x| \to \infty$ (an obvious requirement if there are no external sources of growth inhibitor). If we introduce the abbreviations

$$\alpha = \sqrt{\frac{\lambda}{D}} , \qquad \phi = \alpha \frac{1}{2} L ,$$

then the solutions are

$$C(x) = \frac{P}{\lambda} \left(1 - e^{-\phi} \cosh(\alpha |x|) \right) , \qquad |x| \leq \frac{1}{2} L \qquad (2.13)$$

and

$$C(x) = \frac{P}{\lambda} \sinh \phi e^{-\alpha |x|} , \qquad |x| > \frac{1}{2} L . \qquad (2.14)$$

Since $C'(x) < 0$ for $x > 0$, as is easily verified, it follows that $C(x)$ decreases monotonically from its central value of

$$C(0) = \frac{P}{\lambda} \left(1 - e^{-\phi} \right) \qquad (2.15)$$

to its value at the edges of

$$C\left(\pm\frac{1}{2}L\right) = \frac{P}{2\lambda}\left(1 - e^{-2\phi}\right). \tag{2.16}$$

Now if we suppose, with Glass, that there exists a switch-like mechanism such that if the concentration equals or exceeds some critical concentration θ, growth ceases in that region and continues otherwise, then for growth to cease throughout the tissue slab,

$$C\left(\frac{1}{2}L\right) \geq \theta. \tag{2.17}$$

(If $C(L/2) < \theta$ there will be continued growth in at least the outer regions of the slab if $C(0) > \theta$; and throughout the tissue if $C(0) < \theta$).

In terms of the dimensionless parameter $n = P/(2\lambda\theta)$ inequality (2.17) becomes

$$\ln\left(\frac{n}{n-1}\right) \leq 2\phi$$

corresponding to a limiting stable tissue of width

$$L_s = \sqrt{\frac{D}{\lambda}}\ln\left(\frac{n}{n-1}\right). \tag{2.18}$$

See Figure 2.2. L_s is clearly defined for $n > 1$; growth eventually ceases as L approaches L_s. Glass speculated that the "singular region" defined in parameter space by $n \leq 1$ corresponds to the converse of controlled stable growth, namely uncontrolled, unstable growth. This is a very basic definition of cancer: cellular proliferation defying the normal control mechanisms. While claiming in essence to be no more than a metaphor for cancer at this level of description (given the lack of biological input insofar as cellular replication is concerned), this approach has been and continues to be an intriguing and suggestive avenue to a complex phenomenon, that may well require many different but complementary levels of description to enable even a partial understanding to be obtained [ADe].

More realistic geometries necessitate the replacement of the operator d^2/dx^2 in Eq. (2.12) with

$$\frac{1}{r}\frac{d}{dr}\left(r\frac{d}{dr}\right)$$

in the case of cylindrical symmetry, or

$$\frac{1}{r^2}\frac{d}{dr}\left(r^2\frac{d}{dr}\right)$$

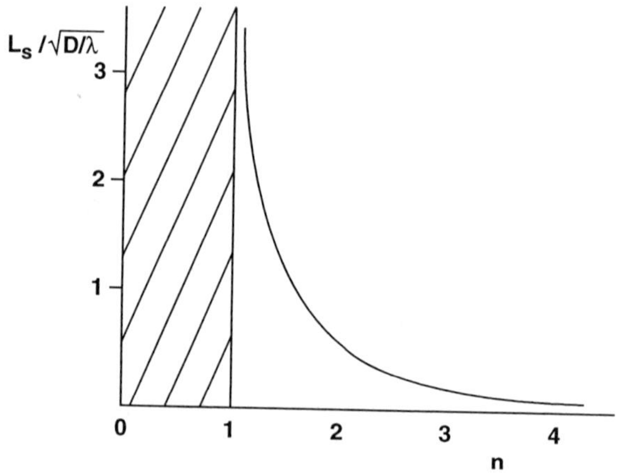

Figure 2.2 — Graph of the stable limiting tissue size L_s vs. n, based on Eq. (2.18). The shaded area corresponds to limitless growth on the basis of this model.

in the case of spherical symmetry, where r is a radial coordinate.

Similar considerations apply in terms of boundary conditions for the tissue boundary at $r = R$ ($0 \leq r \leq R$ corresponding to the cylindrical "cord" or spherical mass respectively). The stable limiting size in each case is found in terms of an implicit transcendental relation which will not be stated here, but the solutions corresponding to Eqs. (2.13) and (2.14) are as follows:

$$\begin{cases} C(r) = \dfrac{P}{\lambda}\left(1 - \dfrac{I_0(\alpha r)}{M(\alpha R)}\right), & r \leq R \\ C(r) = \dfrac{P}{\lambda}\dfrac{I_1(\alpha R)K_0(\alpha r)}{M(\alpha R)K_1(\alpha R)}, & r > R \end{cases} \tag{2.19}$$

for cylindrical symmetry, where I_0, I_1, K_0, K_1 are modified Bessel functions of the first and second kinds (of orders zero and one) respectively. The term $M(\alpha R)$ is defined as

$$M(\alpha R) = \frac{1}{K_1(\alpha R)}\left[I_1(\alpha R)K_0(\alpha R) + I_0(\alpha R)K_1(\alpha R)\right] \tag{2.20}$$

and, for spherical symmetry

$$\begin{cases} C(r) = \dfrac{P}{\lambda}\left(1 - \dfrac{(R\alpha + 1)\sinh(\alpha r)}{\alpha r \sinh(\alpha R)(1 + \coth(\alpha R))}\right), & r \leq R \\ C(r) = \dfrac{P}{\lambda}\dfrac{\alpha R \cosh(\alpha R) - \sinh(\alpha R)}{\alpha r}e^{-\alpha r}, & r > R, \end{cases} \tag{2.21}$$

in terms of hyperbolic functions.

In each case, $C(r)$ is a monotone decreasing function satisfying the boundary conditions discussed above for the tissue slab.

As noted earlier, by introducing somewhat more biologically reasonable boundary conditions at the tissue boundary, Shymko and Glass [SHa] were able to make comparison with their model and experiments on multicellular spheroids [FOd]. The governing derivative boundary condition at the surface defined by $r = R$ for the spherically symmetric case was modified to be

$$D\frac{dC}{dr} = -pC \qquad \text{at} \qquad r = R, \tag{2.22}$$

where p is the permeability of the tissue surface (and assuming that the growth inhibitor is so diluted once it passes through the tissue walls that its concentration is essentially zero). Under these circumstances the interior solution for $r \leq R$ (the only one of interest to them) is, in the present notation.

$$C(r) = \frac{P}{\lambda}\left(1 - \frac{R\sinh(\alpha r)}{r\sinh(\alpha R)\left(1 + \eta\coth(\alpha R) - \dfrac{\eta}{\alpha R}\right)}\right), \qquad r \leq R, \tag{2.23}$$

where

$$\eta = \frac{(\lambda D)^{\frac{1}{2}}}{p}.$$

The authors delineated parameter regions for (i) unstable (or unlimited) growth throughout the tissue (ii) unstable growth with mitosis confined to a peripheral region of the tissue, and (iii) stable, limited growth. A very interesting discussion of the implications of the model and experimental data on cellular and geometric control of tissue growth is presented in this paper, and the reader is urged to consult it for further details. Subsequent developments of this model have focused on non-homogeneous source terms [ADb,c], [CHa], and incorporation of necrosis as a possible source of inhibitor [ADo].

A related set of papers appeared recently. In [BRa], maximum principles for parabolic and elliptic operators were used to examine, in general terms, models of the type discussed above. The authors proved, in particular, under fairly general conditions, that $C(I)$ is nonnegative, unique, and decreases monotonically in the open interval $(0, R)$, where R is the radius of the spheroid (in one, two or three dimensions). Furthermore, they proved that as the tissue size increases, the concentration at any fixed point also increases. Chaplain and Britton [CHa] examined the effect of a smooth, quadratically decreasing source term for the growth inhibitor, and compared their results with existing theoretical work and experimental data. This source term was also used by Chaplain et al. [CHb] in their consideration of nonlinear, spatially dependent diffusion in a spheroid. They demonstrated that a non-uniform source function is not the only way to produce qualitatively correct growth inhibitor concentration profiles, i.e. mathematically it is not possible to distinguish between the effects of non-linear diffusion and a non-linear source term. It would appear that more experimental work on the precise mechanisms governing cell cycle kinetics is desirable in order to elucidate the underlying tissue heterogeneity.

2.3.4 Time-evolutionary diffusion models

As stated by Greenspan [GRa], the objective of the type of diffusion model he developed is to infer the major internal process affecting tumor growth from the most easily obtained in-vitro data which are assumed to be

i) measurements of the outer nodule radius $R_0(t)$ as a function of time, and

ii) a cross-section of the final dormant state which provides the limiting radius $R_0(\infty)$ and the limiting necrotic core radius $R_i(\infty)$.

In this model there develops in general a three-layer structure consisting of a central necrotic core, $r \leq R_i(t)$, a layer of viable nonproliferating cells, $R_i(t) \leq r \leq R_g(t)$, and an outer shell where all mitosis occurs, $R_g(t) \leq r \leq R_0(t)$. (No account is taken of the cell age or stage of cycle). Greenspan lists many assumptions explicit or implicit in the model: we only state the most important here. They are as follows:

i) the tumor nodule is spherically symmetric at all times; r and t are the only independent variables;

ii) cells die when the nutrient concentration $\sigma(r, t)$ falls below some critical level σ_i;

iii) nutrient is consumed by living cells only; the consumption rate may depend on $\sigma(r, t)$ and on the cell proliferation rate;

iv) necrotic cellular debris continually disintegrates into simpler chemical compounds that are freely permeable through the cell membranes. The cell volume lost in this way is replaced by cells pushed inward by the forces of adhesion and tension (see comments on this below);

v) the source of growth inhibition may be one of the following (or a combination of them):

  a) reduced nutrient concentration in the tumor interior. This is somewhat plausible from surface area to volume requirements;

  b) a chemical (of concentration β) may be produced somewhere within the tumor which inhibits mitosis without causing cell death. The source of this inhibitor may be metabolic waste from necrotic debris, or a by-product of metabolism from the living cells;

vi) the tumor is in a state of diffusive equilibrium at all times (nutrient diffusion time small with respect to the typical growth time);

vii) there are a sufficiently large number of cells present in order that the growth process may be considered a continuous one;

viii) the proliferation rate of cell volume by mitosis is described by a source distribution of mitosis and inhibitor $S(\sigma, \beta)$, describing the rate at which cell volume is produced per unit volume of living cells;

ix) the necrotic core "loses" cell volume at a rate that at any time is proportional to the core volume.

(The stability of such a spheroid, initially spherically symmetric, to nonsymmetric perturbations was considered elsewhere by Greenspan [GRc], and an extension will be discussed below).

The basis of growth equation describing the evolution of the outer nodule radius can be described in the following manner:

$$A = B + C - D - E \,, \tag{2.24}$$

$$A = \frac{4}{3}\pi\left(R_0^3(t) - R_i^3(t)\right), \tag{2.25}$$

$$B = \frac{4}{3}\pi R_0^3(0)\,, \tag{2.26}$$

$$C = 4\pi \int_0^t dt' \int_{\max(R_i(t'),R_g(t'))}^{R_0(t')} S(\sigma,\beta) r^2\, dr\,, \tag{2.27}$$

$$D = \frac{4}{3}\pi R_i^3(t)\,, \tag{2.28}$$

$$E = \frac{4}{3}\pi \int_0^t 3\lambda R_i^3(t')\, dt'\,, \tag{2.29}$$

where A is the total volume of living cells at any time t, B is the initial volume of living cells at time $t = 0$, C is the total volume of cells produced in $t > 0$, D is the total volume of necrotic debris at time t, E is the total

volume lost in necrotic core in $t > 0$, $R_g(t)$ is an intermediate "growth radius", and λ is a constant of proportionality.
Hence, Eq. (2.24) becomes

$$R_0^3(t) = R_0^3(0) + 3\int_0^t dt' \int_{\max(R_i,R_g)}^{R_0} S(\sigma,\beta) r^2\, dr - 3\int_0^t \lambda R_i^3\, dt' ,$$

or in time-differentiated form:

$$R_0^2 \frac{dR_0}{dt} = \int_{\max(R_i,R_g)}^{R_0} S(\sigma,\beta) r^2\, dr - \lambda R_i^3 . \tag{2.30}$$

The mitosis source term $S(\sigma, \beta)$ is obtained from the solutions of the respective spherically-symmetric time-independent diffusion equations for $\sigma(r)$ and $\beta(r)$, i.e. in general

$$\frac{1}{r^2}\frac{d}{dr}\left(r^2 D(\sigma)\frac{d\sigma}{dr}\right) = f(\sigma) , \tag{2.31}$$

with a corresponding equation for $\beta(r)$. In practice, the diffusion coefficients and sink/source terms have been chosen to have relatively simple forms for analytical convenience in the absence of any biological evidence to the contrary. Note that $\beta(r)$ is the same as $C(r)$ in the models discussed in Section 2.3.2; we have adopted in each case the notation of the authors concerned.

One feature common to all these prevascular models is that the geometry is spherically symmetric: this is mathematically convenient, for in this ideal situation the net resultant of any intercellular forces within the colony is radially directed. Under these circumstances, no more precise examination of local cell dynamics is needed. However, it is clear that in practice such spherical symmetry is likely to be very rare, and even if this is initially the case, subsequent growth of a small tumor cell colony is unlikely to maintain this symmetry. Chaplain [CHc] has contributed to the understanding of this situation, based in part on earlier work by Greenspan [GRc], and here we draw on the salient features of his work.

There is one caveat to be made, and it applies to all models in which it is assumed that gross internal forces may be characterized by a pressure distribution, non-uniformities in which affect cell motion. Recent experiments on multicellular spheroids (Jain, [JAc]) failed to measure any pressure at all within the spheroids prior to vascularization. Once a spheroid or metastasis has been vascularized, the resultant pressure distribution must reflect the external systemic blood pressure, and by regarding the vascularization to correspond in some sense to a spatially smooth pressure distribution (as in [ADf]) the analysis in these models is still useful. Another prevalent assumption, also already noted, is that internal cell adhesion, like molecular attraction, produces a "surface tension" at the outer boundary of the nodule that maintains compactness and counteracts internal expansive pressures. While it is known that such multicellular spheroids are held together by a variety of junctions (see [CHc]), this postulated quasi-balance of forces (and associated surface area/volume considerations) is not sufficient to explain the stable limiting size of such a spheroid in vitro. Experimental work by Freyer [FRa,b] and others suggest that tumor growth inhibitors have at least some role to play in this regard. This is addressed to some extent by the previously mentioned work of Greenspan [GRa,b] and its extensions (e.g. [MAb], [ADd]).

With this in mind, we are in a better position to appreciate the strengths and weaknesses which characterise models of growing tumor colonies and their stability. An excellent introduction to models of this type can be found in Jones and Sleeman [JOa], who identify the basic assumptions of Greenspan's (1976) model [GRc], and re-derive the governing equations. Thus formulated, the problem falls into the class known as moving boundary value problems, in which the outer surface is represented by the general expression

$$\Gamma(x, y, z, t) = 0\,. \tag{2.32}$$

The interior pressure p and exterior relative nutrient concentration σ satisfy

$$\nabla^2 p = S_i \tag{2.33}$$

inside $\Gamma = 0$ and

$$\nabla^2 \sigma = 0 \tag{2.34}$$

outside $\Gamma = 0$, where S_i is a constant representing the rate of volume loss per unit volume within the colony (due to necrosis, and the freely permeable necrotic debris being replaced by previously living cells via the compaction mechanism postulated above). Various other boundary and initial data are necessary to complete the statement of the mathematical problem. A prime concern is instability: do small perturbations to an initial equilibrium configuration continue to grow in time; or do they stabilize (as far as a linear analysis is concerned)? The simplest case mathematically is that of initial spherical symmetry, for which Eq. (2.32) becomes the simpler expression $r = R(t)$, which satisfies

$$\frac{dR}{dt} = -\frac{dp}{dr} + \lambda\sqrt{\sigma}\,. \tag{2.35}$$

Since the time variable enters the system only in determination of the tumor radius, the preceding system of equations can be solved explicitly for p and σ:

$$p = \frac{S_i}{6}(r^2 - R^2) + \frac{\alpha}{R}, \tag{2.36}$$

$$\sigma = \sigma_\infty - \frac{2\mu\sigma_\infty R^2}{\mu r R + r\sqrt{\mu^2 R^2 + 4\sigma_\infty}}. \tag{2.37}$$

The substitution of these formulae into (2.35) yields a single ordinary differential equation for $R(t)$:

$$R'(t) = -\frac{1}{3} S_i R + \frac{2\lambda\sigma_\infty}{\mu R + \sqrt{\mu^2 R^2 + 4\sigma_\infty}}. \tag{2.38}$$

This last equation can be integrated to yield an unwieldy closed form solution which will not be quoted here since only the qualitative character of $R(t)$ is of interest.

The tumor (cell colony) grows initially at a linear rate and asymptotes to the steady state radius

$$R_\infty = \frac{3\lambda}{S_i}\left(\frac{\sigma_\infty}{1 + \dfrac{3\lambda\mu}{S_i}}\right)^{\frac{1}{2}}, \tag{2.39}$$

in a time-scale regulated mainly by the rate of volume loss of necrotic debris (this equation can be obtained by setting the right hand side of (2.38) to zero).

In these expressions α is a constant relating the pressure and the boundary curvature $1/R$, σ_∞ is the external nutrient concentration, μ and λ are constants associated with nutrient diffusion and cell proliferation rate respectively.

Growth is judged unstable to infinitesimal perturbations if any such disturbance amplifies at an exponential rate (exceeding that of the radius $R(t)$). In this circumstance, the instabilities radically alter the shape of the colony and can even lead to fracturing into two or more pieces. The tumor becomes unstable if and when it reaches a critical size beyond which surface tension is overcome by pressure forces. The precise criterion for this is obtained from the analysis that follows.

We now consider the growth of a spherical tumor (cell colony) which is subject to small deviations that are always inevitably present in a real environment. Originally, for simplicity, Greenspan [GRc] took the perturbations from complete sphericity to be axially symmetric i.e. independent of the azimuthal angle ϕ in spherical polar coordinates (r, θ, ϕ). For completeness, Chaplain [CHc] included the azimuthal dependence in his analysis.

To this end, we let $\bar{p}(r,t)$, $\bar{\sigma}(r,t)$ and $R(t)$ denote the basic state of motion given by Eqs. (2.36–2.38) and $\varepsilon\tilde{p}(r,\theta,\phi,t)$, $\varepsilon\tilde{\sigma}(r,\theta,\phi,t)$ and $\varepsilon\xi(\theta,\phi,t)$ the perturbations therefrom. The total pressure distribution and nutrient concentration are then represented by

$$\begin{cases} p(r,\theta,\phi,t) = \bar{p}(r,t) + \varepsilon\tilde{p}(r,\theta,\phi,t) \\ \sigma(r,\theta,\phi,t) = \bar{\sigma}(r,t) + \varepsilon\tilde{\sigma}(r,\theta,\phi,t)\,, \end{cases} \tag{2.40}$$

and the equation of the moving surface is now given by

$$\Gamma(r,\theta,\phi,t) = r - R(t) - \varepsilon\xi(\theta,\phi,t) = 0\,. \tag{2.41}$$

These expressions are substituted into the relevant equations above and all terms are developed as power series in ε, including the mean curvature and the unit normal vector of the distorted surface. It follows that

$$\nabla^2\tilde{p} = 0\,, \qquad r \le R(t)\,, \tag{2.42}$$

$$\nabla^2\tilde{\sigma} = 0\,, \qquad r \ge R(t)\,, \tag{2.43}$$

with $\tilde{\sigma} \to 0$ as $r \to \infty$.

On $r = R(t)$ we have

$$\frac{\partial\xi}{\partial t} = -\left(\frac{\partial^2\bar{p}}{\partial r^2}\xi + \frac{\partial\tilde{p}}{\partial r}\right) + \frac{\lambda}{2\sqrt{\bar{\sigma}}}\left(\xi\frac{\partial\bar{\sigma}}{\partial r} + \tilde{\sigma}\right), \tag{2.44}$$

$$\frac{\partial^2\bar{\sigma}}{\partial r^2}\xi + \frac{\partial\tilde{\sigma}}{\partial r} = \frac{\mu}{2\sqrt{\bar{\sigma}}}\left(\xi\frac{\partial\bar{\sigma}}{\partial r} + \tilde{\sigma}\right), \tag{2.45}$$

$$\frac{\partial\bar{p}}{\partial r}\xi + \tilde{p} = -\frac{\alpha}{2R^2}\left[\frac{\partial}{\partial\eta}\left((1-\eta^2)\frac{\partial\xi}{\partial\eta}\right) + 2\xi + \frac{1}{\sin^2\theta}\frac{\partial^2\xi}{\partial\phi^2}\right], \tag{2.46}$$

where

$$\eta = \cos\theta\,.$$

Modal solutions of this homogeneous system are given by

$$\tilde{p} = A_n(t)r^n P_n^m(\cos\theta)\cos(m\phi)\,, \tag{2.47}$$

$$\tilde{\sigma} = \frac{1}{r^{n+1}}B_n(t)P_n^m(\cos\theta)\cos(m\phi)\,, \tag{2.48}$$

$$\xi = C_n(t)P_n^m(\cos\theta)\cos(m\phi)\,, \tag{2.49}$$

where $n = 0, 1, 2, 3, \ldots,\ 0 \le m \le n$ and $P_n^m(\cos\theta)$ are the associated Legendre polynomials defined by

$$P_n^m(\cos\theta) = \sin^m\theta \frac{d^m}{d(\cos\theta)^m} P_n(\cos\theta)$$

(in the case $m = 0$ these reduce to the Legendre polynomials $P_n(\cos\theta)$ and the whole analysis corresponds to Greenspan's, where there is no azimuthal dependence).

The result of replacing $\bar{p}, \bar{\sigma}$ and their derivatives by explicit expressions obtained from Eqs. (2.36) and (2.37) is the fundamental equation governing the growth of infinitesimal instabilities:

$$C_n'(t) = (n-1) f(n, R) C_n(t)\,, \tag{2.50}$$

where

$$f(n, R) = \frac{S_i}{3} - \frac{\alpha n(n+2)}{2R^3} + \frac{\dfrac{\lambda\mu}{2}}{(n+1) + \dfrac{\mu R}{4\sigma_\infty}\left[\mu R + (\mu^2 R^2 + 4\sigma_\infty)\right]^{\frac{1}{2}}}\,. \tag{2.51}$$

The disturbance amplifies or decays according to whether the product $(n-1)f(n, R)$ is positive or negative. The tumor development is unstable if small perturbations can amplify — otherwise it is stable. For $n = 0$, the time dependent coefficient in $-f(0, R)$ in Eq. (2.50) is always negative so that this mode is definitely stable. For $n = 1$, $C_1(t)$ is a constant, which is compatible with the fact that this mode represents a translation of axes.

The modes $n \ge 2$ are genuinely unstable when $f(n, R) > 0$. Moreover, since $f(n, R)$ is a decreasing function of the index n for $n \ge 1$, the mode $n = 2$ is the first that can become unstable and it must always be a component of any growing disturbance. The minimum critical radius R_c at which the developing tumor can become unstable is then given by

$$f(2, R_c) = 0\,. \tag{2.52}$$

If $R_c > R_\infty$, the steady state radius of the tumor (see Eq. (2.39)), then the tumor is stable during its entire growth and attains its symmetric equilibrium configuration.

If however $R_c < R_\infty$, then the tumor becomes unstable at some definite time in its growth when small disturbances amplify and change both the structure and the shape of the tumor. In this case, the changing pressure distribution overcomes the surface tension before spherical equilibrium is reached.

The onset of stability in the mode $n = 2$ is manifested as a pinch in the outer surface around the equatorial region. As the tumor grows and increases in size, other modes become unstable and more radical changes in configuration may occur, which can be used to model the tumor invading the surrounding tissues.

On the basis of this model Chaplain discusses two topics of crucial interest in tumorgrowth: (i) local invasion of the surrounding tissues, and (ii) the spread of tumor cells by the lymph and circulatory systems. Noting that the classification of tumors into benign and malignant categories really represents the extremes of a spectrum of tumor growth, he makes the following observations about local invasion for carcinomas in particular:

At the boundary of a carcinoma, single tumor cells and irregular columns or projections of cells infiltrate into the surrounding tissues, extending from the central mass like the legs of a crab. As they proliferate, the invading cells compress the tissue cells and interfere with their blood supply, and highly specialized cells such as the parenchymal cells of internal organs are destroyed. Fibrovascular tissue is more resistant and its growth is stimulated by the tumor cells which thus secure a supporting stroma and blood supply.

Growth occurs most readily along lines of least resistance such as planes of loose connective tissue. Denser tissue, for example fibrous fasciae, the walls of arteries, cartilage and compact bone, are relatively resistant to invasion and while this is largely explained by their structure, there is evidence that constituent pieces of cartilage can both interfere with the growth of cancer cells and inhibit angiogenesis.

Local invasion is very important, not only because it increases the difficulty of excising a carcinoma completely, but also for its effects. In particular, invasion in and around the walls of hollow viscera or gland ducts very commonly causes their obstruction, while involvement of nerves may cause pain. The sooner a carcinoma gives rise to local effects of this sort, the greater the chance of diagnosis and complete removal.

This invasive power of cancers may be attributed to three main factors:

- the abnormal motility and amoeboid movement of some cancer cells;
- the secretion of lytic enzymes e.g. hyaluronidase which dissolve the ground substance and digest formed tissue elements and damage cell membranes;
- the reduced adhesiveness of cancer cells to one another.

When considered alongside two other important features of malignant tumors i.e. a large rate of cell production and extensive necrosis, it can be seen from (2.51), that high modes of instability are possible.

Recalling the form (2.51) for $f(n, R)$, it may be seen that the combination of a high value for S_i (extensive necrosis), a high value for λ (fast proliferation rate) and a small value for the surface tension parameter α (reduced cell-to-cell adhesiveness) leads to the possibility of an instability being dominated by a high mode number n. The mode n that actually dominates the instability is selected by the function $R(t)$ which sets the amplification rate and the time available for each perturbation to amplify, while the selection of the $m-$mode, c.f. $P_n^m(\cos\theta)$, will be determined by external influences such as the denseness of the surrounding tissue and the external distribution of the enzymes secreted by the tumor. Some possible dominant modes are shown in Figure 2.3.

At the other end of the spectrum, there are benign tumors. Generally these show little or no necrosis, have a slower rate of cell proliferation than malignant tumors and are very often surrounded by a fibrous capsule. Even when no such capsule exists, the margin between the tumor and the surrounding tissues remains sharp, without evidence of local invasion. Again upon consideration of the function $f(n, R)$, this time with a low value for S_i (little sign of necrosis), a low value for λ (slower cell proliferation rate) and a high value for α, the surface-tension parameter, (modelling the effect of the fibrous capsule), we see that the possibility of domination by a high mode number n is very small. Indeed, the presence of the capsule, which keeps the tumor a compact spherical mass, effectively rules out the growth of any small instability except perhaps the mode $n = 0$, which is simply associated with radial growth. This models the non-invasive nature of benign tumors.

For tumors of an intermediate nature i.e. combining some of the properties of both malignant and benign tumors, the choice of mode number n will not be as clear-cut, depending upon a more complicated interplay between the parameters involved and the external influences. This will vary upon the degree of malignancy from tumor to tumor.

In addition to invading surrounding tissues, tumor cells also invade the walls of lymphatics and blood vessels in and around the tumor. This gives rise to the possible spread of the tumor to other parts of the body where secondary tumors or metastases then form.

Smaller lymphatics, whose walls consist of little more than an endothelium with loose intercellular junctions and an incomplete basement membrane, are readily invaded by carcinoma cells which may either become detached and carried in the lymph to the next draining lymph node, or may remain attached at the site of invasion and proliferate within the lymphatic system to form a continuous column of tumor which distends and obstructs the lumen.

Carcinoma cells also invade the walls of small vessels, particularly venules, in and around the tumor, and single cancer cells or small groups of cells frequently become detached and are carried away in the venous blood where they are likely to become impacted as emboli in the next microvascular network.

There is clinical and experimental evidence that rough handling of a malignant tumor promotes the escape of tumor cells into the blood and

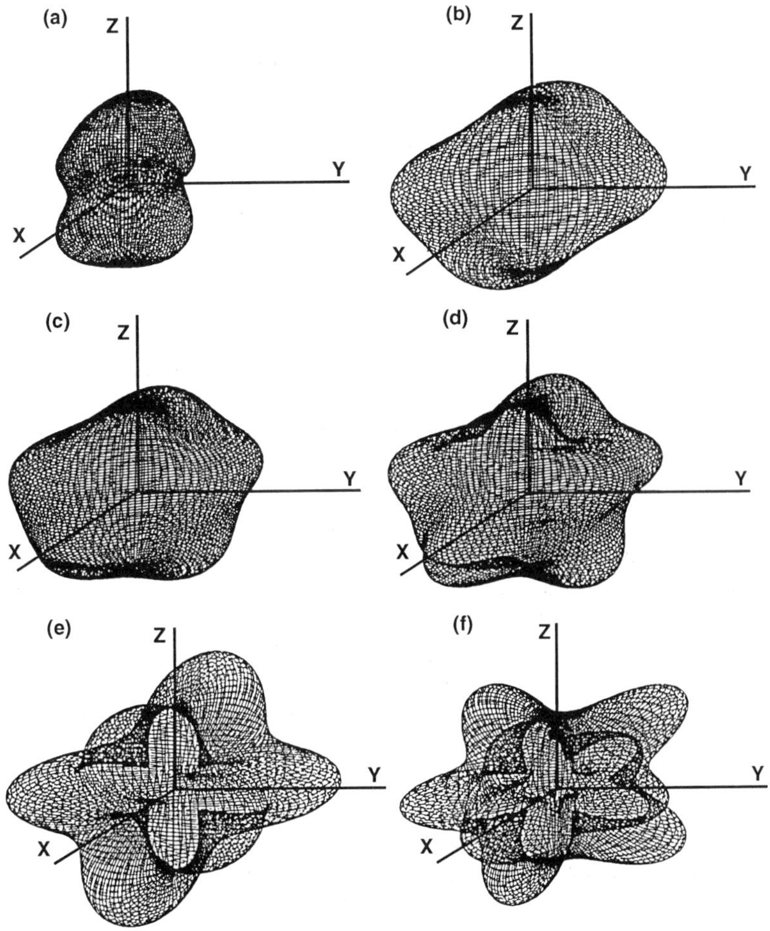

Figure 2.3 — Various modes of instability of the Greenspan–Chaplain model. (After[CHc]).

increases the risk of metastasis. Like the primary tumor, metastases are locally invasive and their cells also enter the lymphatics and blood vessels and cause further dissemination by these routes.

The theory developed for this model enables the locus of an individual cell to be followed (in principle) as it moves about on the surface of the tumor. It transpires that for a dominant high mode number (corresponding to an instability for highly malignant tumors) cells on the surface have a fairly substantial movement in both angular directions (θ and ϕ). Given the greatly reduced cell to cell adherence for malignant tumors and the surface tension distribution according to this model, there is the possibility that single cells or clumps of cells may become detached and carried away, for example, in the bloodstream. In general it appears on the basis of this model that the more malignant the tumor is, the more mobile the cells will be on the surface and the more likely metastasis will be to occur.

A further comment is worth making here. It is tantalizing to speculate, as has been done in other biological contexts [GDa], that what is called invasiveness here can be described as a series of transformations to successively higher energy levels of some generalized surface energy. The onset of instability may be supposed to correspond to a minimum of the total surface energy, subject to certain constraints arising from the organization of the live, proliferating cells on the tumor surface. At the time of writing, little has been done in this area, but the interested reader is referred to Chaplain [CHc] for further details.

Further work by Chaplain and Sleeman [CHd,e] on tumor growth involves the use of results and techniques from (i) nonlinear elasticity theory, and (ii) differential geometry. Their mathematical model describes the growth of a solid tumor using membrane and thick-shell theory. A central feature of the model is the characterization of the material composition of the model through the use of a strain-energy function, thus permitting a mathematical description of the degree of differentiation of the tumor explicitly in the model. Conditions are given in terms of the strain-energy function for the processes of invasion and metastasis occurring in a tumor, being interpreted as the bifurcation modes of the spherical shell (modeling the tumor essentially as this). The results are compared with actual experimental results and with the general behavior shown by benign and malignant tumors. Finally, the authors use these results in conjunction with aspects of surface morphogenesis of tumors (in particular, the Gaussian and mean curvatures of the surface of a solid tumor) in an attempt to produce a mathematical formulation and description of the important medical processes of staging and grading cancers.

Specifically, if (u, v) are the Cartesian coordinates of a point on a plane, mapped isotropically onto a surface $\underline{x}(u, v)$, the Gaussian curvature κ is defined in particular as

$$\kappa = -\frac{1}{\lambda^2} \nabla^2(\log \lambda) \,,$$

where $\lambda(u, v)$ is the linear scale factor of the surface growth at the point (u, v). Recalling that the Laplacian of a function provides an approximate measure of the difference between the average value of the field at a point, and the actual field value at the point, regions for which $\kappa > 0$ (i.e. superharmonic growth rates, $\nabla^2(\log \lambda) < 0$) correspond to regions of the tumor surface where the growth rate is greater than average in the neighborhood of a point. Conversely, $\kappa < 0$ corresponds to subharmonic growth rates, smaller than the average in such a neighborhood.

It may be that the mean curvature H is an indirect way to measure the local surface tension on the tumor surface, since in terms of the principal curvatures κ_1 and κ_2,

$$H = \frac{1}{2}(\kappa_1 + \kappa_2)$$

(the Gaussian curvature can also be written as the product $\kappa_1\kappa_2$). The surface tension locally will be proportional to this mean curvature

$$T = \alpha H$$

and on the basis of this, Chaplain and Sleeman conjecture that there exists a minimum local surface tension $T^*(= \alpha H^*)$ such that if $T \geq T^*$, there is no invasion and/or metastasis; otherwise invasion and/or metastasis will occur. Obviously these ideas are preliminary, but they may form the basis of a significant mathematical component to the medical processes of staging and grading cancers.

A very recent development of these models, by Byrne and Chaplain [BYa] concerns the evolution of a single tumor, prior to the onset of necrosis, with particular attention focused on the existence and stability of steady-state tumor configurations, in which there is a balance between cell proliferation and cell death or apoptosis (i.e. programmed cell death). Modifications to the tumors growth characteristics induced by the presence of an inhibitor are analysed, with a view to assessing the efficacy of certain cancer treatments. For simplicity of exposition, a single nutrient species and single inhibitor species are considered, so that the model comprises two coupled reaction-diffusion equations for each species and an integro-differential equation which describes the evolution of the tumor boundary.

In the light of considerable evidence in its favor, Byrne and Chaplain note that it is highly likely that apoptosis is the cause of the observed volume loss in solid spheroids in vivo and should, therefore, be included in any mathematical model describing their evolution. To date, only McElwain and Morris [MCb] have incorporated apoptosis into mathematical model, by assuming a constant cell (or, equivalently, nutrient) loss rate in mitosing regions. Under certain conditions, their model admits *dormant* states which do not possess necrotic cores. The dormant states possess a two-layer structure: an outer, proliferating rim, enveloping a layer in which the rates of nutrient consumption and cell proliferation fall. By contrast, the model proposed in [BYa] admits mono-layer dormant solutions, which correspond to a tumor comprising only viable, proliferating cells, in which the flux and consumption of nutrient are in equilibrium. The authors show that this feature is crucial to the existence of nontrivial steady configurations, for which the central necrotic core is absent. Without this cell-loss term, no such solutions exist and the familiar results are recovered, with exponential growth of the tumor predicted throughout phase I. (A phase I tumor is defined to be a tumor comprising only active proliferating cells with no regions of necrosis evident).

Another feature of this model, previously unaddressed, is that multiple scale analysis is employed: we have already noted that the diffusion time scale of nutrients and inhibitors in spheroids, (of the order of minutes) is much shorter than the typical tumor doubling time (hours or even days). These disparate time scales can be exploited to gain insight into the transient behavior of tumors. In dimensionless variable the mathematical system they consider is

$$\varepsilon\frac{\partial\sigma}{\partial t}=\frac{1}{r^2}\frac{\partial}{\partial r}\left(r^2\frac{\partial\sigma}{\partial r}\right)+\Gamma(\sigma_\beta-\sigma)-\lambda\sigma-\gamma_1\beta\,,\tag{2.53}$$

$$\varepsilon\frac{\partial\beta}{\partial t}=\frac{D}{r^2}\frac{\partial}{\partial r}\left(r^2\frac{\partial\beta}{\partial r}\right)-\gamma_2\beta\,,\tag{2.54}$$

$$\frac{\partial R}{\partial t}=\frac{s}{R^2}\int_0^R(\sigma-\tilde{\sigma})\left(1-\frac{\beta}{\tilde{\beta}}\right)r^2\,dr\,,\tag{2.55}$$

subject to boundary and initial conditions

$$\begin{aligned}&\frac{\partial\sigma}{\partial r}(0,t)=\frac{\partial\beta}{\partial r}(0,t)=0\,,\\&\sigma(R,t)=\sigma_R(t)\,,\quad\sigma(r,0)=\sigma_0(r)\,,\\&\beta(R,t)=\beta_R(t)\,,\quad\beta(r,0)=\beta_0(r)\,,\quad R(0)=1\,.\end{aligned}\tag{2.56}$$

The variables σ, β and R refer to the nutrient concentration, inhibitor concentration and outer radius respectively. The small parameter ε (with ε small compared with 1) is the ratio of the diffusion time to the doubling time; σ_β, $\tilde{\beta}$ (all constants) are the nutrient concentration in the vasculature, and limiting nutrient and inhibitor concentrations respectively. $s\sigma$ is a first-order cell proliferation rate, and Γ (also constant) is the rate of nutrient transfer per unit length of vasculature; $\lambda\sigma$ is the nutrient depletion or consumption rate, and $\gamma_1\beta, \gamma_2\beta$ represent simple forms chosen to represent sinks of nutrient and inhibitor respectively. In the resulting study of this system, both analytical and numerical, an important parameter arises:

$$\Lambda = \frac{1}{3}\,\frac{\tilde{\sigma} - \dfrac{\Gamma\sigma_\beta}{\Gamma+\lambda}}{\sigma_{R_s} - \dfrac{\Gamma\sigma_\beta}{\Gamma+\lambda}},$$

where R_s is the value of R in the inhibitor-free, steady state model ($\varepsilon = 0$). In particular, Byrne and Chaplain show that if $\Lambda > \frac{1}{3}$ then the trivial solution is asymptotically stable, and no nontrivial tumors exist. Conversely, if $0 < \Lambda < \frac{1}{3}$, then the trivial solution is unstable and a nontrivial tumor configuration exists which is stable. For an avascular tumor ($\Gamma = 0$), this result reduces to give $0 < \tilde{\sigma} < \sigma_R$ as necessary conditions for the existence and stability of nontrivial tumor configurations. From this they deduce an important role played by apoptosis in obtaining nontrivial solutions: in the absence of apoptosis, with $\tilde{\sigma} = 0$, the trivial solution is the only steady solution. Where they exist, the steady solutions possess a quasi two-layer structure: in the outer region there is a net proliferation of cells, towards the centre of the tumor there is a net loss of cells, but the net result of the two effects, averaged over the tumor, yields an equilibrium configuration.

In the light of their detailed examination of the model, Byrne and Chaplain draw the following conclusions. Under normal circumstances the tissue environment is hostile to the malignancy ($\Lambda > \frac{1}{3}$) and the tumor-free trivial state is the only stable configuration that can be sustained. A change in the tissue environment brought about by, for example, stress, illness or disease, tranforms the system into one which is more conducive to tumor growth ($0 < \Lambda < \frac{1}{3}$, for the inhibitor-free case). Depending on the physical laws governing nutrient consumption, cell proliferation, etc., the tumor may develop rapidly and without bound until compressional forces from the external surroundings of the host organ check its growth (unstable growth). Equally, it may grow to a finite size (existence and stability of nontrivial solution) which is relatively harmless to the individual and can be sustained until either the tumor becomes vascularized as a result of angiogenesis, or until some change in the external surroundings destabilizes the dormant configuration. The implications of this for cancer therapies are intriguing and certainly worthwhile pursuing.

2.4 A Predator-Prey Approach

In [DLa], a deterministic predator prey model was presented which described the cell population dynamics of a solid tumor in the presence of a specifically reactive lymphocyte population stimulated by and antagonistic to the tumor. In this relatively simple model of immune response, the lymphocytes produced by the host are regarded as predators and the tumor cells are regarded as prey. Since the growth kinetics of multicell spheroids are similar to in-vivo tumors, the model here may apply to the early vascular stage of growth of these spheroids when inserted into laboratory mammals. In [ADg] the basic model was modified to include, in a primitive manner, the effects of vascularization. The resulting nonlinear system of equations contains six parameters, each of which may be regarded as a bifurcation parameter when the remainder are held constant.
In what follows (see [DLa], [REa]):

L = number of free lymphocytes on the tumor surface,
C_f = number of cancer cells within the spherical tumor and on its surface that are not bound by a lymphocyte,
C_0 = number of cancer cells comprising the tumor,
C_s = total number of cancer cells (bound and unbound) on the cancer surface,
L_c = maximum number of lymphocytes that can be attained (saturation level).

Since within the tumor no cancer cell is bound by a lymphocyte, the following relationship exists:

$$C = C_f - C_0 + C_s \, . \tag{2.57}$$

The assumptions inherent in this model differ from those in [DEa] only insofar as additional terms representing the effects of vascularization on growth rates of free lymphocytes and cancer cells are concerned; this is, however, a significant difference as it enables this model to account (in a phenomenological manner) for modifications of the population dynamics due to enhanced nutrient supply within the tumor.

Assumption 2.4.1. *Only cells on the tumor surface are vulnerable to attack.*

Assumption 2.4.2. *The lymphocyte death rate is a first-order process, with rate constant* λ_1.

Assumption 2.4.3. *The growth rate of surface lymphocytes is given by* $aC_0 f(L)$*, where* a *is a constant.*
Specifically,

$$f(L) = L\left(1 - \frac{L}{L_c}\right). \tag{2.58}$$

Assumption 2.4.4. *In the absence of lymphocytes, the growth rate of cancer cells is a first-order process with rate constant* λ_2*.*

Assumption 2.4.5. *The elimination rate of cancer cells is proportional (with constant of proportionality* b*) to the product of the number of free lymphocytes and unbound cancer cells on the tumor surface.*

Assumption 2.4.6. *The tumor remains spherical at all times.*

Assumption 2.4.7. *There are no differences in cell numbers per unit volume within the tumor.*

Assumption 2.4.8. *There is an equilibrium relation between the free and bound lymphocytes.*

Assumption 2.4.9. *The rate of change of the free lymphocyte population is reduced by an amount proportional to the surface area of the tumor that is penetrated by the vascular network.*

Assumption 2.4.10. *The rate of change of the total number of cancer cells is enhanced by an amount proportional to the volume of the tumor that is occupied by the vascular network.*

In these last two assumptions we further posit that the specified surface area/volume penetration is proportional to the tumor surface area/volume respectively. This can be modified somewhat, but is not unreasonable biologically and certainly provides some additional mathematical simplification.

Governing equations

We first note that Assumptions 2.4.6 and 2.4.7 imply

$$C_s = gC^{2/3}, \tag{2.59}$$

where g is a positive constant. Assumption 2.4.8 implies that

$$C_s = C_0 = KC_0L \tag{2.60}$$

in terms of the equilibrium constant K for lymphocyte-cancer cell interaction. Thus it follows that

$$C_0 = \frac{gC^{2/3}}{1 + KL} \cdot \tag{2.61}$$

From (2.57), therefore

$$C_f = C - \frac{gKLC^{2/3}}{1 + KL} \cdot \tag{2.62}$$

We are now in a position to write down the complete pair of predator-prey equations for the system, namely:

$$\frac{dL}{dt} = -\lambda_1 L + aC_0\left(1 - \frac{L}{L_c}\right) - \hat{\beta}_1 C^{2/3} , \tag{2.63}$$

$$\frac{dC}{dt} = \lambda_2\left(C - \frac{gC^{2/3}KL}{1 + KL}\right) - \frac{bgKLC^{2/3}}{1 + KL} + \beta_2 C , \tag{2.64}$$

where $\hat{\beta}_1$ and β_2 are constants representing the "efficiency" of penetration of the tumor surface area and volume respectively. In terms of the new variables and parameters

$$x = KL , \qquad y = KC , \qquad x_c = KL_c ,$$
$$\alpha_1 = agK^{-2/3} , \qquad \alpha_2 = gk^{1/3}(\lambda_2 + bK^{-1}) , \qquad \beta_1 = \hat{\beta}_1 K^{1/3} ,$$

these equations become, respectively,

$$\frac{dx}{dt} = -\lambda_1 x + y^{2/3}\left(\frac{\alpha_1 x(x_c - x)}{x_c(1 + x)} - \beta_1\right) \equiv F(x, y) , \tag{2.65}$$

$$\frac{dy}{dt} = (\lambda_2 + \beta_2)y - \frac{\alpha_2 x y^{2/3}}{1 + x} \equiv G(x, y) . \tag{2.66}$$

The domain restrictions are $0 \leq x \leq x_c$; $y \geq 0$, and $\alpha_1 > 0$, $\alpha_2 > 0$, $\beta_1 \geq 0$, $\beta_2 \geq 0$, $\lambda_1 > 0$, $\lambda_2 > 0$. Critical or equilibrium points occur when

$$F(x, y) = 0 = G(x, y) . \tag{2.67}$$

Obviously $(0, 0)$ is such a point, and is unstable (see the discussion below). If x and y are both non-zero, then eliminating y between the Eqs.

(2.67) yields the following expression for the x-location of remaining critical points:

$$k_1 = \frac{x^2(x_c - x)}{x_c(1+x)^3} - \frac{k_2 x}{(1+x)^2} \equiv \psi(x_c, k_2; x)\,, \tag{2.68}$$

where

$$k_1 = \frac{\lambda_1(\lambda_2 + \beta_2)^2}{\alpha_1 \alpha_2^2} \tag{2.69}$$

and

$$k_2 = \frac{\beta_1}{\alpha_1}\,. \tag{2.70}$$

Qualitatively, we may understand the solutions of (2.68) by examining the intersection of the horizontal line $y = k_1$ with the graph of $y = \psi(x)$. In Figure 2.4, $\psi(x)$ is illustrated for several values of k_2, including that corresponding to no vascularization ($k_2 = 0$). The maximum value of $\psi(x)$ occurs at

$$x_m = \alpha^{-1}\left(1 + \sqrt{1 - \alpha k_2}\right), \tag{2.71}$$

where

$$\alpha = 1 + \frac{3}{x_c} - k_2\,.$$

Clearly a restriction on k_2 for x_m to be real is that $\alpha k_2 \leq 1$. The expression for $\psi(x_m)$ is complicated and we do not write it here; it is sufficient for our purposes to make several observations. First, in the absence of vascularization ($k_2 = 0$)

$$x_m = \frac{2x_c}{x_c + 3} \quad \text{and} \quad \psi(x_m) = \frac{4x_c^2}{27(1+x_c)^2}\,. \tag{2.72}$$

Secondly, as k_2 increases away from zero, x_m decreases, as of course does $\psi(x_m)$. Eventually there is a critical value of k_2 above which $\psi(x) \leq 0$ for all $x \in [0, x_c]$, again placing a constraint on acceptable values of this parameter. Thirdly, it is clear that increasing β_1 and β_2 (with other parameters constant) will increasingly separate the two graphs whose intersection we seek.

There are zero, one or two points of intersection depending on whether k_1 exceeds, equals or is exceeded by $\psi(x_m)$ respectively. The topological dynamics of these critical points remain the same, it is readily seen, in the $k_2 \neq 0$ case as in the $k_2 = 0$ case (though of course the critical points are functions of all the parameters in general). Thus, when $k_1 > \psi(x_m)$ the only critical point is $(0, 0)$: it is unstable, for any initial non-zero value of (x, y) the trajectories approach (x_c, ∞), i.e. uncontrollable tumor growth.

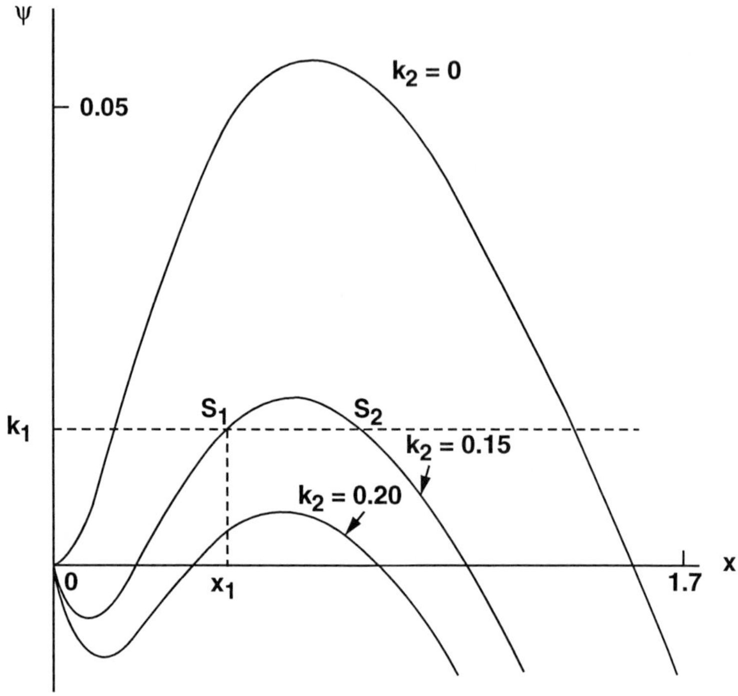

Figure 2.4 — The function $\psi(x_c, k_2; x)$ for various values of k_2; the intersections $\psi = k_1$ define the equilibrium points $S_1(x_1, y_1)$ and $S_2(x_2, y_2)$. $x_c = 1.5$ here.

If $k_1 = \psi(x_m)$ then the second critical point is $(x_m, \psi(x_m))$. Here again, this is unstable with trajectories approaching (x_c, ∞); for a more detailed discussion of the trajectories see [DEa]. Finally, if $k_1 < \psi(x_m)$ there are two points of intersection, $S_1(x_1, y_1)$ and $S_2(x_2, y_2)$; S_2 is a saddle point and therefore unstable, but S_1 may be a center, node or focus and either stable or unstable. (It was the point S_1 that was the focus of attention in [ADg].)

Note that increasing λ_1, λ_2, β_1 or β_2 or decreasing α_1 or α_2 favors tumor survival (by tending S_1 non-existent). Decreasing λ_1, λ_2, β_1 or β_2, or increasing α_1 or α_2 may favor a stationary state of oscillation of the system (i.e. limit cycle). In the expression for k_1 we also note that variations in α_2, λ_2 or β_2 may have more significant influence on the dynamics of the system than comparable variations in λ_1 or α_1.

As noted above, the ultimate behavior of the system studied here is determined by whether or not in expression (2.68), k_1 is greater than, equal to or less than the maximum value of $\psi(x_c, k_2; x)$, i.e. $\psi(x_m)$, where x_m is given by Eq. (2.71). Phase plane analysis indicates that in the first two situations all trajectories move towards (x_c, ∞), i.e. unbounded tumor cell proliferation. Reasons why this may occur are most easily seen from the expressions (2.69) and (2.70) for k_1 and k_2 respectively, in conjunction with Figure 2.4. **Increasing** (i) the lymphocyte death rate λ_1, (ii) the growth rate of cancer cells λ_2, (iii) the degree of vascularization of the tumor (β_1 and β_2), or **decreasing** (iv) the growth rate of surface lymphocytes a, (and hence α_1) or (v) the elimination rate of cancer cells b, (and hence α_2) tend to increase k_1 and k_2, moving the system towards (x_c, ∞). On the other hand **decreasing** (i)–(iii) and **increasing** (iv)–(v) reduce k_1 and k_2, rendering more it likely that the condition $k_1 < \psi(x_m)$ will occur. Indeed, parameter ranges exist for which this will occur, and in these regimes the possibility exists for periodic oscillations of lymphocyte and tumor cell populations to occur in the form of limit cycle behavior.

Clearly k_2 is more sensitive to variations in the quantities $(\lambda_2 + \beta_2)$ and α_2 than to variations in λ_1, and α_1 (changing the latter only affects the tumor indirectly; changing the former affects the tumor directly). As pointed out in [DLa], should oscillations occur, their significance will depend on their location in the phase plane and upon their amplitude. If they are such that the host can tolerate the maximum levels of tumor and lymphocyte cells (i.e. the amplitude is small enough), and the limit cycle is stable, then survival of both populations is possible. The periods of such oscillations will determine how realistic such models might be for studies of tumor remission, for example.

Although not explicitly identified here, the possibility exists for anomalous behavior to occur. This was first noted in [DLa] and the incorporation of terms corresponding to the vascularization of the tumor will not change the qualitative nature of the phenomenon. Examples of such anomalous behavior are uncontrolled tumor growth (ultimately) arising from a **reduction** in the number of tumor cells or an **increase** in the number of lymphocytes. This can occur according to the model when the limit cycle is such that a perturbation to the trajectory moves it out of one region into another which has (x_c, ∞) as the inexorable limit. Such perturbations of course, being external to the system, may correspond to surgery, with consequent agressive tumor cell proliferation, or therapy of some kind designed to reduce the tumor cell population. Infusion of lymphocytes in some treatment modalities may also have this highly undesirable consequence. Indeed, as early as 1971, Prehn [PRa] found that an increase in the number of lymphocytes could enhance the likelihood of tumor survival under certain circumstances.

Further developments are possible along other lines. In [DLa] a modification of the basic model allowed for lymphocytes to enter the system at a steady rate, by adding a constant source term $\lambda_1 x_0$ to the right hand side of Eq. (2.63). The dynamics, even in the avascular case, are then much more complicated because there may be more equilibrium points. In a sequel to that paper [REa], the authors introduced a delay in the formation of killer lymphocytes. The introduction of a second stage allows tumor development from even a single cell (i.e. "de novo" tumor growth). Thus the lymphocytes are not active as soon as they are produced, but mature at a fixed rate. In addition, the saturation term for lymphocytes was represented by exp $(-L/L_c)$ rather than $(1 - L/L_c)$. Finally, noting that a tumor is frequently vascularized (as assumed here), Assumption 2.4.1 was modified to include all tumor cells, not merely those on the surface, because lymphocytes may now have access to the entire tumor volume. However, the presence of a vascular network will undoubtedly enhance the proliferation rate of tumor cells also (represented by the term $\beta_2 y$ in (2.66) in the present model). Furthermore, the present model also contains the above modified assumption insofar as it corresponds to a reduction of the term λ_1 in Eq. (2.65).

More recently, an entirely different approach to the dynamics of tumor-host immune interactions has been formulated, based on the modeling of cellular interactions after the fashion of nonlinear statistical mechanics [BLa]. The philosophy behind this method of modeling is entirely complementary to the deterministic type of model adopted here, and it would be of interest to pursue the interconnections between two approaches, particularly in the light of Section 5 of [BLa], and related comments made in [ADe].

2.5 A Model of Tumor Cell/Immune System Interaction

Cancer is a complex phenomenon consequent on the breakdown of the normal cellular interaction and control of replication. The transformation of a normal cell can be broadly described as follows [LEa], [WHa], [HEa]. In normal tissues, the pattern of organization is determined by a sophisticated interplay of long- and short-range interactions between cells. These interactions are mediated by genetically coded proteins, and they control the mechanisms involved in cellular replication. There are many factors likely to be of importance in all this — metabolic, hormonal, genetic, immunological, geometric, environmental, etc. Any disturbance in this genetic control (e.g. due to environmental factors) may yield a cell or cells with a different type of response to the cellular interactions taking place in its local milieu. A malignant transformation will produce cells that are characterized by a high proliferative advantage. There are mechanisms of defense against such "predator" cells which under normal circumstances will destroy the abnormal cells or at least control their subsequent development. One such mechanism involves the immune system and the phenomenon of immunosurveillance. Thus, in general terms, certain cells of a tissue may lose their physiological function (due to environmental or other carcinogenic agents, or viral oncogenes) and become malignant. They subsequently tend to invade the host organism by rapid proliferation (and, if successful, with subsequent vascularization and metastasis). Generally, the organism tries to counteract their action by sending specialized "killer cells" into the "battlefield". The result is a competition between malignant and killer cells (amongst other things; and as discussed in Section 2.4 for a particular model), the outcome of which will decide whether the cancer is rejected or becomes dominant.

More specifically, the immune system produces undifferentiated immune stem cells in the bone marrow. These subsequently differentiate into B- and T- lymphocytes, and are released into the organism as a whole. When the B-cells encounter the antigen (foreign "invader") they differentiate further into large cells that proliferate and secrete chemical substances capable of neutralizing the antigen (antibodies). On the other hand, the T-cells, after further differentiation in the thymus, regulate the action of the B-cells by both activation (or enhancement) and inhibition (or suppression). They are also involved in immune responses that are directly cell-mediated. This function-cytotoxic activity is shared by other cellular species of the immune system, such as macrophages. There is a sequence of increasingly sophisticated mathematical models in the literature that concerns such cell-mediated responses. Early theoretical studies were carried out in [PIa,b] (see also [BEb]). These works did not address the spatio-temporal problem of antibody-antigen dynamics, but are nevertheless extremely important to an understanding of (to quote Bell [BEa]) a "simplest possible" model of immune response. Lefever and Garay [LEb] also developed a model of local cellular interactions in tumors, and under some reasonable simplifying assumptions obtained a local balance equation for the number x of target (cancer) cells. They summarized much of the data on cytotoxic and rejection parameters for the various neoplastic cell populations. This is important, because once the malignant cell production rate is inhibited, and the T-cell cytotoxicity ensures tumor rejection, tumor recurrence is certainly possible as long as a single neoplastic cell exists.

The next development along these lines was provided by Prigogine and Lefever [PGa]. They included spatial (1-dimensional) variations in a **set** of local balance equations for the cancer cells (dead and alive) and effector cells. This formulation leads directly to the concept of reaction-diffusion equations, which have received considerable attention in the last several decades (for an early account, see Fife [FIa]). Most of their subsequent analysis in that paper pertains to the scalar case which arises when the effector cells diffuse much faster than the cancer cells "propagate" by cellular replication, and when the dead cells are eliminated rapidly. The governing equation is nevertheless extremely rich in its structure, and it is this richness of structure that we address here in summary fashion.

A type of reaction-diffusion analysis related to [PRa] above has also been carried out by Lefever and Erneaux [LEc]. They incorporated nonlinear terms and used perturbation techniques to construct slowly-varying travelling wave solutions to a system of four coupled reaction-diffusion equations. They also examined the sensitivity of the system to environmental fluctutations, and the dependence of bistability on these fluctuations. Cellular environments depend, as we have noted above, on a plethora of factors (genetic, metabolic, geometric, hormonal, immunological, membranous, radiation, temperature, etc.) which can be expected to fluctuate somewhat over time (at best they may be constant on average). The authors showed that even in the presence of large, extremely rapid and completely incoherent (memoryless) noise (like Gaussian white noise) the stationary state of the tumor growth model remains remarkably coherent. Furthermore, by increasing the variance of the noise, it is possible to induce bistability in a system which displays none (for certain parameter ranges) under constant environmental conditions. Clearly, this may modify the mechanism of tumor growth — indeed, tumor rejection seems facilitated [LEd]. More recently, Qi [QIa] has re-examined some of the above models by Lefever and co-workers. He has reduced his system to one in two variables x and p, representing the density of living and dead cancerous cells, respectively. Obviously the dynamics of this system can be very complex as the parameter domains vary: we will be content in this section to survey the response of a spatio-temporal system with one dependent variable (x); this model may be extended to include [ADh] various growth terms chosen both for their suggestive behavior as growth factor modifications, and for their analytic simplicity. More recent work in this area can be found in [LEe].

As we have noted, tumor growth is a function not only of the tumor cells themselves and their environment, but also upon their interactions with each other and normal cells. Most notably, there is much interest with regard to "Transforming Growth Factors" (TGF's: see [GSa], [ADj]). Sporn and Todaro [SPa] and Sporn and Roberts [SPb] have proposed two pathways for the involvement of growth factors in cellular growth control. Thus, an **autocrine** control loop corresponds to a type of self-stimulation, whereby a cell secretes a hormone-like substance for which the cell itself has surface receptors [BJa]. Recently, this concept has been extended to include inhibitory control mechanisms also [ROa]. The other type of control loop is **paracrine**, in which local release of growth factors affects other types of cells in the surrounding microenvironment. The primary effect of paracrine factors is an increase of the organism's ability, at a local level, to support the tumor. Thus, the tumor manipulates its environment to its own advantage (see the chapter by Michelson in this book).

An important related aspect of the above discussion is that of cancer metastasis. Once a tumor cell enters the blood stream or lymphatic system, it runs a major risk, as we have noted, of being wiped out by an immune system on the lookout for such cells. Tumor cells may escape this danger, however, by losing the cell surface molecules [MXa] that are needed for recognition by some immune cells. Tumor cells may also "protect themselves" against immune attack by forming aggregates. If these avoidance processes are successful, there is still no guarantee that all of the cells arriving at a potentially new organ site are capable of growing there, however. The response may well be related to the presence of growth factors produced by that cells microenvironment. Metastatic cells may become responsive to the growth factor(s) by switching on the gene(s) encoding the receptor(s) for it (them). As pointed out in [MXa], any or all of the adaptions that tumor cells must undergo to become metastatic might provide points of attack for therapies aimed at preventing or treating disseminated cancer.

To be somewhat quantitative in the light of these general points, consider a volume element containing a total number of N cells. N represents a saturation level for the cancer cells in that local volume element. The population of tumor cells is denoted by $X(\hat{r}, t)$, while the cytotoxic or "effector" cells are in one of two states: free (E_0) or bound (E), i.e. having recognized and bound a target cancer cell. The role of the cytotoxic cells is to limit the size of the tumor population by recognizing and destroying them. The rate constant for cellular replication of the tumor cells is λ. The recognition-binding process of the X population cells by the E_0 effector cells (rate constant k_2) is followed [LEa] by the lysis of the former and the dissociation of the complex E into E_0 and some non-replicating cellular product P (rate constant k_2). The total number of effector cells is assumed constant in time (for a justification of this and other assumptions see [LEb]). Schematically, the above mechanisms can be represented as follows

$$X \xrightarrow{\lambda} 2X \qquad \text{(proliferation)}$$

$$E_0 + X \xrightarrow{k_1} E \xrightarrow{k_2} E_0 + P \text{ (binding and lysis)}.$$

As far as the various parameter domains are concerned, we will be guided by the detailed and well-justified data in [LEd]. Typically,

i) $0.2/\text{day} < \lambda < 1.5/\text{day}$;
ii) $10^{-2} < \beta < 10$;
iii) $10^{-1} < \theta < 5$;
iv) $0.1 < k_1 N, \qquad k_2 < 20$

where $N \equiv 10^6$ cells/mm^3 for solid cancers.

Lefever and Garay [LEd] also noted that the scale of increasing cytotoxic activity for different active effector cells is: activated macrophages <

immune T-lymphocytes and natural killer cells < allosensitized T lymphocytes (corresponding to the above parameter ranges).

For the population density of malignant cells X, the governing equation is

$$\frac{\partial X}{\partial t} = \lambda f(X) - k_1 E_0 X + D\frac{\partial^2 X}{\partial \hat{r}^2}, \tag{2.73}$$

where D is the coefficient of diffusion and λ is a rate constant for $f(X)$ where

$$f(X) = X\left(1 - \frac{X}{N}\right), \tag{2.74}$$

where N is a "local" saturation limit or carrying capacity. Thus f represents a logistic type growth rate, and represents a "normal" growth term. Extensions of this model to include other types of growth rate terms can be found in [ADh]. The equation for the population density E_0 of free cytotoxic cells is

$$\frac{dE_0}{dt} = -k_1 E_0 X + k_2 E. \tag{2.75}$$

Since lysis is expected to be much faster than the other processes in the volume element considered [PGa], the quasi-steady state approximation $dE_0/dt = 0$ is invoked, implying

$$E = \frac{k_1 E_t X}{k_1 X + k_2}, \tag{2.76}$$

whence Eq. (2.73) becomes

$$\frac{\partial X}{\partial t} = \lambda f(X) - \frac{k_1 k_2 E_t X}{k_1 X + k_2} + D\frac{\partial^2 X}{\partial \hat{r}^2}. \tag{2.77}$$

The following changes of variable

$$x = \frac{k_1 X}{k_2}, \quad \tau = \lambda t, \quad \theta = \frac{k_2}{k_1 N}, \quad \beta = \frac{k_1 E_t}{\lambda}, \quad \hat{r} = \left(\frac{D}{\lambda}\right)^{\frac{1}{2}} r,$$

reduce (2.77) to

$$\frac{\partial x}{\partial \tau} = g(x) - \frac{\beta x}{1+x} + \frac{\partial^2 x}{\partial r^2}, \tag{2.78}$$

where $g(x) = x(1 - \theta x)$.

A convenient and evocative description of the steady states of the governing partial differential equation can be made in terms of the so-called free energy function $V(x)$, extrema of which define the homogeneous states of the system. This function is of particular importance in the study of phase coexistence of tumoral/non-tumoral regimes and subsequent nucleation in dimensions greater than one. In terms of $V(x)$, the steady states of Eq. (2.78) are solutions of the Hamiltonian type system

$$H = \frac{1}{2}\left(\frac{dx}{dr}\right)^2 + V(x)\,, \tag{2.79}$$

where H is a spatial invariant determined by the boundary conditions chosen, and the "potential energy" or "free energy" referred to above is

$$V(x) = \int_0^x g(\alpha)\,d\alpha - \beta x + \beta \ln(x+1)\,. \tag{2.80}$$

The homogeneous steady states of Eq. (2.78) are the extrema of $V(x)$, which in general admits at most two physically acceptable values, i.e. x_s, where

$$g(x_s) = \frac{\beta x_s}{1+x_s}\,. \tag{2.81}$$

We refer to the situation when $x_s = 0$ as the null tumoral or "cancer free" state. Clearly, this exists for all values of θ and β. However, this cancer-free state is unstable for $\beta < 1$; it is stable for $\beta > 1$. The non-zero steady state for $\theta > 1$ is given by [PGa], [ADh]

$$x_s(\beta) = \frac{1-\theta+\sqrt{(1+\theta)^2 - 4\theta\beta}}{2\theta}\,. \tag{2.82}$$

This exists only for $\beta < 1$ (see Figure 2.5b). In terms of the quantity β_c, where

$$\beta_c = \frac{(1+\theta)^2}{4\theta}\,, \tag{2.83}$$

this steady state is stable with respect to small departures from x_s.

If $\theta < 1$, there exists for $\beta \in (1, \beta_c)$ the phenomenon of bistability: two non-zero (i.e., cancerous) steady states exist (see Figure 2.5a). The upper branch in $(0, \beta_c)$ is stable, the lower is unstable. If $\beta < 1$, only the stable upper branch is present. If $\beta > \beta_c$, we recover the stable cancer-free state only. The bistability is defined by

$$x_s(\beta) = \frac{1-\theta \pm 2\sqrt{\theta(\beta_c - \beta)}}{2\theta}\,. \tag{2.84}$$

Phase-plane analysis of the governing equations yields the likelihood (under appropriate conditions) of traveling wavefront solutions, carrying

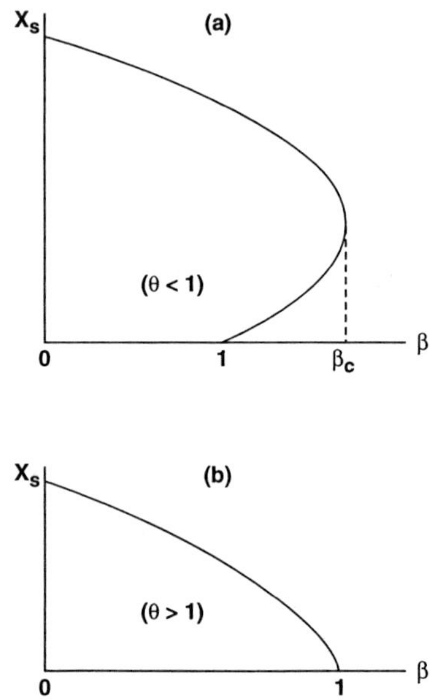

Figure 2.5 — Steady states $x_s(\beta)$ for (a) $\theta < 1$, (b) $\theta > 1$.

one stable steady state into another stable or unstable one. Lower bounds on the wave speeds may be obtained in standard fashion [MUa]. The wave can be progressive ($c > 0$) or regressive ($c < 0$) depending on the available difference of free energy $V(x)$ between the steady states, and in principle the sign of c can change as the various biological parameters are modified appropriately. Analytic solutions for the waveform and speed have been obtained for approximate "source terms" in the governing equations and this provides insight into the dependence of the wave speed on the location of the steady states. Estimates of wave speeds can be made for a certain range of diffusion coefficient, as are estimates (neglecting spherical geometric effects) of a tumor "nucleus" size at coexistence (see [ADh]). Sherratt [SRa,b] has studied wave problems in this context in considerable detail.

As is frequently the case in mathematical modeling [MUa], [BDa] a simplified one-dimensional model can give useful insights and parameter limitations for a more realistic fully three-dimensional problem. Many of the characteristics of the simpler system are present in more complex ones (usually modified by geometric factors). However, there is a limitation that needs to be noted: the spherically symmetric radial version of Eq. (2.78) will contain an additional term $2r^{-1}(\partial x/\partial r)$ on the right-hand side. This will preclude in general the existence of plane wave solutions $\phi(r - c\tau)$ for constant c. However, although $c = c(r)$ in general it is clear that for sufficiently large r (provided that $x(r)$ can be considered "slowly varying" in some appropriate sense) this term will usually become small compared to the others.

There is an alternative, somewhat indirect way of gaining insight into this problem. Consider the dimensional Eq. (2.77) written in the following form

$$\frac{\partial X}{\partial t} = \lambda M(X) + D\nabla^2 X\,, \tag{2.85}$$

where

$$\nabla^2 \equiv r^{-n}\frac{\partial}{\partial r}\left(r^n \frac{\partial}{\partial r}\right), \qquad n = 0, 1, 2\,,$$

and $M(X)$ is a general growth term.
Linearizing about $X = 0$ gives

$$\frac{\partial X}{\partial t} = \lambda M'(0)X + D\nabla^2 X\,. \tag{2.86}$$

In one dimension ($n = 0$) a progressive wave of the form $X(r,t) = \phi(r - ct) = \phi(\eta)$ must satisfy

$$D\phi'' + c\phi' + \alpha\phi = 0\,, \tag{2.87}$$

where $\alpha = \lambda M'(0)$.

A necessary and sufficient condition for a non-negative solution ϕ to exist is that $c^2 \geq 4\alpha D$ (there being no restriction if $\alpha \leq 0$). However, the fundamental solution to (2.85) for a unit delta function source at the origin is

$$X(r,t) = \frac{1}{(4\pi D t)^{n/2}} \exp\left(at - \frac{r^2}{4Dt}\right), \tag{2.88}$$

so corresponding to a particular cancer cell density $\bar{X}(r,t)$, it must follow that

$$\frac{r^2}{t^2} = 4D\alpha - 2Dn\,\frac{\log t}{t} - \frac{\text{constant}}{t}\,. \tag{2.89}$$

We may associate a "wave" of advance of the initial population with speed arbitrarily close to $2\sqrt{D\alpha} = 2\sqrt{\lambda M'(0)D}$ for sufficiently large times. Note that (2.88) only depends weakly (i.e. in the asymptotic correction) on n.

As noted by Kendall [KEa], even when $\alpha < 0$, the quantity $2\sqrt{D\alpha}$ still carries the connotation of a wave of advance. For given r, the maximum cell population will occur when

$$\frac{r^2}{t^2} = 4D|\alpha| + \frac{2nD}{t}. \tag{2.90}$$

Again, the maxima move outward from the origin with speed asymptotically equal to $2\sqrt{\lambda|M'(0)|D}$.

It is also important to note that for the range of diffusion coefficient values ($10^{-11} - 10^{-9}$ cm^2/sec) the effects of the "reaction" terms are considerable. It can be shown that a tumoral perturbation may grow to a size of 1cm in as little as 50–500 days: this is compared to a pure diffusion timescale of $L^2/D \sim 10 - 1000$ years!

2.6 Models, Metaphors and Similes: Some Alternative Paradigms

In this section the discussion deliberately will be of a more speculative nature than elsewhere: it sometimes happens that thinking about a phenomenon or process along a new direction leads to new insights into the nature of that process (but sometimes it just confuses the issue!). Clearly, a tumor, or even a multicellular spheroid represents a complex system, even if it is considered to be isolated from its environment. As noted in the chapter by Michelson and Leith, we are dealing with a network of signals and reactions, concentrations and gradients, at several levels of description. Even if one could write down all the governing equations for a single cell in relation to its neighbors, the task of solving such equations and interpreting the solutions would be Herculean. Once the interaction with the immune system is incorporated, the classical applied mathematical approach is seen to be inappropriate, to say the least, at the cellular level (though extremely valuable and informative, as we have seen, at the spheroid/tumor level). Perhaps it was this that led to the remark [BLa] that a new type of mathematics might be necessary to better understand tumor/immune system dynamics at this level. We explore the possibility that (i) an existing area of mathematics, catastrophe theory, and (ii) the concept of tunneling, employed to great effect in quantum mechanics (but not exclusively so), may each serve as a metaphor or simile for some of the fundamental processes on the cellular level that are basic to tumor initiation and growth.

Appendix I deals with catastrophe theory and the reader is encouraged to consult this before embarking on the rest of this section. It is appropriate to define the terms simile and metaphor here: a simile is a statement that one thing is like another; in a metaphor the comparison between two different things is implied. A quote from Daniel Stein is also relevant if we are considering using catastrophe theory and tunneling mechanisms as metaphors for cancer growth and development, or even as a failure of the immune system:

"Aside from the obvious fact that atoms and molecules must still obey physical laws whether within biological systems or without, mathematical models of interacting biological components, whether atoms in a protein, neurons in a brain, or species in an ecosystem, can provide useful qualitative insights as long as the questions asked and conclusions drawn are carefully circumscribed. Physicists and mathematicians are not about to provide a comprehensive picture of any of these problems anytime soon, but may still shed some light on certain of their aspects through inspired modeling." [STa].

Certainly, we may hope to add cancer biology/tumor growth to the examples given by Stein.

2.6.1 The tunneling phenomenon

The so-called time-independent Schrödinger equation can be cast in a standard form

$$\frac{d^2\psi}{dx^2} + \big(E - V(x)\big)\psi = 0 \tag{2.91}$$

(where by a redefinition of x the coefficient of the derivative term is unity). In quantum mechanics the quantity $|\psi(x)|^2$ is a measure of the probability that the "particle" of energy $E > 0$ will be found at location "x", given the particular potential $V(x)$ is present. These ideas have been utilized greatly in quantum mechanics of course (for an introduction see [BAa], [MEa] for example), but also in non-quantized field theories (e.g. in oceanography, astrophysics, geophysics, electrical engineering etc. where one is interested in the "leakiness" of waveguides, effectiveness of wave trapping, resonant modes of oscillation, etc.; see [ADk–n]). Such waves (recalling the wave-particle duality at the quantum scale) can penetrate into regions that are forbidden for "classical" particles of the same energy. To illustrate this phenomenon, we briefly describe the interaction, via Eq. (2.91), of a wave with a potential barrier defined by

$$\begin{aligned} V(x) &= V > 0\,, \qquad 0 < x < a \\ &= 0\,, \qquad \text{otherwise}\,. \end{aligned}$$

If we define $k = \sqrt{E}$ and $K = \sqrt{V - E}$, then a wave (corresponding to a particle of energy $E < V$) incident on the potential barrier from the left has the following form (dictated by requiring solutions of Eq. (2.91) to be continuously differentiable and bounded in $(-\infty, \infty)$):

$$\psi(x) = \begin{cases} Ae^{ikx} + Be^{-ikx}, & x < 0 \\ Ce^{-Kx} + De^{Kx}, & 0 < x < a \\ AS(E)e^{ik(x-a)}, & x > a, \end{cases} \tag{2.92}$$

where the coefficients A, B, C and D are constants. By requiring that $\psi(x)$ and $\psi'(x)$ be continuous at $x = 0$ and $x = a$, relationships between these coefficients are easily established. The form of the solution corresponds to a combination of both incident and reflected waves (or streams of particles) for $x < 0$, and transmitted waves (or again, particles in the quantum mechanical sense) for $x > a$. It is well known that the quantity $AS(E)$ must be non-zero in order to satisfy the boundary conditions, meaning that the wave or quantum particle has a non-zero probability of being found to the right of the step. This phenomenon is called *tunneling*. $S(E)$ is often called the transmission amplitude (or tunneling matrix element). For $E < V$ it can be shown that

$$S(E) = \frac{2ikK}{2ikK\cosh(Ka) + (k^2 - K^2)\sinh(Ka)}. \tag{2.93}$$

A related quantity $T(E)$ $(= |S(E)|^2)$ can be regarded as the energy transmission coefficient:

$$T(E) = \frac{4E(V-E)}{4E(V-E) + V^2\sinh^2(Ka)}. \tag{2.94}$$

$T(E)$ is a monotonically increasing function of E for $E < V$. It is the phenomenon of tunneling that in essence is responsible for radioactive decay of α-particles from an atomic nucleus; it also occurs in solid state physics (e.g. in a so-called tunneling junction composed of two metals separated by a thin insulating layer). Furthermore, the *time-dependent* tunneling of a wavepacket can be discussed. This and its connection with the time-independent problem discussed here is addressed in [SCa]. Related quantum mechanical ideas have been applied recently to a model of chemotherapy [ADi].

2.6.2 Some speculation

How then, may we utilize the concepts of tunneling and catastrophe as alternative paradigms for cancer development and immune response? For simplicity, we discuss these topics separately at first and then attempt to tie the threads together.

Consider first the scattering problem as applied to cancer development: let the independent variable x represent a continuous variation from normal cells (x small with respect to 0, say) through benign ($x > a$) to malignant cells (x large with respect to a). The barrier may be considered to represent the "resistance" of a cell to neoplasia, i.e. to becoming cancerous. Let the quantity $|\psi|^2$ represent the probability that a cell of certain "metastatic" or carcinogenic potential E (which must necessarily be defined) will be located at some $x \in (-\infty, \infty)$ given a "resistance" potential barrier $V(x)$.

Alternatively, the barrier may in some way represent the efficiency of the immune system, with $x < 0$ corresponding to an antigen being "trapped" or destroyed by the cumulative effectiveness of the system, and $x > a$ corresponds to immune "escape". Again, for $x > a$, let $|\psi|^2$ represent the probability that a certain antigen is able to escape the effects of the immune system. In each case (i.e. neoplasia and the effectiveness of the immune system in general) the barrier height and to some extent the width (or some combination of both) will determine the effectiveness of the status quo.

We concentrate on the problem of carcinogenesis within this paradigm, since this is perhaps better suited to such speculation, containing as it does the immune system (or its failure) implicit within it. As in quantum mechanics, it may be of significance to regard non-cancer as a metastable state, i.e. the "particle" is trapped for a long time by the barrier or some potential well, but eventually "tunnels" through to the outside, $x > a$, corresponding to the "decay" of the non-cancerous state to a cancerous one. The timescale T for this to occur is proportional to $|\psi|^{-2}$ for any given location x.

We can also regard the transition from state A to state B as a *catastrophe* in which the system, initially occupying one minimum V_A of the potential function is "persuaded" by varying control parameters to occupy another minimum V_B (see Figure 2.6). This process is discussed in more detail in Appendix I. Clearly, when V_A and V_B both exist, separated by a local maximum (unstable), tunneling may also occur (in principle) between the two minima. This is a completely different means of transferring the system from state A to state B; it does not involve any variation of the control parameters.

There is a third possible situation which is more correctly associated with stochastic fluctuations, either of the energy associated with the "particle", or of the barrier itself. In the first instance, a sufficiently large energy fluctuation may cause the particle to surmount the barrier; in the second instance if the potential is fluctuating, a "downward" fluctuation may be sufficient to enable the particle to move to state B. This is another way of looking at the catastrophic jump, replacing smooth variation of control

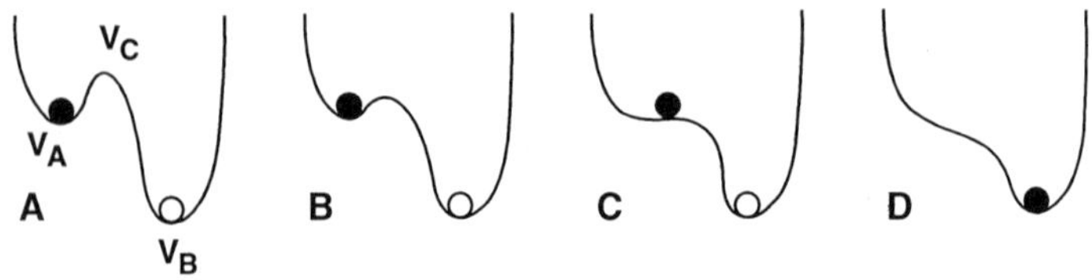

Figure 2.6 — Schematic representation of equilibrium positions V_A, V_B (both stable) and V_C (unstable). The position of the "system" during the ABCD transition is indicated in black. The position during the reverse transition DCBA is in white. (Based on [EKa]).

parameters by fluctuations due to "noise" (see also [LEd]).

We have already noted that we are dealing with metastable states, i.e. with long but finite lifetimes. In order to change from one such configuration to another, the system has to pass through a sequence of less favorable (less probable) configurations, namely a "barrier", possibly of the type discussed in Section 2.6.1. By whatever means we choose to describe this process, the system will spend very little time "en route", so to speak, which explains why so many evolutionary processes in a system appear to be "punctuated"; "missing links" are hard to find (e.g. reactants and products are easily observed in a chemical reaction, but intermediate transition states are not [STa]).

Are ideas such as these of value in thinking about the nature of the complex phenomena we call cancer, and the immune response? This remains to be seen; as these ideas are developed in a more tangible way (in a specific context), the degree to which they accommodate known phenomena and predict new phenomena will be a measure of how far "metaphor" has become "model".

2.7 References

[ADa] Adam J.A., A simplified mathematical model of tumor growth, *Math. Biosci.*, **81** (1986), 229–244.

[ADb] Adam J.A., A mathematical model of tumor growth: II. Effects of geometry and spatial non-uniformity on stability, *Math. Biosci.*, **86** (1987), 183–211.

[ADc] Adam J.A., A mathematical model of tumor growth: III. Comparison with experiment, *Math. Biosci.*, **86** (1987), 213–227.

[ADd] Adam J.A. and Maggelakis S.A., Diffusion regulated growth characteristics of a prevascular carcinoma, *Bull. Math. Biol.*, **52** (1990), 549–582.

[ADe] Adam J.A., On complementary levels of description in applied mathematics. II. Mathematical models in cancer biology, *Int. Jnl. Math. Ed. Sci. Tech.*, **19** (1988), 519–535.

[ADf] Adam J.A. and Noren R., Equilibrium model of a vascularized spherical carcinoma with central necrosis: some properties of the solution, *J. Math. Biol.*, **31** (1993), 735–745.

[ADg] Adam J.A., The effects of vascularization on lymphocyte-tumor cell dynamics: qualitative features, *Math. Comp. Modelling - Special issue on modeling and simulation problems on tumor/immune system dynamics*, Bellomo N. ed., **23** (1996), 1–10.

[ADh] Adam J.A., The dynamics of growth-factor-modified immune response to cancer growth: one dimensional models, *Math. Comp. Modelling*, **17** (1993), 83–106.

[ADi] Adam J.A. and Panetta J.C., A simple mathematical model and alternative paradigm for certain chemotherapeutic regimes, *Math. Comp. Modelling*, **22** (1995), 49–60.

[ADj] Adam J.A., Solution uniqueness and stability criteria for a model of growth factor production, *Appl. Math. Lett.*, **5** (1992), 89–92.

[ADk] Adam J.A., Asymptotic solutions and spectral theory of linear wave equations, *Phys. Repts.*, **86** (1982), 217–316.

[ADl] Adam J.A., Critical layer singularities and complex eigenvalues in some differential equations of mathematical physics, *Phys. Repts.*, **142** (1986), 263–356.

[ADm] Adam J.A., A linear scattering problem in magnetohydrodynamics: transmission resonances in a magnetic slab, *Astrophys. Sp. Sci.*, **133** (1987), 317–337.

[ADn] Adam J.A., Non-radial stellar oscillations: a perspective from potential scattering. I. Theoretical foundations, *Astrophys. Sp. Sci.*, **220** (1994), 179–233.

[ADo] Adam J.A. and Maggelakis S.A., A mathematical model of tumor growth. IV. Effects of a necrotic core, *Math. Biosci.*, **97** (1989), 121–136.

[BAa] Baym G., **Lectures on Quantum Mechanics**, Benjamin (1989).

[BDa] Bender E.A., **An Introduction to Mathematical Modeling**, Wiley (1978).

[BEa] Bell G.I., Predator-prey equations simulating an immune response, *Math. Biosci.*, **16** (1973), 291–314.

[BEb] Bell G.I., Some models for the interaction between cells of the immune system, in **Systems Theory in Immunology**, Brini C., Doria G., Koch G., and Strom R. eds., Lecture Notes in Biomathematics, Vol. 32, Springer-Verlag (1979), 66–74.

[BJa] Bajzer Z. and Vuk-Pavlovic S., Quantitative aspects of autocrine regulation in tumors, *Crit. Rev. Oncog.*, **2** (1990), 53–73.

[BJb] Bajzer Z., Marusic M., and Vuk-Pavlovic S., Conceptual frameworks for mathematical modeling of tumor growth dynamics, *Math. Comp. Modelling - Special Issue on Modelling and Simulation Problems on Tumor-Immune System Dynamics*, Bellomo N. ed., **23** (1996), 31–46.

[BLa] Bellomo N. and Forni G., Dynamics of tumor interaction with the host immune system, *Math. Comp. Modelling*, **20** (1994), 107–122.

[BNa] Burton A.C., Rate of growth of solid tumors as a problem of diffusion, *Growth*, **30** (1966), 159–176.

[BRa] Britton N.F. and Chaplain M.A.J., A qualitative analysis of some models of tissue growth, *Math. Biosci.*, **113** (1993), 77–89.

[BUa] Bullough W.W., Mitotic and functional homeostasis: a speculative review, *Cancer Res.*, **25** (1965), 1683–1727.

[BUb] Bullough W.W. and Deol J.U.R., The pattern of tumor growth, *Symp. Soc. Exp. Biol.*, **25** (1971), 225–275.

[BYa] Byrne H.M. and Chaplain M.A.J., Growth of non-necrotic tumors in the presence and absence of inhibitors, *Math. Biosci.*, **130** (1995), 151–181.

[CAa] Casciari J.J., Sotiochos S.V., and Sutherland R.M., Mathematical modelling of microenvironment and growth in EMT6/Ro multicellular tumor spheroids, *Cell Prolif.*, **25** (1992), 1–22.

[CHa] Chaplain M.A.J. and Britton N.F., On the concentration profile of a growth inhibitory factor in multicell spheroids, *Math. Biosci.*, **115** (1993), 233–243.

[CHb] Chaplain M.A.J., Benson D.L., and Maini P.K., Nonlinear diffusion of a growth inhibitory factor in multicell spheroids, *Math. Biosci.*, **121** (1994), 1–13.

[CHc] Chaplain M.A.J., The development of a spatial pattern in a model for cancer growth, in **Experimental and Theoretical Advances in Biological Pattern Formation**, Othmer H.G., Maini P.K., and Murray J.D. eds., Plenum Press (1993), 45–60.

[CHd] Chaplain M.A.J. and Sleeman B.D., A mathematical model for the growth and classification of a solid tumor: a new approach via nonlinear elasticity theory using strain-energy functions, *Math. Biosci.*, **111** (1992), 169–215.

[CHe] Chaplain M.A.J. and Sleeman B.D., Modelling the growth of solid tumors and incorporating a method for their classification using nonlinear elasticity theory, *J. Math. Biol.*, **31** (1993), 431–473.

[CHf] Chaplain M.A.J., Avascular growth, angiogenesis, and vascular growth in solid tumors: the mathematical modelling of the stages of tumor development, *Math. Comp. Modelling - Special issue on modeling and simulation problems on tumor/immune system dynamics*, Bellomo N. ed., **23** (1996), 47–88.

[CRa] Craig I.J.D. and Brown J.C., **Inverse Problems in Astronomy**, Adam Hilger (1986).

[DEa] Deakin A., Model for the growth of a solid in-vitro tumor, *Growth*, **39** (1975), 159–165.

[DEb] Deakin M.A.B., Applied catastrophe theory in the social and biological sciences, *Bull. Math. Biology*, **42** (1980), 647–679.

[DLa] Delisi C. and Rescigno A., Immune surveillance and neoplasia - I. A minimal mathematical model, *Bull. Math. Biol.*, **39** (1977), 201–221.

[EDa] Edelstein-Keshet L., **Mathematical Models in Biology**, Random House (1988).

[EKa] Ekeland I., **Mathematics and the Unexpected**, University of Chicago Press (1988), Chapter 3.

[FIa] Fife P.C., Mathematical aspects of reacting and diffusing systems, in *Lecture Notes in Biomathematics*, **28** (1979), Springer-Verlag.

[FKa] Franko A.J. and Sutherland R.M., Oxygen diffusion distance and the development of necrosis in multicell spheroids, *Radiat. Res.*, **79** (1979), 439–453.

[FOa] Folkman J., Tumor angiogenesis, *Adv. Cancer Res.*, **19** (1974), 331–358.

[FOb] Folkman J. and Greenspan H.P., Influence of geometry on control of cell growth, *Biochim. Biophys. Acta*, **417** (1975), 211–236.

[FOc] Folkman F. and Klagsbrun M., Angiogenic factors, *Science*, **235** (1987), 442–447.

[FOd] Folkman J. and Hochberg M., Self-regulation of growth in three dimensions, *J. Exp. Med.*, **138** (1973), 745–753.

[FRa] Freyer J.P., Regulation of growth saturation and development of necrosis in EMT6/Ro multicellular spheroids by the glucose and oxygen supply, *Cancer Res.*, **46** (1986), 3504–3512.

[FRb] Freyer J.P., Role of necrosis in regulating the growth saturation of multicellular spheroids, *Cancer Res.*, **48** (1988), 2432–2439.

[GDa] Goodwin B.C. and Trainor L.E.H., A field description of the cleavage process in embryogenesis, *J. Theor. Biol.*, **85** (1980), 757–770.

[GFa] Griffel D.H., **Applied Functional Analysis**, Ellis Harwood (1981).

[GHa] Ghosh Roy D.N., **Methods of Inverse Problems in Physics**, CRC Press (1991).

[GLa] Glass L., Instability and mitotic patterns in tissue growth, *J. Dyn. Syst. Meas. Control*, **95** (1973), 324–327.

[GOa] Goldacre R.J. and Sylven B., On the access of blood-borne dyes to various tumor regions, *Br. J. Cancer*, **16** (1962), 306–322.

[GRa] Greenspan, H.P., Models for the growth of a solid tumor by diffusion, *Stud. Appl. Math.*, **51** (1972), 317–340.

[GRb] Greenspan H.P., On the self-inhibited growth of cell cultures, *Growth*, **38** (1974), 81–95.

[GRc] Greenspan H.P., On the growth and stability of cell cultures and solid tumors, *J. Theor. Biol.*, **56** (1976), 229–242.

[GSa] Goustin A.S., Loef E.B., Shipley G.D., and Moses H.L., Growth factors and cancer, *Cancer Res.*, **46** (1986), 1015–1018.

[HEa] Henkart P.A., Mechanism of lymphocyte-mediated cytotoxicity, *Ann. Rev. Immunol.*, **3** (1985), 31–58.

[JAa] Jain R.K. and Wei J., Dynamics of drug transport in solid tumors: distributed parameter model, *J. Bioeng.*, **1** (1977), 313–330.

[JAb] Jain R.K., Barriers to drug delivery in solid tumors, *Sci. Amer.*, **271** (1994), 58–65.

[JAc] Jain R.K., Comment made by him during a lecture at the International Center for Mathematical Sciences, February 1995.

[JOa] Jones D.S. and Sleeman B., **Differential Equations and Mathematical Biology**, George Allen and Unwin (1983).

[KEa] Kendall D.G., A form of wave propagation associated with the equation of heat conduction, *Proc. Camb. Phil. Soc.*, **44** (1948), 591–594.

[KIa] King W.E., Schultz D.S., and Gatenby R.A., Multi-region models for describing oxygen tension profiles in human tumors, *Chem. Eng. Commun.*, **47** (1986), 73–91.

[LAa] Laird A.K., Dynamics of tumor growth. Comparison of growth rates and extrapolation of growth curve to one cell, *Br. J. Cancer*, **19** (1965), 278–291.

[LEa] Lefever R. and Garay R.P., A mathematical model of the immune surveillance against cancer, in **Theoretical Immunology**, Bell G.I., Perelson A.S., and Pimbley G. eds., Marcel Dekker (1978), 481–518.

[LEb] Lefever R. and Garay R.P., Local description of immune tumor rejection, in **Biomathematics and Cell Kinetics**, Vallerron A.J. and MacDonald P.D.M. eds., Elsevier (1978), 333–344.

[LEc] Lefever R. and Erneux T., On the growth of cellular tissues under constant and fluctuating environmental conditions, in **Nonlinear Electrodynamics in Biological Systems**, Ross W. and Lawrence A. eds., Plenum Press (1984), 287–305.

[LEd] Lefever R. and Horsthemke W., Bistability in fluctuating environments. Implications in tumor immunology, *Bull. Math. Biol.*, **41** (1979), 469–490.

[LEe] Lefever R., Hiernaux J., Urbain J., and Meyers P., On the kinetics and optimal specificity of cytotoxic reactions mediated by $T-$lymphocyte clones, *Bull. Math. Biol.*, **54** (1992), 839–873.

[LVa] Levins R., **Evolution in Changing Environments**, Princeton University Press (1968), 7.

[MAa] Maggelakis S., Type α and type β transforming growing factors as regulators of cancer cellular growth: a mathematical model, *Math. Comp. Modelling*, **18** (1993), 9–16.

[MAb] Maggelakis S. and Adam J.A., Mathematical model for prevascular growth of a spherical carcinoma, *Math. Comp. Modelling*, **13** (1990), 23–38.

[MCa] McElwain D.L.S. and Ponzo P.J., A model for the growth of solid tumor with non-uniform oxygen consumption, *Math. Biosci.*, **35** (1977), 267–279.

[MCb] McElwain D.L.S. and Morris L.E., Apoptosis as a volume loss mechanism in mathematical models of solid tumor growth, *Math. Biosci.*, **39** (1978), 147–157.

[MCc] McElwain D.L.S., Callcott R., and Morris L.E., A model of vascular compression in solid tumors, *J. Theor. Biol.*, **78** (1979), 405–415.

[MEa] Messiah A., **Quantum Mechanics**, North-Holland (1961).

[MKa] Müller-Klieser W.F. and Sutherland R.M., Influence of convection in the growth medium on oxygen tensions in multicell tumor spheroids, *Cancer Res.*, **42** (1982), 237–242.

[MKb] Müller-Klieser W.F. and Sutherland R.M., Oxygen tensions in multicell spheroids of two cell lines at different stages of growth, *Br. J. Cancer*, **45** (1982), 256–264.

[MKc] Müller-Klieser W.F. and Sutherland R.M., Frequency distribution histograms of oxygen tensions in multicell spheroids, in **Oxygen Transport to Tissue**, Bicker H.I. and Briley D.F. eds., Plenum Press (1983), Vol. IV, 497–508.

[MRa] Marusic M., Bajzer Z., Freyer J.P., and Vuk-Pavlovic S., Modeling autostimulation of growth in multicellular tumor spheroids, *Int. J. Biomed. Comput.*, **29** (1991), 149–158.

[MRb] Marusic M. and Bajzer Z., Generalized two-parameter equation of growth, *J. Math. Anal. Applics.*, **179** (1993), 446–462.

[MRc] Marusic M., Bajzer Z., Freyer J.P., and Vuk-Pavlovic S., Analysis of growth of multicellular tumor spheroids by mathematical models, *Cell Prolif.*, **27** (1994), 73–94.

[MRd] Marusic M., Bajzer Z., Vuk-Pavlovic S., and Freyer J.P., Tumor growth in-vivo and as multicellular spheroids compared by mathematical models, *Bull. Math. Biol.*, **56** (1994), 617–631.

[MUa] Murray J.D., **Mathematical Biology**, Springer-Verlag (1989).

[MXa] Marx J.L., How cancer cells spread in the body, *Science*, **244** (1989), 47–48.

[OLa] Old L.J., Tumor necrosis factor, *Sci. Amer.*, **258** (1988), 59–75.

[PEa] Perelson A.S. and Kauffman S.A. eds., **Molecular Evolution on Rugged. Landscapes: Proteins, RNA and the Immune System**, Addison-Wesley (1991).

[PGa] Prigogine I. and Lefever R., Stability problems in cancer growth and nucleation, *Comp. Biochem. Physiol.*, **67B** (1980), 389–393.

[PIa] Pimbley G.H., Periodic solutions of predator-prey equations simulating an immune response, I, *Math. Biosci.*, **20** (1974), 27–51.

[PIb] Pimbley G.H., Periodic solutions of predator-prey equations simulating an immune response, II, *Math. Biosci.*, **21** (1974), 251–277.

[PRa] Prehn R.T., Stimulatory effects of immune reactions upon the growth of transplanted tumors, *Cancer Res.*, **55** (1994), 908–914.

[QIa] Qi A.-S., Multiple solutions of model describing cancerous growth, *Bull. Math. Biol.*, **50** (1988), 1–17.

[REa] Rescigno A. and Le Lisi C., Immune surveillance and neoplasia–II. A two-stage mathematical model, *Bull. Math. Biol.*, **39** (1977), 487–497.

[ROa] Roberts A.B., Anzano M.A., Wakefield L.M., Roche N.S., Roche D.F., Stern D.F., and Sporn M.B., Type beta-transforming growth factor: a bifunctional regulator of cellular growth, *Proc. Nat. Acad. Sci.*, (1985), 119–121.

[SCa] Schiff L.I., **Quantum Mechanics**, McGraw-Hill (1968).

[SHa] Shymko R.M. and Glass L., Cellular and geometric control of tissue growth and mitotic instability, *J. Theor. Biol.*, **63** (1976), 355–374.

[SPa] Sporn M.B. and Todaro G.J., Autocrine secretion and malignant transformation of cells, *New Engl. J. Med.*, **303** (1980), 878–880.

[SPb] Sporn M.B. and Roberts A.B., Autocrine growth factors and cancer, *Nature*, **313** (1985), 745–747.

[SRa] Sherratt J.A. and Nowak M.A., Oncogenes, antioncogenes and the immune response to cancer, *Proc. Roy. Soc. Lond.*, **B 248** (1992), 261–271.

[SRb] Sherratt J.A., Cellular growth control and traveling waves of cancer, *SIAM J. Appl. Math.*, **53** (1993), 1713–1730.

[STa] Stein D.L., What can physics do for biology?, in [PEa], 39–46.

[SUa] Sutherland R.M., McCredie J.A., and Inch W.R., Growth of multicellular spheroids in tissue culture as a model of nodular carcinomas, *J. Natl. Cancer Inst.*, **46** (1971), 113–120.

[SUb] Sutherland R.M. and Durand R.E., Radiation response of multicellular spheroids: an in-vitro tumor model, *Curr. Top. Rad. Res.*, **11** (1976), 87–139.

[SUc] Sutherland R.M. and Durand R.E., Growth and cellular characteristics of multicell spheroids, *Rec. Res. Canc. Res.*, **95** (1985), 24–49.

[SUd] Sutherland R.M., Cell and environment interactions in tumor microregions: the multicell spheroid model, *Science*, **240** (1988), 177–184.

[SWa] Swan G.W., **Some Current Mathematical Topics in Cancer Research**, University Microfilms International (1977).

[SWb] Swan G.W., The diffusion of inhibitor in a spherical tumor, *Math. Biosci.*, **108** (1992), 75–79.

[TAa] Tannock I.F., The relation between cell proliferation and the vascular system in a transplanted mouse mammary tumor, *Br. J. Cancer*, **22** (1968), 258–273.

[THa] Thom R., **Structural Stability and Morphogenesis: An Outline of a General Theory of Models**, Addison-Wesley (1989).

[VAa] Vaupel P., Hypoxia in neoplastic tissue, *Microvasc. Res.*, **13** (1977), 399–408.

[VAb] Vaupel P., Oxygen supply to malignant tumors, in **Tumor Blood Circulation. Angiogenesis, Morphology and Blood Flow of Experimental and Human Tumors**, Peterson H.I. ed., CRC Press (1980), 144–168.

[VAc] Vaupel P., Namz R., Múller-Klieser W.F., and Grunewald W.A., Intracapillary $Hb0_2$ saturation in malignant tumors during normoxia and hyperoxia, *Microvasc. Res.*, **17** (1979), 181–191.

[VYa] Vaidya V.G. and Alexandro F.J., Evaluation of some mathematical models for tumor growth, *Int. J. Bio-Med. Comp.*, **B** (1982), 19–35.

[WHa] Wheldon T.E., **Mathematical Models in Cancer Research**, Adam Hilger (1988).

[WOa] Woodcock A.E.R., Cellular differentiation and catastrophe theory, *Ann. N.Y. Acad. Sci.*, **231** (1974), 60–76.

[WOb] Woodcock A.E.R., Catastrophe theory and cellular determination, transdetermination and differentiation, *Bull. Math. Biol.*, **41** (1979), 101–117.

[ZEa] Zeeman E.C., **Applications of Catastrophe Theory**, Tokyo University Press (1973).

2.8 Appendices

2.8.1 Appendix I – Comments on catastrophe theory

General description

The mathematical classification of stable mappings and their singularities was developed by Thom [THa] and applied extensively by many others, principally Zeeman [ZEa] (but see also [WOa,b]). These pure mathematical methods have been applied to the analysis of problems in fields as diverse as biology, sociology, physics, economics and engineering. It should be pointed out however, that these applications have not been without controversy, particularly in the so-called "soft" sciences [DEb]. Nevertheless, in general catastrophe theory has been recognized by the mathematical sciences community as a valid and useful contribution to the complementary levels of description that are so necessary for a complete understanding of "real world" phenomena. In this sense we may properly regard it as a "model". Like all models (or mathematical metaphors and similes) it is based on assumptions, and there are domains outside of which it is of questionable validity. Provided we remain aware of the limitations inherent in this or any model we should not go too far astray!

In catastrophe theory (as in quantum mechanics), the phenomenon under study is assumed to be governed by a potential function of some kind (think of a particle in a well — the shape and depth of the well is governed by the potential — see Figures 2.6–2.8). The stable states of the system (biological, economic, etc.) — those states observed to occur — are regarded as minima of this potential. If the potential function has multiple minima, more than one stable state may be accessible to the system (e.g. normal/cancerous, benign/malignant, good prognosis/poor prognosis). Changing the control parameters in an experiment may alter the form of the governing potential function so as to change the positions, relative heights, or total number of local minima. Thus the observed state of a system **may change in a discontinuous way as the controls are changed smoothly**. These observed discontinuous changes in state are called **catastrophes** [EKa].

The potential function

Let us imagine that the state of the system can be expressed in terms of the variables $x_1, x_2, x_3, \ldots, x_n$. These variables could represent anything depending on the system of interest; they might represent the concentrations of n chemicals in a cell, or the "state" of n cells in a mass of tissue

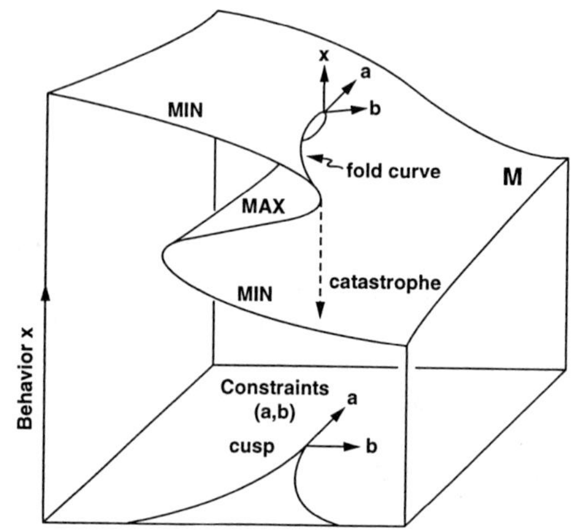
x
a
b
MIN
fold curve
M
MAX
catastrophe
MIN
Behavior x
Constraints
(a,b)
a
cusp
b

(a)

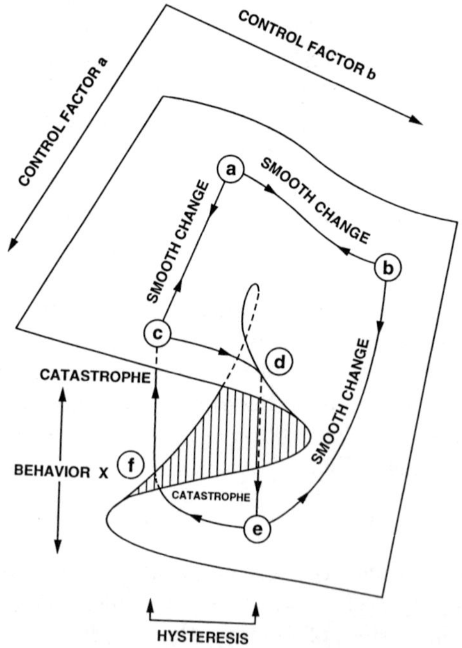
CONTROL FACTOR a
CONTROL FACTOR b
a
SMOOTH CHANGE
SMOOTH CHANGE
b
c
d
SMOOTH CHANGE
CATASTROPHE
BEHAVIOR X
f
CATASTROPHE
e
HYSTERESIS

(b)

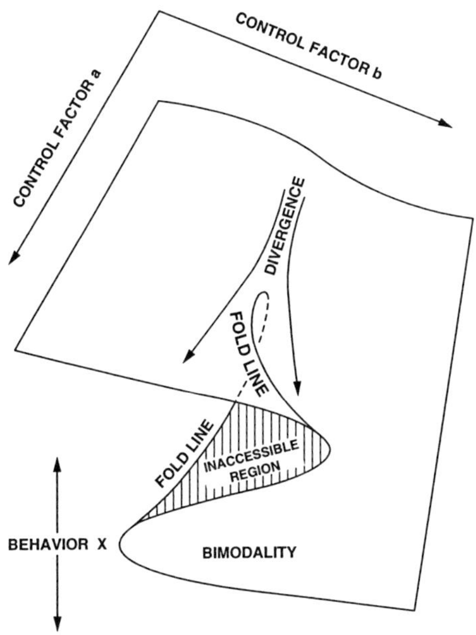

(c)

Figure 2.7 — (a,b,c) The generic form of the cusp catastrophe; (a) and (b) are the control variables, x is the behavior variable, illustrating the various phenomena discussed in Appendix I.

(n can be as large as we please — it might be 10,000 to describe the states of a cell in the embryo, or 10,000,000,000 to describe neuronal activity in the brain, or even infinite-dimensional). Alteration of $x_1, \ldots, x_n$ causes the configuration of the system to change, and making them vary with time will permit a description of the evolution of the system to be made (in principle). It will be necessary to insist, however, that small variations in the x_i ($i = 1, \ldots, n$) are accompanied by small changes in the system configuration. In addition to the x_i we allow the existence of some parameters $a_1, a_2, \ldots, a_k$ which characterize the nature of interactions between various parts of the system or the system and its environment (prognostic indices, radiation intensity levels, metastatic potential, etc.). A slight adjustment of the environment will result in small deviations of $a_1, \ldots, a_k$ from their original values. At this point, the system will either be modified a little (in some definable sense) or transformed dramatically. In the latter case a (mathematical) catastrophe has been said to occur and the set of values of $a_1, \ldots, a_k$ for which this happens is called the *catastrophe set.* The quantities $x_1, \ldots, x_n$ are known as the *state or internal variables* while the parameters $a_1, \ldots, a_k$ are also known as the *external or control variables.* To proceed further it is necessary to assume that there exists a (gradient) potential function

$$V(x_1, \ldots, x_n; \quad a_1, \ldots, a_k)$$

which, for fixed values of $a_1, \ldots, a_k$ defines the possible states of the system as the values of $x_1, \ldots, x_n$ vary, provided that

$$\frac{\partial V}{\partial x_1} = 0\,, \quad \frac{\partial V}{\partial x_2} = 0\,, \quad \ldots\,, \quad \frac{\partial V}{\partial x_n} = 0 \tag{A.1.1}$$

for each $i = 1, \ldots, n$.
Often (but not always) the potential V will be related to some measure of the "energy" of the system-hence the name. When $x_1, \ldots, x_n$ satisfy (A.1.1) above, they define an *equilibrium state.*

Geometric description

The so-called *elementary catastrophes* are known by very picturesque names. In increasing order of complexity (defined by the number of state and control variables) they are the FOLD, CUSP, SWALLOW-TAIL, BUTTERFLY, HYPERBOLIC UMBILIC, ELLIPTIC UMBILIC and PARABOLIC UMBILIC catastrophes respectively. The equilibrium surface for each catastrophe contains, in some form or other, the proceeding simpler catastrophe surfaces. In particular, when two control variables (a_1, a_2) are available, the **cusp** is the appropriate catastrophe to utilize. This may be of sufficient complexity to appear relevant to the cancer problem, while at the same time being relatively simple to describe and understand. In what follows we designate the control variables (ultimately to be identified experimentally) as $a_1 = a$ and $a_2 = b$. There is no loss of generality in identifying only one state variable (x) explicitly [JOa].

The generic case of the cusp catastrophe arises from a potential of the form

$$V(x) = \frac{1}{4}x^4 + \frac{1}{2}ax^2 + bx\,. \tag{A.1.2}$$

The minima of $V(x)$ occur when

$$x^3 + ax + b = 0 \tag{A.1.3}$$

and

$$3x^2 + a > 0 \,. \tag{A.1.4}$$

We now assume that the system of interest is governed by the potential $V(x)$ and is subject to the control variables a and b. Three situations may arise (see Figure 2.8) depending upon the sign of the number

$$N = \frac{1}{4}b^2 + \frac{1}{27}a^3 \,. \tag{A.1.5}$$

If $N > 0$ then $V(x)$ has one minimum. If $N = 0$, $V(x)$ has one minimum and a point of inflection. If $N < 0$, $V(x)$ has two distinct local minima and one local maximum. By analogy with the particle in the well, we associate minima (upper and lower sheets of the surface in Figure 2.8) with STABLE equilibria and the maximum (middle sheet) with an UNSTABLE equilibrium. This identification can be rigorously justified.

Before proceeding further with a description of the catastrophe surface, it is of interest to note that the equation of the "catastrophe set" $N = 0$ may easily be obtained from the condition $V'(x) = 0$ (Eq. (A.1.3)) and the condition for the roots to coalesce: $V''(x) = 0$, i.e.

$$3x^2 + a = 0 \,. \tag{A.1.6}$$

Eliminating x yields the equation $N = 0$, which is just the equation of the cusp (the projection of the folded surface in the (b, a) plane.
If the control variable a is held fixed at $a = A < 0$ and variable b is varied, then for

$$|b| < \left(- \frac{4}{27}A^3 \right)^{\frac{1}{2}} = c \tag{A.1.7}$$

the unique minimum is on the lower sheet. Thus, as the parameter b changes through the interval $(-c, c)$, the system must at some point jump from the upper to the lower sheet. The set of all such points of discontinuity is called the bifurcation set of the system. Similarly, if one fixes $b = B$ and varies the parameter a, then as one crosses the curve (in the sense of increasing a)

$$a = \left(- \frac{27}{4}B^2 \right)^{\frac{1}{3}} \tag{A.1.8}$$

the number of local minima changes from two to one. Again, bifurcation can occur.

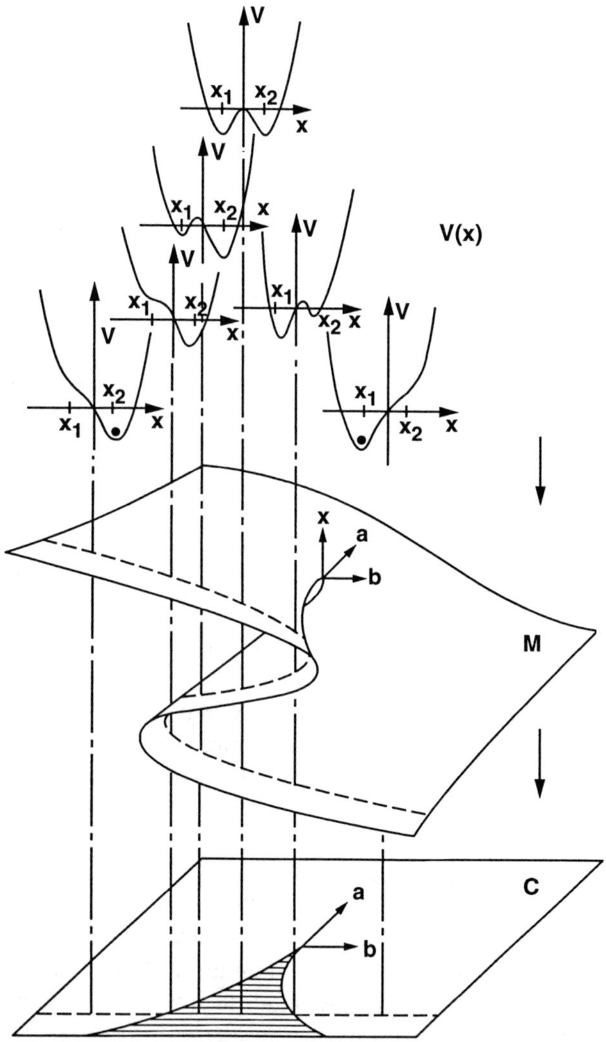

Figure 2.8 — The generic form of the cusp catastrophe, whose potential is $V(x) = \frac{1}{4}x^4 + \frac{1}{2}ax^2 + bx$. The uppermost level of the diagram displays the potentials corresponding to different settings of the constraints. The middle level represents the surface of extrema of $V(x)$, while the lower plane shows the constraint space, (b, a)-space, together with the cusp (hatched region). The bifurcation set must lie somewhere within this cusp. (Based on [ZEa]).

Properties of the cusp catastrophe

There are five interrelated qualitative features associated with this catastrophe surface. It is not necessarily the case that they will all be manifested if the model applies, but if none appear to them the model is surely vacuous! These features are:

i) Bimodality
ii) Discontinuity
iii) Hysteresis
iv) Divergence
v) Inaccessibility

These properties refer to selected behaviors of the system which may not all occur under normal circumstances. If conditions are perturbed, however, the system may move to a configuration that exhibits other properties in this list. A system that evolves smoothly but irregularly to one or the other of two possible final states (bimodality and divergence) might jump catastrophically (discontinuously) between these states if an appropriate new perturbation is applied.

Bimodality may occur when observations tend to cluster around two statistical measures. Tumors, for example, can be benign or malignant, (and prognosis can be either good or bad). Bimodality is basically a static property which we incorporate as a given feature.

Discontinuity refers to a large behavioral change resulting from a small change in control variables, as has been discussed earlier.

Hysteresis occurs when a system has a delayed response to a changing stimulus. A plot of response against stimulus will follow one path when the stimulus increases and another when it decreases.

Divergence occurs when initial conditions which are in some sense "nearby" evolve to widely separated final states. Two patients with similar histories of cancer and identical treatment modalities may respond in radically different fashion. Cell differentiation is another example (indeed, Thom originally developed the theory to study morphogenesis).

Inaccessibility refers to the existence of the unstable middle sheet of the folded surface. The represents those equilibria which are rarely, if ever observed, and are completely destroyed when perturbed (e.g. a coin balanced on edge).

Some general comments on modeling

In most biological systems we are not in a position to write down the equations that govern its evolution (where the word evolution is not necessarily meant in the temporal sense). There may be thousands or millions of them! Catastrophe theory may assist us by allowing us to use observations directly to suggest the generic types of equations we are seeking. (It is much easier to work backwards from the answer!) We do not have to know in advance what approximations we may make. Instead, we can determine which ones we must make if the model is to be consistent with the observations. This may lead to a greater understanding of the way the system works, by connecting certain internal features of it to the observed phenomena in ways which otherwise might be difficult to discover. Of course, there is also the possibility that the model is useless to us, and in that situation we must cut our losses and look for pastures new.

Lest it should appear that in the application of catastrophe theory to a system we are trying to get something for nothing, it is perhaps worthwhile to add some further comments. Firstly, there is a great amount of work "behind the scenes", so to speak, as far as catastrophe theory is concerned. The theorems proved by Thom and others are very "deep" and have an austere beauty not only in their own right, but also in connection with the power, applicability and relative simplicity of the seven elementary catastrophes. Secondly, a complete model of the system contains (usually) an enormous amount of information, and so requires a great deal of input . In attempting to apply catastrophe theory to a particular system, we are in effect seeking the answer to one or two specific questions (e.g. is the prognosis good or bad for this patient?). A relatively small amount of information (which may still be a lot!) may suffice. In this sense, catastrophe theory is an efficient technique if it can tell us what we want to know with the minimum of data and standard theoretical background as input.

Thirdly, in some applications (e.g. in sociology) the governing family of potential functions is used strictly as a phenomenological tool. However, when augmented by other arguments (be they statistical or otherwise in nature), catastrophe theory can be used as a predictive tool to account in a quantitative manner for the changes in a given system as the constraints on a system are changed.

2.8.2 Appendix II – Solution existence, uniqueness, stability and bifurcation and the inverse problem

Many of the systems examined in connection with reaction-diffusion equations have properties that are similar to those described by the model

$$\frac{\partial u}{\partial t} - \frac{\partial^2 u}{\partial x^2} = h(x,u)\,, \quad 0 \le x \le 1\,, \quad t > 0$$

$$u(0,t) = 0 = u(1,t)\,, \quad t > 0 \qquad (A.2.1)$$
$$u(x,0) = u_0(x)\,, \quad x \in (0,1)\,,$$

where the diffusion constant has been chosen without loss of generality to be unity. One basic question that may be asked is: will the process ever settle down to an equilibrium? If so, an equilibrium solution u_e will satisfy

$$\frac{d^2u_e}{dx^2} + h(x, u_e) = 0\,, \qquad u_e(0) = u_e(1) = 0\,. \qquad (A.2.2)$$

If Eq. (A.2.2) has a solution, this is a candidate to be a steady-state solution of Eq. (A.2.1), i.e.

$$\lim_{t\to\infty} u(x,t) = u_e(x)\,.$$

Consider now a common nonlinear function (in a biological context) $h(x,u)$, i.e. the logistic form

$$h(x,u) = ru\left(1 - \frac{u}{\theta}\right), \qquad 0 \le u \le \theta\,, \qquad (A.2.3)$$

with only implicit x-dependence. It can be shown (using the contraction mapping theorem, see [GFa]) that (A.2.2) possesses a unique solution if $r < 3\sqrt{10}$. However, since $u_e \equiv 0$ satisfies Eq. (A.2.2), it is clearly the unique (trivial) solution for this range of r. This in turn suggests that

$$\lim_{t\to\infty} u(x,t) = 0$$

for system (A.2.1). What happens if the linear growth rate r exceeds $3\sqrt{10}$? Clearly, $u_e = 0$ is still a valid solution, so we might expect the **uniqueness** of solutions to fail. This would mean that there is at least one **non-zero** equilibrium solution for this problem; physically it will correspond to a balance between diffusion (tending to "dissipate" the solution towards zero) and nonlinear growth (causing the solution to grow). For this particular solution, these statements may be verified in detail by phase-plane analysis; furthermore an exact solution of (A.2.2) and (A.2.3) can be found in terms of elliptic integrals. This is not in general possible, and it is under these circumstances that the power of the theorems becomes apparent. To exemplify this further, we return to the time-dependent problem (A.2.1). We can write it in terms of the operator $\mathcal{L}(u)$, such that

$$\frac{\partial u}{\partial t} = \mathcal{L}(u) \equiv \frac{\partial^2 u}{\partial x^2} + h(x,u)\,. \qquad (A.2.4)$$

For a certain class of operators P (of which $\mathcal{L}$ is a member; see [GFa]) if all the eigenvalues λ of the linearized operator $\tilde{P}(u_0)$ satisfy

$$Re(\lambda) \leq \tilde{a} < 0 \qquad \text{for some} \qquad \tilde{a} \neq \tilde{a}(\lambda),$$

then the equilibrium solution u_0 of the equation

$$\frac{\partial u}{\partial t} = P(u) \tag{A.2.5}$$

is stable.

For

$$P(u) = \frac{d^2u}{dx^2} + ru\left(1 - \frac{u}{\theta}\right), \tag{A.2.6}$$

$$\tilde{P}(u) = \frac{d^2u}{dx^2} + ru\,, \tag{A.2.7}$$

and the eigenvalues of $\tilde{P}$ are

$$\lambda_n = r - n^2\pi^2\,, \qquad n = 1, 2, 3, \dots\,.$$

Clearly the equilibrium solution is stable if $r < \pi^2 \approx 9.87$, and unstable otherwise. We have already noted that the equilibrium is unique if $r < 3\sqrt{10} \approx 9.49$, which is in error by less than 4% from the value of π^2. Since the bound $r < 3\sqrt{10}$ is based on sufficiency, rather than necessity for uniqueness, we are led to ask if there is a connection between the **loss of stability** and the **loss of uniqueness**: the answer is yes! In fact, as r increases, the trivial zero solution becomes unstable precisely at the point where a non-zero solution appears. The property of stability is transferred to the new non-zero solution. This process is well illustrated by the "model" eigenvalue problem

$$\frac{d^2u}{dx^2} + \left(\lambda - 2\int_0^1 |u(x)|^2\,dx\right)u = 0\,, \tag{A.2.8}$$

where

$$u(0) = 0 = u(1)\,.$$

This represents a type of weighted eigenvalue problem, and though highly idealized, is similar to a problem arising in solid-state physics. The system has a solution of the form

$$u(x) = \alpha \sin n\pi x\,, \qquad n = 1, 2, 3, \dots\,, \tag{A.2.9}$$

where

$$\lambda - |\alpha|^2 = n^2\pi^2 \,. \qquad (A.2.10)$$

$\alpha = 0$ is a solution for all values of λ; for given $m, \alpha = \pm(\lambda - m^2\pi^2)^{\frac{1}{2}}$ is a real solution for $\lambda > m^2\pi^2$, etc. so the points $\lambda = m^2\pi^2$, $m = 1, 2, 3, \ldots$ are points of bifurcation from zero.

Another topic of importance is that of *inverse problems*, but we can do no more here than illustrate them with a simple example: the reader is encouraged to examine the detailed discussions in [GHa] and [CRa], which although set in the contexts of mathematical physics and astronomy respectively, do address the lack of uniqueness problem with clarity (especially [CRa]).

Our example is taken from elementary calculus, though in fact is pertains to much more general problems of the type discussed in Section 2.3.4, (see Eq. (2.31) for example). According to the so-called second fundamental theorem of calculus, if $f(x)$ is an integrable function of its argument on any appropriate domain, and if

$$g(x) = \int_c^x f(\xi)\,d\xi \qquad (A.2.11)$$

c being any constant, then

$$g'(x) = \frac{d}{dx}\int_c^x f(\xi)\,d\xi = f(x) \qquad (A.2.12)$$

or

$$f(\xi) = \frac{dg}{dx}|_{x=\xi} \,. \qquad (A.2.12')$$

We have, in effect, "inverted" the "integral equation" (A.2.11) to obtain $f(\xi)$. A question of extreme importance for both theoretical and practical (i.e., numerical) exploitation of this result is the following: how sensitive is $f(\xi)$ in (A.2.12′) to small variations in the form of $g(x)$? The answer in general is **very sensitive**, and the implications of this for observational astronomy are well brought out in [CRa]: clearly this problem is not limited to that field alone, but can occur in any situation in which one seeks to "invert" data or obtain information from explicit functional relations, e.g. from (2.30). In that equation, given data on the growth rate and radius of a spheroid as a function of time (and possibly the necrotic core radius), one might wish to infer the nature of the source term $S(\sigma, \beta)$. To illustrate the potential difficulty in even a simple problem, consider the functions $g_a(x)$ and $g_b(x)$, related in turn to Eq. (A.2.11), where

$$g_a(x) = 1 - xe^{-x} \qquad (A.2.13)$$

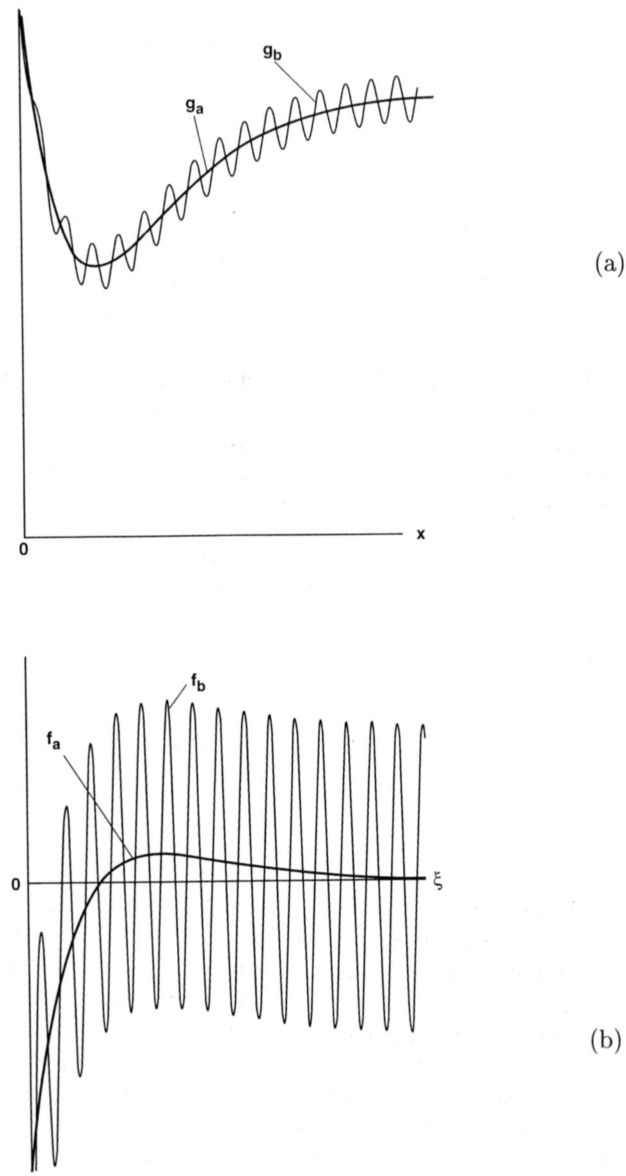

Figure 2.9 — (a),(b) The functions $g_a(x), g_b(x)$ and their respective "inverse" functions $f_a(\xi)$ and $f_b(\xi)$ defined by (A.2.12′). In these figures, based on Eqs. (A.2.13) and (A.2.14), $\omega = 15$ and $\beta = 0.05$.

and

$$g_b(x) = g_a(x) + \beta \sin(\omega x)\,, \tag{A.2.14}$$

where β and ω are both real numbers, with $|\beta|$ small with respect to 1, and $|\omega|$ large with respect to $|\beta|$, i.e. g_b differs from g_a by the addition of a small but highly oscillatory function.

Clearly, from (A.2.12′) the corresponding $f(\xi)$ functions are

$$f_a(\xi) = (\xi - 1)e^{-\xi}$$

and

$$f_b(\xi) = f_a(\xi) + \beta\omega \cos \omega\xi\,.$$

No matter how small is a given value of β (corresponding to very low amplitude "noise") it is clear that if the "noise" is sufficiently oscillatory (or, more precisely, if it contains high frequency Fourier modes) then the additional term swamps $f_a(\xi)$ by a term of magnitude $|\beta\omega|$. This is illustrated in Figure 2.9, and simplistic though it is, should serve as a warning to practitioners of mathematical modeling: is the inverted data believable?

3

Mathematical Modeling of Tumor Growth Kinetics

Ž. BAJZER AND S. VUK-PAVLOVIĆ

Mayo Clinic and Mayo Foundation
Rochester, MN, USA

AND
M. HUZAK

University of Zagreb
Zagreb, Croatia

ABSTRACT. The overall goal of this survey is to develop and present a coherent and integrated interpretation of mathematical models which describe tumor growth. Rigorous description and quantitative understanding of tumor growth kinetics have been a focus of mathematical modelers for more than five decades. Consequently, many models have been proposed, ranging from conceptually and mathematically simple empirical models to complex "functional" models which include kinetics of the cell cycle, cell-cell interactions, cell age distribution, microenvironmental factors, etc. However, these models have been seldom validated against experimental tumor growth curves, largely because of the relative scarcity of appropriate data. On the other hand, contemporary experimental techniques increase the prospects for obtaining high quality data. With this in mind, we summarize the pertinent deterministic models of tumor growth kinetics with special emphasis on model scrutiny against experimental data. Prominent among these models is the Gompertz model which has been remarkably successful in description of growth curves for various tumors. The biological interpretation of this model, originally developed as an actuarial curve, remains unclear and we summarize the relevant interpretations of this model. Also, we discuss two other similarly simple models, the logistic model and the von Bertalanffy model, and then present models of increasing complexity which include elements of the cell cycle and cell-cell interactions. Within the typical kinetic paradigm, these models are based on systems of ordinary differential equations. However, we also consider models defined by partial differential equations which involve age and time.

3.1 Introduction

Mathematical models are ideas and thus are limited only by logic and imagination. The extent to which models conform to reality is determined by testing them against experimental data with the aid of computational and statistical methods. However, data are often restricted physically and technically and these restrictions may preclude rigorous testing of models. Consequently, cancer research is replete today with models that range from detailed and comprehensive (see e.g., [SHa]), but sometimes hardly testable, to the parsimonious, that are more rigorously testable against available data [MAb].

Historically, these two extreme paradigms of model building, the comprehensive and the parsimonious, have been combined in different degrees both to refine ideas for further experimental testing and to discipline the mind when data require. The present volume illustrates such different modeling practices rather well; this chapter dwells mostly on a parsimonious approach rooted in the self-evident concept that models should not depart too far from their basis in quantitative observations. This is not to say that mathematical models are not valuable on their own merit as conceptual and mathematical constructs that reflect our ability to imagine within strict logical structures and still reach relevance and intrinsic beauty. Indeed, models can be judged also by their mathematical content and elegance as they can on the ability to predict the qualitative behavior of the modeled system. For this review, we selected the material on the basis of these model features, too.

Mathematical modeling of tumor growth kinetics is ripe for a fresh systematic review. For reviews from other vantage points, we refer the reader to the rather comprehensive text by Swan [SWa] and to the more recent paper by Calderón and Kwembe [CAa]. A recent issue of the journal *Mathematical and Computer Modeling* has been devoted to the interactions of tumors and the immune system [BLa].

In this review, we consider the growing tumor as a deterministic dynamic system represented by ordinary differential equations. During the last two centuries, physicists and mathematicians developed the theory of deterministic dynamical systems remarkably well. More recently they focused their attention onto global behavior of solutions revealed by analysis of equations without necessarily solving them. In many applications the emphasis has been on the steady (equilibrium) state of the system, rather than on transient phenomena. For tumor growth, the critical part is the period of growth (regression) and not so much the period of true stagnation which even may not be achieved before the death of the host.

The central concept of a dynamical system is the trajectory. For tumor growth the trajectory is the growth curve that describes the change in tumor size with time from the start of proliferation of initial tumor cell(s). The tumor size is expressed by mass or volume or cellularity, depending on what is measured. For modeling, these quantities are sometimes interchanged, based on the assumption that in solid tumors these quantities are proportional to each other. Here we do not challenge this assumption.

We begin this review with mathematical preliminaries referring to some general properties of autonomous differential equations (Section 3.2). Then, in Section 3.2.1, we consider different approaches to specification of differential equations on the basis of fundamental observations. Leaving generalities aside, in Sections 3.3, 3.4, and 3.5, we concentrate on conceptual and mathematical aspects of the three classical tumor growth kinetic models, the Gompertz model, the logistic model, and the von Bertalanffy model. Among them, the Gompertz model has been used most widely and with most success in description of tumor growth curves. Yet, its foundation remains unclear and we provide a critical review, as complete as possible, of different approaches to the understanding of the basis of the empirical Gompertz law (Sections 3.3.1–3.3.7). For several proposed explanations we insisted on mathematical rigor (beyond the level exercised in original papers) and enhanced, we believe, the understanding of arguments (Section 3.3.6). In Section 3.4, we discuss briefly the logistic model and in Section 3.5 we analyze some mathematical aspects of the general von Bertalanffy model and its special cases that include the logistic and the Gompertz model. Section 3.6 is devoted to more complex models which emphasize specific mechanisms of growth, i.e., competition among cell populations (Section 3.6.1), the cell cycle and its regulation by growth factors (Section 3.6.2), and positive feedback mechanisms (Section 3.6.3).

In Section 3.7, we discuss model validation against data. We analyze the notion that different models can fit data similarly well (see e.g., [WIa]) and the assumption that any biologically reasonable model will fit the data given a sufficient number of parameters; we suggest that the mere number of parameters and reasonable assumptions are not always sufficient, but that the applicability is restricted by the mathematical structure of the model, too. In other words, fitting of model functions to a well measured tumor growth curve can discriminate among tumor models better than has been generally assumed [MAb].

3.2 Tumor Growth as a Dynamical System

As pointed out already, it is reasonable to consider a growing tumor as a dynamical system classically described by ordinary differential equations. This is the most widely used framework for modeling kinetics in general, although growth models in biology are formulated successfully also by partial differential equations (see e.g., [ADa] and other chapters in this volume). Here we consider tumor growth kinetics described by ordinary autonomous differential equations under the assumption that growth is an autonomous process in an effectively nonchanging environment. In other words, any change in the environment is promptly countered by the adaptive response of the growing tumor which tends to preserve its basic growth dynamics. From a somewhat different point of view, one can say that the growth dynamics described by a system of sufficiently rich autonomous differential equations contains already all possible outcomes of the interaction between the growing tumor and its environment.

First, in some generality we consider here the simple tumor growth model described by a single, first order, autonomous differential equation

$$y' = f(y) , \qquad y(0) = y_0 > 0 , \tag{3.1}$$

where $y(t) > 0$ is tumor size at time t and $f(y) \in C^1$ is a function describing the growth rate. The above initial condition will be assumed throughout the paper. Inspection of (3.1) leads to the following basic questions: *What kind of behavior can the unique solution of this equation assume? How does this solution correspond to phenomenology of tumor growth?*

The solution of (3.1) has the remarkable property of a monotonic ascending function of time when $f(y_0) > 0$, or a monotonic descending function of time when $f(y_0) < 0$ (see footnote in [BAa], p. 38). In the case of an ascending function, this implies that the stationary (critical) point corresponds to the maximum possible tumor size, y_m, achieved for $t \to \infty$. Similarly, in the case of a descending function, the stationary point achieved for $t \to \infty$ is $y_s \geq 0$. Any other root of equation $f(y) = 0$ cannot belong to the range of function $y(t)$.

From this analysis we conclude that the model given by (3.1) describes continuous tumor growth which asymptotically approaches the finite value y_m or infinity (that corresponds to the unattainable unrestricted growth). On the other hand, (3.1) can describe continuous tumor regression from size $y = y_0$ to extinction ($y = 0$) at some finite time or when $t \to \infty$. It is essential to emphasize here that the solution of (3.1) cannot describe oscillatory tumor growth with regressions and relapses. This can be achieved when $f(y)$ is separately defined in time intervals characterized by monotone increases or decrease of y. Strictly speaking, in this case $f(y)$ is actually time-dependent and (3.1) is only partially autonomous.

The solution $y(t)$ represents a sigmoidal ascending curve characteristic of tumor growth if a unique inflection point exists. This condition can be achieved for some simple functions $f(y)$ (see Sections 3.2.1, 3.3, 3.4, and 3.5). It is conceivable that functions $f(y)$ exist which yield solutions with multiple inflection points resulting in "multisigmoidal" curves. Such curves would describe tumor growth with recurrent stagnation phases.

More complex models of tumor growth kinetics are described by systems of ordinary autonomous first-order differential equations

$$\begin{cases} y' = f(y, x_1, \ldots, x_n)\,, \\ x_i' = f_i(y, x_1, \ldots, x_n)\,, \end{cases} \tag{3.2}$$

for $i = 1, \ldots, n$ and with initial conditions $y(0) = y_0 > 0$, $x_i(0) = x_0$.

Here $x_1, \ldots, x_n$ are variables describing various factors responsible for tumor growth (e.g., levels of available nutrients, growth factor activity, size of quiescent cell population, etc.). The functions f and f_i and the variables x_i are chosen to represent growth mechanisms of particular interest. For mathematical simplicity the functions f and f_i are chosen to be continuous in the appropriate domain with continuous partial first order derivatives. In this way, the solution of the system is unique and one can analyze stability of stationary solutions on the basis of a Jacobian matrix (cf. [BEa]).

Unlike the simple model given by (3.1), the system of two differential equations ($n = 1$) can describe smooth oscillatory tumor growth. In other words, the solution of (3.1) can exhibit several maxima and minima. In the case of three autonomous ($n = 2$) differential equations, for a certain domain of model parameters one can expect the peculiar chaotic behavior.

3.2.1 Construction of growth rate functions

Inasmuch equations (3.1) and (3.2) provide one among possible general frameworks for tumor growth kinetics, there is no further advance without specifying model functions f, f_i that represent tumor growth mechanisms. Which among these mechanisms is the most important, which must be taken into account explicitly and which implicitly are the questions that bring to mathematical modeling the elements of art. In the following text we present two general approaches to the construction of model functions.

First we consider the classical chemical kinetics paradigm based on mass conservation. For tumor growth, this paradigm can be expressed in its simplest form by

$$y(t + \Delta t) = y(t) + G\big(y(t)\big)\Delta t - D\big(y(t)\big)\Delta t\,. \tag{3.3}$$

The tumor size (mass) at time $t + \Delta t$ is equal to the size at time t enlarged by $G\big(y(t)\big)\Delta t$ (generation of mass) during the small time interval Δt, and diminished by $D\big(y(t)\big)\Delta t$ (degradation of mass) during the same time interval. The functions $G(y) > 0$ and $D(y) > 0$ are the growth and degradation rates, respectively, assumed to depend on tumor size only. This assumption views tumor growth as an autonomous process supported by an effectively nonchanging environment. Within the limit of $\Delta t \to 0$, (3.3) becomes a differential equation

$$y' = G(y) - D(y)\,, \qquad y(0) = y_0 > 0\,. \tag{3.4}$$

Growth stagnates for the solution of $G(y) = D(y)$ that belongs to the range of $y(t)$. Conditions necessary for establishment of a sigmoidal (ascending) growth curve include:
a) $G(y_0) > D(y_0)$;
b) only one solution $y_m > y_0$ of $G(y) = D(y)$ exists as does only one solution $y_i > 0$ of $dG(y)/dy = dD(y)/dy$, and
c) $y_i < y_m$.
In the latter case, y_m is the maximal tumor size achieved asymptotically and y_i is the tumor size at the inflection point. The stated conditions can be met easily if both $G(y)$ and $D(y)$ are monotonic ascending functions. In a typical chemical kinetics paradigm, these functions are given by the power function, ky^n, where k is the rate constant and n is the order of the process. We discuss specific models based on this idea in Sections 3.4, 3.5 and 3.6.

Another approach to construction of model functions is rooted in more biological reasoning. The fundamental idea is that tumor growth results from exponential cell proliferation (often called "Malthusian growth") described by

$$y' = \alpha y\,, \qquad \alpha > 0\,. \tag{3.5}$$

This equation describes unrestricted growth leading to infinite tumor size, a notion not supported by observation. Initially, tumor growth behaves approximately according to (3.5), but eventually it becomes stagnant due to restrictions within the tumor itself and to those imposed by the environment. Thus, exponential growth must be modified to include terms that restrict growth. This can be achieved by multiplying y on the right-hand side of (3.5) with a function $F(y) > 0$ satisfying $\lim_{y\to y_m} F(y) = 0$. The corresponding differential equation is

$$y' = \alpha\, y F(y)\,. \tag{3.6}$$

Biologically, the function $F(y)$ can be interpreted as a growth fraction, i.e., as the ratio of proliferating cells in the tumor versus total cell population, or more generally, the ratio of growing tumor mass versus total tumor mass. The consequence of this interpretation requires that $F(y) \le 1$ and that parameter α be interpreted as the growth rate constant for the hypothetical unrestricted growth.

The maximal tumor size, y_m, predicted by the model is often designated as *carrying capacity*, $K > 0$, of the environment for tumors *in vitro* or of the host for tumors *in vivo*. It is useful to introduce K explicitly into the model (see e.g., [ARa])

$$y' = \alpha\, y\, g\left(\frac{y}{K}\right), \qquad y(0) = y_0 > 0\,. \tag{3.7}$$

According to our general conclusions about the behavior of solutions of (3.1) and, consequently, of (3.7), a tumor can reach the carrying capacity only asymptotically implying

$$\lim_{t\to\infty} y(t) = K\,, \qquad g(1) = 0\,. \tag{3.8}$$

Furthermore, the solution of (3.7) will represent a sigmoidal curve if there is a unique solution $y_i < K$ of the equation

$$K\, g\left(\frac{y}{K}\right) + y\,\frac{d}{dy} g\left(\frac{y}{K}\right) = 0\,.$$

Mathematically, the simplest realization of the function g (with no free model parameters) is a linear function: $g(z) = 1 - z$. Such a selection for the growth fraction leads to the well known logistic model [VEa], much used in population dynamics. We further discuss this model in Section 3.4 and here note only that it represents sigmoidal growth and that it too can be interpreted in terms of (3.4) whereby the growth rate is a linear process, $G(y) = \alpha y$, and the degradation rate is a second order process, $D(y) = \alpha y^2/K$.

Mathematically, both considered approaches (yielding (3.4) or (3.7)) are equivalent and one can easily transform one equation into the other. However, from the vantage point of modeling and interpretation, the two approaches are quite different. The same differential equation can yield an intuitively acceptable interpretation in one approach, while it can lack a transparent interpretation in the other.

The paradigms of mass conservation and growth fraction can obviously be used in development of more elaborate models yielding systems of equations (3.2). There the task of constructing model functions becomes more complex and the mathematical simplicity becomes more necessary. For example, the growth rate of a cell population y dependent on the available nutrition level x_1 is modeled kinetically as a second order process: kyx_1 (cf. [VAc]). In other words, simple proportionality to both variables is assumed. The question may be posed whether one can identify a more fundamental and systematic approach to growth modeling within the framework of equations (3.2), an approach that would reflect the observed real phenomena and still offer reasonable mathematical tractability. In this respect, we find as most promising the work of M. Savageau on the "S-systems", standing for "synergistic and saturable" systems [SAa], [SAb], [SAc]. It seems that this work, although developed over more than the past 25 years, has not been sufficiently recognized and applied. Here we present a brief account of S-systems as a framework for growth modeling.

The basic idea is the kinetic paradigm mathematically expressed as

$$\begin{cases} y' = G(y, x_1, \ldots, x_n) - D(y, x_1, \ldots, x_n)\,, \\ x_i' = R_i^+(y, x_1, \ldots, x_n) - R_i^-(y, x_1, \ldots, x_n)\,, \quad i = 1, \ldots, n\,. \end{cases} \tag{3.9}$$

Here the functions R_i^+ and R_i^- stand for any forward or backward kinetic rate, respectively, describing the change of system variables x_i. In principle, some of these variables may also represent true concentrations of biologically important substances responsible for growth control. As before, the functions G and D represent the growth rate and the degradation rate specifying growth of the biological mass under study.

Essentially, using the principle of allometry [HUa], Savageu [SAa] arrived at the following expression for any of the rates involved in the system of equations (3.9), designated generally by R_j

$$R_j(y, x_1, \ldots, x_n) = a_j y^{\alpha_j} \prod_{i=1}^{n} x_i^{\beta_{ij}}\,, \tag{3.10}$$

where $a_j > 0$ and β_{ij} are real constants. In words, the rates are characterized by the power law with exponents that can be any real number. Such a system of differential equations is called an S-system. Some specific models of tumor growth kinetics considered below are special cases derived directly from (3.9) with (3.10). Other models can be transformed into that form. Namely, Savageau and Voit [SAc] have shown that S-systems are canonical for the class of autonomous differential equations (3.2) with functions f

and f_i comprised of sums and products of elementary functions, or nested functions of elementary functions. Any differential equation of this class can be transformed into an S-system with additional nonlinear algebraic equations considered as constraints.

The S-systems have other useful properties, e.g., they permit explicit expressions for nonzero stationary states; these expressions are obtained by logarithmic transformation of (3.10) yielding linear algebraic equations. Also, the S-systems permit explicit determination of conditions for local stability [SAc]. A strategic convenience for studies of S-systems is the availability of ESSYNS, an algorithm for numerical solution of S-systems which is 10 to 100 times faster than classical algorithms [IRa]. Finally, and most importantly, the S-systems are appropriate models for various biological phenomena [SAb].

After this very general discussion, we now turn to specific "classical" models of tumor growth that still have not been fully explored.

3.3 The Gompertz Model

At its conception in 1825 [GOa], this model had nothing to do with growth, but rather it dealt with human mortality. Gompertz found empirically that the distribution $P(\tau)$ of human age τ for a community is given by

$$P(\tau) = pe^{-e^{a-b\tau}} = pA^{B^{\tau}}, \tag{3.11}$$

with constants a, p, and b, where $p > 0$, $b < 0$, and $A, B > 0$, respectively. More than a hundred years later, Wright [WRa] and Winsor [WIa] realized that the Gompertz empirical law can also be used to describe growth in size of organisms (in this case b becomes positive and $P(t)$ is the size of organism at age t). Since then a number of authors fitted the Gompertz formula to growth data for animals and organisms with remarkable success. Older literature refers to the Gompertz model as to the Gompertz "law of growth". (The distinction between a law of nature and a mathematical model is subtle and we will not discuss it here, but will use both terms interchangeably.) Already in 1934, Casey [CEa] fitted the Gompertz model to tumor growth data and was followed by numerous authors (e.g., [LAa], [LAb], [LAd], [SIa], [SUa], [NOa], [BSa], [MAb], [MAe], [BSb]). Based on many thorough analyses, the general conclusion has been that the Gompertz law successfully describes tumor growth. The question appears as to *why such an empirical formula with no obvious interpretation reflects growth so faithfully and universally.* It is even more puzzling why it is so successful in describing *tumor* growth. *Are there any inherent, though not obvious fundamental assumptions which yield such a highly applicable model?* Many authors have tried to solve this intriguing problem. Here we discuss approaches developed more specifically to address this problem in the context of tumor growth. By the same token, this gives us the opportunity to present several elaborate tumor growth models interesting on their own merit.

3.3.1 Gompertz model as a simple dynamical system

First we wish to relate the Gompertz formula to the dynamic system models of tumor growth (3.1). In the paradigm of chemical kinetics (3.4), equation

$$y' = k_+ y - k_- y \ln y\,, \qquad y(0) = y_0 > 0\,, \tag{3.12}$$

has the Gompertz growth formula as the unique solution. The growth rate $k_+ y$ reflects the Malthusian law with clear interpretation, but the degradation rate lacks any such interpretation.

Xiaoli Xu attempted to understand the Gompertz growth on the assumption that the growth rate and the degradation rate are both proportional to tumor size (the author considers volume) [XUa]. Formally, this would yield the equation $y' = (k_+ - k_-)y$, which corresponds to unrestricted Malthusian law. However, Xu postulates that growth is described by

$$y' = k_+ y - k_- y^{1+\eta}\,,$$

where η tends to zero from above yielding (3.12). This limiting process was not performed rigorously, although it could have been [MAa]. We discuss this issue further within the context of the generalized logistic model and the von Bertalanffy model (Sections 3.4 and 3.5). Let us only note here that the basic idea is intuitively appealing as it views the Gompertz model as a simple kinetic paradigm where rates are defined by a power law that includes an exponent arbitrarily close to one, but never exactly one. The notion of such an exponent leads to the idea of tumors as fractal structures.

In the growth fraction paradigm (3.7), the equation equivalent to (3.12) is obtained for $g(z) = -\ln z$, i.e.

$$y' = -\alpha\, y \ln\left(\frac{y}{K}\right), \qquad y(0) = y_0 > 0\,. \tag{3.13}$$

Thus, the growth fraction $g(z)$ is the simplest possible elementary transcendental function which obeys $g(z) \in [0, 1)$ for $z \in (0, 1]$ with $g(1) = 0$. Besides the simplicity argument, there is no obvious interpretation of the growth fraction function. The solution of (3.13) and (3.12) reads

$$y = y_0 e^{\ln(K/y_0)(1-e^{-\alpha t})} = K e^{-\ln(K/y_0) e^{-\alpha t}} = y_0 e^{(k_+/k_- - \ln y_0)(1-e^{-k_- t})} . \tag{3.14}$$

As expected from (3.13) for a fixed y_0 and the carrying capacity K, at a certain time t the tumor is larger for a larger growth rate constant α. Besides this trivial statement, it is difficult to find any deeper interpretation of the mode of growth definition by the parameters. However, comparison of (3.12) and (3.13) yields interesting relations among parameters

$$k_- = \alpha , \qquad k_+ = \alpha \ln K . \tag{3.15}$$

These relations suggest that the inherent growth rate constant α (the rate constant for unrestricted growth, i.e., for $K \to \infty$) is equal to the degradation rate constant k_- and yet α is also proportional to the Malthusian growth rate constant k_+. This indicates that the *Gompertzian growth is regulated by the parameter α which controls both growth and degradation.* The same phenomenon can be seen more clearly from the formulation of the Gompertz model within the framework of two differential equations.

3.3.2 Gompertz model as an S-system

If we start from (3.13) and declare the growth fraction a new time dependent variable

$$x = g\left(\frac{y}{K}\right) = \ln\left(\frac{K}{y}\right), \tag{3.16}$$

the solution (3.14) satisfies also the system of equations:

$$y' = \alpha x y , \tag{3.17}$$

$$x' = -\alpha x , \tag{3.18}$$

with initial conditions $y(0) = y_0$ and $x(0) = \ln(K/y_0)$.

Here it is clear that the parameter α is at the same time the inherent growth rate constant and the rate constant for the temporal decrease of the growth fraction. This certainly is a peculiarity of the Gompertz model which supports the idea that the single parameter α controls an inhibitory feedback mechanism operating in tumors. Beyond this and beyond the transparent structure of (3.17) and (3.18) that have a simple interpretation, other fundamental insights are not apparent.

Another possibility to present the Gompertz model as a system of two differential equations is based on the introduction of the effective growth rate $x_1' = \alpha x$ as a variable, as suggested in [LAc]

$$\begin{cases} y' = x_1 y\,, \\ x_1' = \alpha x_1\,. \end{cases}$$

This system of equations is interpreted as describing exponential growth with exponential retardation. However, this can be inferred from (3.11) directly.

In his discussion of growth models, Savageau [SAa] pointed out that the system (3.17–3.18) is a special case of the S-systems. Therefore, to some extent the model shares the universality and foundations of such systems.

3.3.3 Gompertz model and quiescence

Still staying within the framework of dynamic systems described by (3.2), we consider an interesting recent model of tumor growth proposed by Gyllenberg and Webb [GYa] and further applied to the analysis of periodic chemotherapy treatment [GYb]. The authors based the model on cell population dynamics and used cellular quiescence to explain its Gompertzian character. The model is given by equations

$$P' = \Big[\beta - \mu_P - r_o(N)\Big]P + r_i(N)Q\,, \tag{3.19}$$

$$Q' = r_o(N)P - \Big[r_i(N) + \mu_Q\Big]Q\,, \tag{3.20}$$

with $N(t) = P(t) + Q(t)$ where $P(t)$ is the number of proliferating cells at time t, $Q(t)$ is the number of quiescent cells and $N(t)$ is the total number of cells. The constant $\beta > 0$ is the cell division rate, and constants $\mu_P > 0$ and $\mu_Q > 0$ are the death rates for proliferating cells and for quiescent cells, respectively. The function $r_o(N)$ is the rate of transition of proliferating cells into quiescence and the function $r_i(N)$ is the rate of return of quiescent cells into proliferation.

Based on their qualitative analysis, the authors discuss the appearance of necrotic cores in larger tumors, the apoptosis of quiescent cells and the case of quiescent cells resuming proliferation. Apart from this analysis, the authors show that the Gompertz model is a special case of their model. Here we develop a more general derivation of that corollary to unveil some additional features.

First, in conformity with (3.2) we introduce $x = P$, $y = N$, and recast (3.19–3.20) into

$$y' = (\beta - \mu_P)x - \mu_Q(x - y)\,, \tag{3.21}$$

$$x' = \big[\beta - \mu_P - r_o(y)\big]x - r_i(y)y\,. \tag{3.22}$$

Now, it is required that the right-hand side of (3.21) be equal to the right-hand side of (3.12) (the Gompertz model). From the equation obtained, we express x as a function of y. The time derivative of the obtained x is then made equal to the right-hand side of (3.22). Using again the right-hand side of (3.12) for the derivative of y, after a few algebraic steps, we obtain the relation:

$$cr_i(y) + r_o(y) - k_- \ln y = \beta - \mu_P \,, \tag{3.23}$$

and

$$\begin{aligned} c &= \frac{1}{(d-\mu_q)} - 1 \,, \\ d &= \mu_Q + \frac{k_-}{2} + \sqrt{\left(\mu_Q + \frac{k_-}{2}\right)^2 + \mu_Q^2} \,. \end{aligned} \tag{3.24}$$

Gyllenberg and Webb considered only the special case of (3.23) for $r_i(y) = 0$, $r_o(y) = 1 + \ln y$, $k_- = \beta - \mu_P = 1$. The relation (3.23) demonstrates that (3.21) and (3.22) are compatible with the Gompertz model if the form of only one transition rate (r_i or r_o) is specified; the other is then determined from (3.23). The specification of one rate is almost arbitrary. Consequently, when the Gompertz model is applied to the total cell population, it contains rather limited specific information about the dynamics of proliferating and quiescent cell compartments. Gyllenberg and Webb noted that their model is consistent also with the logistic growth model (*via* another specification of transition rates).

In the final analysis, it appears that the rather general model by Gyllenberg and Webb justifies the Gompertz model within the framework of biologically well founded assumptions, but does not reveal in what sense the Gompertz model is unique. On the other hand, by the fact that the Gompertz model is a special case of their model, Gyllenberg and Webb automatically validated their model by the wealth of tumor growth data successfully fitted by the Gompertz formula. We think that this is an important feature, because, surprisingly enough, some rather complex models with more free parameters than the Gompertz model could not fit all tumor growth data [MAa], [MAe]. This will be further discussed in Section 3.7. Now we present another analysis of the Gompertz model based on cell kinetics and depart into the realm of partial differential equations.

3.3.4 Gompertz model and cell kinetics

Frenzen and Murray [FRa] developed a rather elaborate argument to justify the Gompertz formula on the basis of a cell kinetics model proposed and studied earlier by Rubinow [RUa]. The model describes a cell population where each cell is characterized by a degree of maturation described by a maturity variable, $\mu \in [0,1]$. The value of μ increases with time, but varies from cell to cell. When a certain cell is characterized by $\mu = 1$, it divides into two daughter cells. The cell population is described by the cell density function $n(\mu, t)$ with respect to maturity (i.e., $n(\mu, t)d\mu$ represents the number of cells in the maturity interval $[\mu, \mu + d\mu]$). Conservation of mass leads to the following partial differential equation

$$\frac{\partial n}{\partial t} + \frac{\partial (nv)}{\partial \mu} = -\lambda n\,, \tag{3.25}$$

where $-\lambda n$ is the loss term and $v = d\mu/dt = v(\mu, t)$ is the maturation velocity (which can depend on various biologically relevant parameters). The authors consider the time scale on which $\lambda \approx 0$, i.e., when cell death is improbable. They specify maturation velocity as $v = \nu f(t)$, where ν varies from cell to cell and $f(t) \geq 0$ determines collectively the evolution of maturation velocity of every cell. By further specifying the boundary conditions, and after a laborious derivation, the authors arrive at the solution for the total number of cells defined by

$$N(t) = \int_0^1 n(\mu, t)\, d\mu\,. \tag{3.26}$$

The solution for growth over few population doubling was compared to the growth dynamics of the microorganism *Tetrahymena geleii* [PRa]. The agreement of the theory and experiment was remarkably good: $N(t)$ closely followed the data which exhibited a multisigmoidal growing curve. For growth over many population doublings, the model with an exponential decay of maturation velocity predicted the growth curve which agreed (within approximately 5%) with the Gompertz curve created by parameters derived from the model. Such a result is contrasted with the sharp disagreement of the Gompertz curve and the growth curve proposed by Rubinow [RUa], where maturation velocity of any individual cell is constant. In that sense, the model of Frenzen and Murray is much closer to reality. However, the question remains whether the Frenzen–Murray model is close enough to provide an indisputable justification of the Gompertz model, rather than of some other model, e.g., the logistic model. The possible answer to this question may come if one can find explicit expressions for maturation velocity that lead analytically to the Gompertz model and the logistic model and then possibly reject one of the models on the ground of some biological or even mathematical argument.

3.3.5 Gompertz model and entropy

For a long time it has been speculated that the term $y\ln(y/K)$ in the Gompertz model (3.13) can be related to entropy of the system [SWa]. Calderón and Kwembe [CAa] have developed a simple justification of the Gompertz model based on such speculations. Here we present their argument paying more attention to the clear exposition and mathematical rigor which we feel is lacking in the corresponding part of the otherwise good paper.

The authors open their discussion with the statement that tumor growth depends on the interplay between proliferation and quiescence — the very same starting point as that of Gyllenberg and Webb. However, they consider the probability $p(t) = P(t)/P_m$ that the cell is in the proliferative state at time t and the corresponding probability $q(t) = Q(t)/Q_m$ that it is in the quiescent state. Since tumors grow to finite size, it is possible to introduce $P_m = \max_{t>0}[P(t)]$ and $Q_m = \max_{t>0}[Q(t)]$ as maximal numbers of proliferative and quiescent cells, respectively. From the definition of the probabilities it follows

$$p(t) + q(t) = \frac{P(t)}{P_m} + \frac{Q(t)}{Q_m} = 1\,. \tag{3.27}$$

The authors define the entropy of the system as

$$E(t) = -q(t)\ln q(t) - p(t)\ln p(t) \tag{3.28}$$

and further assume (without justification) that the change in probability for quiescent cells is proportional to entropy

$$q'(t) = kE(t)\,. \tag{3.29}$$

Although intuitively this assumption appears based in the reasoning that the transition into quiescence leads into a state of higher disorder, one would like to have more convincing arguments for this notion. Accepting (3.29) and then using (3.27), (3.28) and (3.21), one can obtain

$$\frac{dN}{dt} = C\left[\frac{Q}{Q_m}\ln\frac{Q_m}{Q} + \frac{P}{P_m}\ln\frac{P_m}{P}\right], \tag{3.30}$$

where $N(t)$ is the size of the total population and C is the constant expressed in terms of k, Q_m, P_m. At this point, the authors reasonably assumed that the tumor eventually stops growing and that all cells become quiescent, i.e., that $\lim_{t\to\infty} P(t) = 0$ and, consequently

$$\lim_{t\to\infty} N(t) = \lim_{t\to\infty} Q(t) = Q_m\,.$$

Thus, for large tumors one can approximate (3.30) by

$$\frac{dN}{dt} \approx C \ln \frac{Q_m}{N}, \tag{3.31}$$

which corresponds to the Gompertz model. This whole argument appears simple and obviously suggestive, but to make it fully acceptable one would have to discuss the applicability of the involved approximation for finite times and, as noted, a better founded thermodynamic argument for (3.29).

Most recently, Ling and He [LIa] performed a conceptually interesting (see also [XUb]) and mathematically rigorous entropic analysis of the logistic, the von Bertalanffy and the Gompertz growth models. Without much detail (well presented in the original paper), here we emphasize the main points. Starting from (3.13), Ling and He introduce the normalized equation for $z(t) = y(t)/K = y(t)/y(\infty)$, i.e., $dz/dt = -\alpha z \ln z$. This equation is then used to construct a probabilistic model based on isomorphism, formally implied by the correspondence

$$p \leftrightarrow z\,, \quad \rho \leftrightarrow \frac{dz}{dt}\,, \quad p_0 \leftrightarrow z(0)\,, \quad t \leftrightarrow \tau\,,$$

where $p(\tau)$ is defined as the probability distribution function, $\rho(\tau)$ as a probability density function, and τ is a nonnegative random variable. Thus, the probabilistic model reads

$$\rho(\tau) = -\alpha p(\tau) \ln p(\tau)\,, \qquad p(0) = p_0\,. \tag{3.32}$$

The authors define the change in entropy by the use of the Boltzmann continuous formula,

$$\Delta S = -\int_0^\infty \rho(\tau) \ln \rho(\tau)\, d\tau \tag{3.33}$$

and for ρ, given by (3.32), derive the explicit expression for ΔS in terms of g and p_0. According to the principle of isomorphism, this expression represents the total entropy change involved in the entire evolution of growth as described by the Gompertz model. In further discussion, the authors specifically refer to tumor growth. Based on the analysis of entropy for open systems, it is concluded that the Gompertzian growth, characterized by negative entropy change, corresponds to predominantly negentropic transport from the environment, i.e., external influences (such as available nutrients) dominate over internal influences (such as irreversible processes due to competition). This finding contrasts the results of the analogous analysis for the logistic and the von Bertalanffy model. For these two models the entropy change can be also positive for parameter values smaller than some critical values. Then the authors invoke the phenomenology of early exponential tumor growth, when competition among cells is supposedly negligible, and conclude that the Gompertz model is more appropriate than the other two.

Obviously, there is one critical point in this argument which the authors unfortunately did not address. Namely, when experimental tumor growth data are fitted by the logistic or the von Bertalanffy model, are the respective parameters above or below the critical values?

3.3.6 Gompertz model and tumor heterogeneity

The paper of Kendal [KEa] represents and intriguing attempt to explain the Gompertz model by tumor heterogeneity and by interactions among different cell subpopulations (i.e., proliferating cells, nonproliferating clonogenic cells, and nonproliferating nonclonogenic cells). Tumor heterogeneity is quantitated by assuming that the j-th cell in the population of n cells can adopt one of the q_j possible states ($j = 1, \ldots, n$). Different phases of the cell cycle and different phenotypes specify distinct states. The number of combinations of such states, given by

$$N_c = q_1 q_2 \ldots q_n \, , \tag{3.34}$$

represents the measure of tumor heterogeneity which some authors phenomenologically relate to the tumor growth rate [HEa]. One can then assume the existence of a function $H : N^+ \to N^+$ (with N^+ denoting the set of positive integers) that relates the number of combinations N_c to the number of cells with proliferative potential N_p, i.e., $N_p = H(N_c)$. Accordingly, for the two cell populations with the respective number of combinations of states N_{c1} and N_{c2}, the numbers of cells with proliferative potential are $N_{ri} = H(N_{ci})$, $i = 1, 2$. If these two populations are now considered as one population, the corresponding number of combinations of states is

$$N_c = N_{c1} N_{c2} \tag{3.35}$$

and the corresponding number of cells with proliferative potential is $N_{r1} + N_{r2} = N_r$. On the other hand, $N_r = H(N_c)$, so that the following functional equation is valid

$$H(N_{c1} N_{c2}) = H(N_{c1}) + H(N_{c2}) \, . \tag{3.36}$$

Here, it is tacitly assumed that bringing the two cell populations together did not alter the number of cells with proliferative potential in each population. This assumption (not mentioned in Kendal's paper) can justifiably be questioned because of interactions among cells, but we continue along Kendal's reasoning.

The functional equation (3.36) for $H : N^+ \to N^+$ can be satisfied by various functions. However, since N_r and N_c are large numbers, one can introduce the corresponding continuous positive variables X_r and X_c and define the function $\tilde{H} : R^+ \to R^+$ (with R^+ denoting the set of positive real numbers) which is assumed to satisfy (3.36). Then, it follows that $\tilde{H}$ is uniquely defined by the logarithmic function

$$X_r = \tilde{H}(X_c) = k \ln X_c \,, \tag{3.37}$$

where k is a constant. The author did not consider the transition to continuous variables.

At this point, we introduce the transition to the continuous variable, $X(t)$, for the total number of cells n at time t. Further, we assume that the change of $X(t + \Delta t) - X(t)$ is proportional to the number of cells that actually proliferate within the time interval Δt. This number of cells, in turn, is assumed to be proportional to the number of cells with proliferative potential $X_r(t)$. Consequently

$$X'(t) = akX_r(t) = ak \ln X_c(t) \,. \tag{3.38}$$

Additionally, it is assumed that a and k are constants. This already is similar to the Gompertz equation, but for a full equivalence $X_c(t)$ would have to be related to $X(t)$. Towards this goal, Kendal considered the population of n nonidentical and mutually interacting cells in a tumor. Interactions among cells can only restrict the number of states which each cell can assume in an ideal case of noninteracting cells. Consequently, the number of possible states for each cell decreases with the population size n, because the larger n brings more chances for cell-cell interactions. Thus, Kendal assumes that the number of states attainable by the j-th cell is $q_j = c_j/n$, where $c_j > 0$ is a proportionality constant. It follows that the number of combinations of states is

$$N_c = \frac{c_1 \ldots c_n}{n^n} = \frac{K}{n^n} \,, \tag{3.39}$$

where $K > 0$ is a constant. If now these integer variables are transformed into continuous variables, i.e., N_c is replaced by $X_c(t)$, and n by $X(t)$, equation (3.37) becomes the Gompertz model equation. The fundamental problem in Kendal's argument, not addressed by the author, is that the number of combinations given by (3.39) cannot satisfy the relation (3.35) that is basic to the whole argument. Thus, one concludes that even if all other assumptions involved are impeccable, the relation (3.39) cannot be accepted and the whole argument is, unfortunately, invalid.

3.3.7 Other explanations and analyses of Gompertz model

Only briefly here we mention two other papers related to the analysis of Gompertzian growth; a full presentation of these papers is beyond the scope of this chapter.

Witten investigated senescence in biological systems [WTa]. Using quite original concepts, he derives a mathematical model within the framework of probability theory. In certain instances his model can be approximated by the Gompertz formula. The approximation essentially involves arbitrarily chosen exponential probability density distribution. Such a choice does not appear more fundamental than the similarly arbitrary choices in the arguments presented above. Otherwise, the paper abounds with interesting concepts and analyses.

A methodology completely different from any discussed here is pursued in a recent paper on a cellular automaton model of cancer growth [QIa]. The authors constructed a cellular automaton that involves relevant microscopic mechanisms of tumor growth within the host (including the immune response), and obtained the growth curve which was fitted by the Gompertz formula. The question of how uniquely the Gompertz model fits their automaton model remains unanswered. Also, the authors have not addressed the possibly relevant fact that even the simplest tumor models *in vitro*, derived from a single tumor cell and devoid of any interaction with the organism (e.g., multicell tumor spheroids) also obey the Gompertz growth law [MAb], i.e., that the postulated microscopic mechanisms are not a condition for Gompertzian growth, but that the "program" for this growth law appears inherent in the basic cell kinetics. However, the methodology developed is powerful and can be used to answer numerous relevant questions in tumor growth modeling.

In conclusion of this section, it appears that no explanation of the Gompertz model is sufficiently convincing. However, we are inclined towards simplicity and parsimony: The Gompertz model is an incarnation of a particularly simple dynamics in which the growth rate and the growth fraction decay rate are governed by the same rate constant (Section 3.3.2).

3.4 The Logistic Model

The model characterized by the equation

$$y' = \alpha y\left(1 - \frac{y}{K}\right) = k_+ y - k_- y^2 \,, \tag{3.40}$$

(cf. (3.7) and (3.4)) with the solution

$$y = \frac{y_0 K}{y_0 + (K - y_0)e^{-\alpha t}}, \tag{3.41}$$

has been termed, for reasons somewhat unclear, the "logistic model". In 1838, Verhulst proposed it as a description of population growth [VEa]. The model had been virtually forgotten until Pearl "rediscovered" it years later [PEa]. Since then it has been often used as a point of departure for more advanced population models (see e.g., [MUa]). In 1945, Rashevsky, one of the founders of modern mathematical biology, arrived to the logistic model by considering tumor growth [RAa]. From the perspective of 50 years later it is interesting to quote Rahsevsky's original argumentation:

"Suppose that the rate of growth and of multiplication of each cell is determined by some factor g, the exact physicochemical nature of which is for the present immaterial. Suppose, furthermore, that each cell of an organism exerts an inhibitory effect due to a factor j upon every other cell through the medium of some chemical substance. If we have n cells in an organism, we may consider that the rate of multiplication of each cell is proportional to $ag - b(n-1)j$, where a and b are two coefficients of proportionality, since $(n-1)j$ is the inhibitory effect upon a cell of the other $n-1$ cells. Hence

$$\frac{dn}{dt} = n\big[ag - bj(n-1)\big] = n\big[(ag + bj) - bjn\big]\,."$$

At the time when the concept of cell cycle regulation by growth factors was completely unknown, these words must have sounded almost prophetic. Rashevsky, however, was well aware that this reasoning was too simplistic and that more realistic models were needed. Interestingly, the logistic model was used for fitting to tumor growth data much less frequently than the Gompertz model (see discussion in Section 3.7). On the other hand, the logistic model has been used in kinetic models describing immune response to tumor (see e.g., [KUa], where it has served as a mathematically simple description of immunologically unaffected tumor growth. Similarly, the logistic model has been used in models for chemotherapy optimization [SWb].

The immediate generalization of the logistic model (3.40) is

$$y' = k_+ y - k_- y^\nu\,, \qquad \nu > 1\,, \tag{3.42}$$

with solution

$$y = \left[k - (k - y_0^{1-\nu})e^{k_+(1-\nu)t}\right]^{1/(1-\nu)}, \qquad k = k_+/k_- . \tag{3.43}$$

Function (3.43) is often designated as the Richards function [FLa]. The solution of (3.42) has been thoroughly discussed by Fletcher [FLa]. Interestingly, when this model was fitted to tumor growth data with y_0, k_+, k_-, and ν as free parameters, in most cases it was found that $\nu \approx 1$ [MIa]. Clearly, ν cannot be exactly 1, because then (3.42) would describe unrestricted exponential growth. However, if (3.42) is reparametrized somewhat peculiarly as

$$y' = \left(a + \frac{b}{\nu - 1}\right)y - \frac{b}{\nu - 1}y^\nu = ay - by\frac{y^{\nu-1} - 1}{\nu - 1}, \tag{3.44}$$

then in the limit $\nu \to 1$ one obtains the Gompertz model $y' = ay - by \ln y$. Here we used the general result

$$\lim_{x \to 0} \frac{c^x - 1}{x} = \ln c .$$

This line of derivation is much more rigorous than the one suggested in [XUa]. Now, the result that fitting to data yielded $\nu \approx 1$ can be interpreted as a clear indication that the Gompertz model is a much more adequate description of tumor growth kinetics than is the logistic model.

3.5 Models of von Bertalanffy

The combination of the chemical kinetics paradigm (3.3) and the principle of allometry [HUa] led von Bertalanffy [BTa] to formulate the model of organismic growth represented by the equation

$$y' = k_+ y^\mu - k_- y^\nu, \qquad \mu > 0, \quad \nu > 0 . \tag{3.45}$$

This equation represents a typical S-system and Savageau [SAa] arrived at the same model within his general discussion of S-systems. Equation (3.45) was solved and thoroughly discussed in [MAa]. It was shown that for any μ and ν the solution of (3.45) cannot be expressed in terms of elementary functions, but in terms of the modified beta-function,

$$\beta(x, r, s) = \int_{1/2}^{x} (1 - u)^{r-1} u^{s-1}\, du \tag{3.46}$$

and its inverse.

Several special cases of the general von Bertalaffy model (3.45) have been discussed. The model characterized by $\mu = 2/3$ and $\nu = 1$ is based on the so called "surface rule" and is often named after von Bertalanffy [BTa]. The underlying notion is that the anabolic growth rate is proportional to the surface area (expressed as $y^{2/3}$ where y is interpreted as volume), and the catabolic growth rate is proportional to the volume itself (see also [VAa]).

Another special case of (3.45) is the generalized logistic model with $\mu = 1$, presented by (3.42), and its counterpart with $\nu = 1$:

$$y' = k_+ y^\mu - k_- y\,, \qquad \mu < 1\,. \tag{3.47}$$

The solution of this equation is of the same form as (3.43), because (3.47) can be formally transformed into (3.42) by parameter redefinition, as clearly presented by Fletcher [FLa]. Obviously, model (3.47) contains the von Bertalanffy "surface rule" model. On the other hand, it was shown in [CAa] that (3.47) is a special case of an age-dependent model of tumor growth given by the equation

$$\frac{\partial m}{\partial t} + \frac{\partial m}{\partial a} = -\lambda(a,t)m\,, \tag{3.48}$$

where $m = m(a,t)$ is the size of the cell population of age a at time t, and $\lambda(a,t) > 0$ is the age-specific degradation rate. The basis for (3.48) is the mass conservation law. The solution of (3.48) can be obtained in terms of function $m(0,t)$. Invoking the allometric principle, Calderón and Kwembe assumed that

$$m(0,t) = C[M(t)]^\mu\,, \qquad M(t) = \int_0^\infty m(a,t)\,da\,, \tag{3.49}$$

where $M(t)$ is the total cell population size of any age, and $C > 0$, $0 < \mu < 1$ are constants. Under this assumption one can construct an integral equation for $m(0,t)$. Calderón and Kwembe analyzed the existence and the uniqueness of the solution of that integral equation and the possible routes for its efficient numerical solution. Moreover, they noted that for $\lambda(a,t) = \lambda_0$, the simple integration of (3.48) with respect to a within the limits 0 to ∞ yields

$$\frac{dM}{dt} + m(\infty,t) - C[M]^\mu = -\lambda_0 M\,. \tag{3.50}$$

Under the quite reasonable assumption $m(\infty,t) = 0$, this equation becomes equivalent to (3.47). Thus, the von Bertalanffy model (3.47) is interpretable within the framework of a more general age-dependent model (3.48).

Returning to the general model (3.45), we wish to point out its not-so-obvious relationship to the Gompertz model. Similarly to the generalized logistic model, (3.45) can be reparametrized into

$$y' = ay^{\mu} - \frac{1}{\varepsilon}by^{\mu}(y^{\varepsilon} - 1)\,. \tag{3.51}$$

In the limit $\varepsilon \to 0$, one then obtains the so called "generalized Gompertz model" [MAb]

$$y' = ay^{\mu} - by^{\mu}\ln y\,, \tag{3.52}$$

which, for $\mu = 1$, reduces to the original Gompertz model. In practice, this means that tumor growth data described by the generalized von Bertalanffy model with $\mu \approx 1$, $\nu \approx 1$, are described also by the Gompertz model (see [MAb], [MAe]). Another route from the general von Bertalanffy model to the Gompertz model is based on reparametrization of (3.47), in complete analogy with (3.44).

3.6 Tumor Growth Modeled by Specific Mechanisms

In the hitherto considered models of tumor growth kinetics, the various growth mechanisms have been essentially lumped together either into the overall rates of growth and degradation or into the growth fraction, with each "lumped" quantity described by a simple function. While discussing the foundations of these models, we briefly reviewed some more detailed models which explicitly involve determinants of tumor growth, such as quiescent and proliferating cell populations, cell maturation, and others. Here we discuss other interesting models based on mechanistic considerations. From the mathematical point of view, we limit our discussion to the models expressed by systems of ordinary differential equations (3.2).

3.6.1 Competition among cell populations

The population dynamics of competing species has been described classically by the Lotka–Volterra model (cf. [MUa]). The application of this model to tumor growth was considered particularly by Jansson and Révész [JAa] who modeled the growth of Ehrlich ascites in mice. Their model included competition among three cell types observed in the tumor: (1) diploid cells, (2) tetraploid cells, and (3) aberrant and distinguishable tetraploid cells. Consequently, the model is represented by the system of three Lotka–Volterra-type equations for the respective population sizes

$x_i(t)$, $i = 1, 2, 3$:

$$x_i' = a_i x_i + b_i x_i^2 + (c_{ij} x_j + c_{ik} x_k) x_i \,. \tag{3.53}$$

Here indices i, j, k are cyclic and a_i, b_i, c_{ij}, c_{ik} are model parameters; Jansson and Révész expressed these model parameters through parameters with more closely defined meaning. Apart from the competition term $(c_{ij} x_j + c_{ik} x_k) x_i$, equation (3.53) is logistic in each variable. It is interesting to consider how the authors constructed the exact solution for this system. First, they solved the linear system with only $a_i \neq 0$; this condition corresponds to unrestricted growth. Then they assumed that growth is restricted by a "damping" function $f(t)$, the same for each subpopulation:

$$x_i = x_i^* f \,, \qquad i = 1, 2, 3 \,. \tag{3.54}$$

Here x_i^* is the solution of the linear system. This assumption is equivalent to the assumption that the relative population sizes are unaffected by the experimentally observed growth restriction [JAa], i.e.

$$\frac{x_i}{x_1 + x_2 + x_3} = \frac{x_i^*}{x_1^* + x_2^* + x_3^*} \,.$$

Under assumption (3.54), system (3.53) reduces to a separable differential equation in f that is readily solved. Besides elegant mathematics, the model is biologically well founded and has been validated against data quite thoroughly. From the historical perspective, it is somewhat mysterious that this work has not been pursued further and with more vigor.

Within the framework of the Lotka–Volterra dynamics, Michelson et al. recently focused on qualitative analysis of model equations, rather than on their quantitative validation (for a detailed discussion, see the chapter by Michelson and Leith in this volume [MIb]). Inherent in these models is the problem that equations such as (3.53) contain the competition term involving products of subpopulation sizes, $x_i x_j$ — an approach somewhat lacking in mechanistic insight. In the predator-prey population models, this term represents the direct attack of predator on prey [EDa]. Consequently, the question arises: If the competition among cell populations can be reduced to competition for nutrients, could one explicitly model the intake and uptake of nutrients by cell subpopulations? Recently, Vaidya et al. made an attempt in this direction [VAc]. They considered relationships among normal cells with mass $x_1(t)$, cancer cells with mass $x_2(t)$ and the mass of available nutrients $x_3(t)$ (we retain the original notation). Moreover, they used the essence of the chemical kinetics paradigm to construct the following model equations:

$$x_1' = g_1 x_1 x_3 - d_1 x_1 \,, \tag{3.55}$$

$$x_2' = g_2 x_2 x_3 - d_2 x_2 - I_2 \tanh\left(\frac{x_2}{\varepsilon_2}\right), \tag{3.56}$$

$$x_3' = f_1 - g_1 x_1 x_3 - g_2 x_2 x_3 \,. \tag{3.57}$$

In equation (3.55), the term $g_1 x_1 x_3$ is the anabolic rate for normal cells that includes proportionality to the mass of normal cells and to the available mass of nutrients; the catabolic rate $d_1 x_1$ is modeled as a first order decay of normal cell mass. Analogously, equation (3.56) describes changes in mass of cancer cells, except for the additional catabolic term which accounts for the overall response of the immune system. By the hyperbolic tangent in (3.56), Vaidya et al. modeled triggering of the immune system that initially responds in proportion to the mass of cancer cells, but approaches saturation (characterized by I_2) when x_2 becomes large. For a given I_2, the parameter ε_2 controls the efficiency of the immune system in reducing cancer cell mass. Finally, equation (3.57) describes the constant supply of nutrients (by parameter f_1) and depletion of nutrient mass by "transformation" into the mass of normal cells and cancer cells. In this model, competition between normal cells and cancer cells is clearly related to the availability of nutrients.

Vaidya et al. analyzed the dynamic system (3.55–3.57) globally along the lines of nonlinear dynamic system theory [JCa]. They found three stationary points corresponding to the state of the system with no cancer cells, to the state with no normal cells, and to the state of unstable equilibrium between normal and cancer cells. Also, they discussed in detail two significant bifurcations relevant to the inception and cure of cancer. Interestingly, the interplay between the available nutrients and the immune response lends support to the idea that restricted nutrition can prevent cancer. Besides a qualitative analysis, the authors point out that the model with $I_2 = 0$ can fit tumor growth curves [VAb]. However, a more comprehensive validation of the model against data is still missing. In general, this model provides a parsimonious description of important mechanisms inherent to tumor growth. Clearly, the response of the immune system is very simplified. Much more sophisticated models are discussed in this volume, see [ADb], [BLb], and [KUb].

3.6.2 Cell cycle kinetics and regulation by growth factors

Stimulation and inhibition of proliferation by growth factors and inhibitors is a fundamental feature of the cell cycle. Consequently, it has been postulated that carcinogenesis can be associated with aberrations in the regulatory mechanism of stimulation, e.g., as in the autocrine hypothesis of regulation in cancer growth [SPa], [SPb]. A model of simplified cell cycle kinetics by Piantadosi [PIa] provided the framework for interpretation of some models which included modulation of tumor growth by endogenous tumor inhibitors [WHa], [COa] and stimulators [BAa].

The model by Piantadosi assumes that the total tumor cell population consists of two cell subpopulations, i.e., of the proliferating subpopulation of the size $P(t)$ and the quiescent subpopulation of the size $Q(t)$. Further, the model assumes that the growth rate is characterized by the rate constant α and is proportional to $P(t)$, while the quiescent cells reenter the proliferating subpopulation at the rate $k(t)Q(t)$. Finally, in both subpopulations cells die according to a first-order process characterized by the rate constant ω. These assumptions yield the system of equations

$$P' = kQ - \alpha P - \omega P\,, \tag{3.58}$$

$$Q' = 2\alpha P - kQ - \omega Q\,. \tag{3.59}$$

The factor 2 in (3.59) reflects the biologically founded assumption that each cell divides exactly into two cells. In the case when the rate $k(t)$ is an effective function of the total population only, $y(t) = P(t) + Q(t)$, i.e., $k(t) = r(y(t))$, equations (3.58–3.59) are a special case of equations (3.19–3.20) that represent the Gyllenberg–Webb model (see Section 3.3.3).

Piantadosi did not specify the rate $k(t)$, but rather combined (3.58) to obtain the single equation with an unspecified growth fraction g

$$y' = \alpha\, y\, g - \omega\, y\,, \qquad g = \frac{P}{y}\,. \tag{3.60}$$

It is noteworthy that (3.60) is equivalent to the age-dependent model (3.48) with constant age-specific degradation rate. This becomes clear through the following substitutions:

$$M(t) = y(t)\,, \qquad \lambda(a,t) = \omega\,, \qquad m(0,t) = \alpha y(t) g(t)\,.$$

For the growth fraction, Piantadosi proposed a *de facto* empirical expression:

$$g = g(y) = (1 + \beta y^{\gamma})^{-1/\gamma}\,, \qquad \beta, \gamma > 0\,.$$

Other authors developed models with the growth fraction dependent on mechanisms of inhibition and stimulation of growth by growth mediators. We consider some of these models below.

Cox et al. assumed that cells secrete a growth inhibiting factor which diffuses into the extracellular space [COa]. The concentration $x_1(t)$ of the inhibitor changes as a result of two competing first-order processes

$$x_1' = \sigma\, y - \delta\, x_1\,, \tag{3.61}$$

where $\sigma > 0$ accounts for the rate of inhibitor secretion and $\delta > 0$ represents the rate constant for inhibitor degradation. Further, Cox et al. assumed that each cell contains one receptor that can combine with one inhibitor molecule. When the receptor is unoccupied, the cell belongs to the reproducing subpopulation; when the receptor is occupied, the cell is arrested in the G_0 phase. These assumptions, together with simple binding kinetics, yield

$$x_2' = -k_1 x_1 x_2 + k_2 x\,, \qquad R = x + x_2\,, \tag{3.62}$$

where x_2 is the concentration of unoccupied receptors, x is the concentration of the receptor-inhibitor complex, and R is the total receptor concentration. The constants k_1 and k_2 are the binding rate constant and the dissociation rate constant, respectively. According to the above assumptions on the role of receptor occupancy, the size of the reproducing subpopulation is proportional to the concentration of unoccupied receptor, i.e., $P = \rho x_1$, and the total receptor concentration is proportional to the population size, i.e., $R = cy$. These relations together with (3.61–3.62) yield the system of equations of the general form (3.2):

$$y' = \alpha\, \rho\, x_2 - \omega\, y\,, \tag{3.63}$$

$$x_1' = \sigma\, y - \delta\, x_1\,, \tag{3.64}$$

$$x_2' = -k_1 x_1 x_2 + k_2(cy - x_2)\,. \tag{3.65}$$

This dynamical system has only one nonzero stationary point which corresponds to the finite asymptotic value for y [BAa]. Since the processes described by (3.61) and (3.62) can be considered rapid in comparison to population growth, it was assumed in [COa] that they obey the quasi-steady-state approximation, $\sigma y = \delta x_1$, $k_1 x_1 x_2 = k_2(cy - x_2)$, which then yields

$$y' = \frac{\alpha_1}{1 + \beta y} - \omega\, y\,. \tag{3.66}$$

Comparing (3.65) and (3.60) one concludes that the factor $(1 + \beta y)^{-1}$ is proportional to the growth fraction. Parameter $\beta = \sigma k_1/(k_2\delta)$ includes parameters pertinent to dynamics of growth inhibition, while the parameter $\alpha_1 = \alpha\rho c$ encompasses the inherent growth rate and the susceptibility of cells to inhibition. The model represented by (3.65) is a special case of the Piantadosi model ($\gamma = 1$) [PIa] and is equivalent to the model of Wheldon et al. [WHa] who used the same basic idea that growth is controlled by inhibitory growth factors, but other assumptions by Wheldon et al. differed from those of Cox et al. [BAd].

The observation that growth is controlled also by stimulatory growth factors has been modeled recently along the same lines of receptor-mediated regulation of tumor growth [BAa]. In that work we assumed that together with the receptor for growth inhibitor, each cell bears one receptor for the stimulatory growth factor molecule and that the binding of these molecules obeys simple second-order kinetics. The cell proliferates when the receptor for inhibitor is unoccupied and/or when the receptor for stimulator is occupied. The model is then developed in analogy with the model of Cox et al. yielding

$$y' = \alpha_2\, y \left[\frac{1}{1+\beta y} + \frac{\gamma_1 y}{1+\gamma_2 y}\right] - \omega\, y\,. \tag{3.67}$$

Here the expression within brackets is proportional to the growth fraction. The parameter $\gamma_2 \geq 0$ incorporates parameters essential for dynamics of growth stimulation, parameter γ_1 contains also parameters describing cellular responsiveness to growth inhibitors and stimulators, and parameter α_2 accounts for the inherent growth rate and responsiveness.

The model (3.65) has not been validated against data until recently when it was applied to 15 populations of multicell tumor spheroids, each comprised of a different cell line [MAb]. The results of a thorough statistical analysis showed that the model (3.65) was much less adequate in describing growth curves than the Gompertz model which contains one fewer free parameter. This result demonstrates how important model validation is in the process of modeling. Interestingly, when fitted to the same growth data, even model (3.66) with six free parameters did not show significant improvement over the model (3.65) [BAa]. On the other hand, the Piantadosi model, which contains only one parameter (γ) more than (3.65), fitted the same data very successfully [MAb], [MAe]. One is tempted to conclude that in spite of its elegance and biological foundations, the approach of Cox et al. and Wheldon et al. does not include certain fundamental feature(s) of tumor growth.

We developed another model that described growth of multicell tumor spheroids more adequately and still included a term based on autocrine self-stimulation [MAc]. This model, named the "autostimulation model", is a modification of (3.65) in the sense that the growth fraction explicitly depends on the "level of growth-stimulating biological activity", $x(t)$, resulting from the complex interplay of different growth factors and their receptors. Thus,

$$g = \frac{\phi(x)}{1+\beta y}\,. \tag{3.68}$$

For the sake of simplicity and to keep the number of free parameters at a minimum, the function $\phi(x)$ was chosen to be linear. The growth-stimulating biological activity depends on secretion of growth factors by cells, so that the rate of increase in activity is proportional to the total population, while the rate of decrease results from several processes (degradation within cells, extracellular degradation, diffusion from tumor, etc.) and is modeled as a single n-th order process. The autostimulation model is then given by the following system of differential equations [MAc], [BAb]

$$y' = \alpha_1 y \frac{1+x}{1+\beta y} - \omega y \,, \tag{3.69}$$

$$x' = ax - bx^n \,. \tag{3.70}$$

The effective changes in growth-stimulating biological activity are considered to happen on the same time scale as tumor growth, so that (3.69) cannot be approximated as a quasi-steady-state process. This gives the autostimulation model additional flexibility over the model (3.66), namely the flexibility to describe spontaneous tumor regression after initial growth (see Section 3.2). Also, the autostimulation model was suitable for studies of effects of growth perturbation by agents that can increase and/or decrease stimulation as in hormone-dependent tumors such as estrogen-dependent breast cancer [MAd]. There, withdrawal of estrogen attenuates growth and stimulates the loss of cells deprived of estrogen. Estrogen withdrawal at a given time is described by an immediate and instantaneous change of parameters a, b and ω. We showed by simulations that the effects of estrogen removal on autostimulation could be quantified quite accurately [MAd].

The analysis of stationary points of the system (3.69–3.70) reveals that for $n \geq 2$ one can attain at least one locally asymptotically stable stationary point. For $n = 2$, the model contains the same number of parameters as (3.66). However, the fits of the autostimulation model to tumor spheroid growth curves were statistically satisfactory and much more adequate than those for models (3.66) or (3.65). The autostimulation model was also adequate for description of growth curves of tumors in nude mice and in patients [MAe].

3.6.3 Positive feedback mechanisms in tumors

In 1984, we proposed the idea that stimulation of tumor growth by tumor-borne growth factors can be viewed as a positive feedback mechanism and can be modeled within the framework of control system theory [BAc], [BAa]. The initial mathematical model was developed and applied to a study of positive feedback in murine melanoma B16 [BAc]. The feedback loop included tumor-borne insulin-related growth mediators, glucose in blood, circulating growth hormone and the size of tumor. The size of the tumor increased with the level of growth hormone, which, in turn, correlated with the decrease of glucose concentration. Glucose concentration was found to decrease with the increase of insulin-related growth mediator. The concentration of the mediator was positively correlated to tumor size closing the postulated feedback loop. The mathematical model of this loop was based on exponential and Gompertz-like functions and offered quantitation of the "open-loop gain", a measure of the efficiency of positive feedback. A somewhat simpler, but mathematically more refined model, was applied later to a murine myeloid leukemia *in situ* [BAe]. In its latest version [BAa], this model became rather general, but still mathematically and computationally tractable for quantitation of positive feedback in tumor growth. The only problem was the lack of data required for estimation of model parameters. Such data would include growth curves measured at different levels of external perturbation of stimulatory activity of growth factors together with time-resolved measurement of this activity. Despite the observations of potential clinical correlates, such data are generally difficult to obtain and consequently we sought another approach that is briefly presented below [BAb], [BAa].

We considered the simplest positive feedback: tumor size y increases with activity x of stimulatory growth factors and, in turn, this activity increases with the size of the tumor as an increasing number of cells secrete growth factors. Clearly, this cannot be the only mechanism of tumor growth regulation; growth inhibitory processes must also take place if tumor growth is to remain restricted. The simplest framework to consider the positive feedback via activity x and other mechanisms of growth is the system of two differential equations of the type (3.2):

$$\begin{cases} y' = G_1(x,y)\,, \\ x' = G_2(x,y)\,. \end{cases} \tag{3.71}$$

In the first equation, the dependence of $G_1(x,y)$ on y represents all considered mechanisms of growth (including inhibition) except stimulation *via* activity x which is explicitly modeled by the dependence of $G_1(x,y)$ on x. On the other hand, the stimulatory activity is modeled through $G_2(x,y)$, whereby the dependence on y describes the fact that this activity is influenced by the size of tumor. Thus, the system (3.71) contains the implicit feedback mechanism already. The question arises whether one can characterize the strength of this feedback by a single quantity. One possibility is to evaluate the open-loop gain [RIa], but we prefer a more intuitive concept, the "magnification factor" $\mathcal{M}$ [RIa]. The magnification factor is defined as the factor relating the asymptotic infinitesimal size change $\Delta Y(\infty)$ in the presence of the feedback to the asymptotic size change $\Delta\tilde{Y}(\infty)$ in the absence of the feedback

$$\Delta Y(\infty) = \mathcal{M}\Delta\tilde{Y}(\infty)\,. \tag{3.72}$$

Here, tumor size changes are defined in relation to (3.71) in a nontrivial way which requires a detailed explication. First, we consider functions $Y(t) = h_1(t, \bar{x})$, and $X(t) = h_2(t, \bar{y})$ that satisfy

$$\begin{cases} Y' = G_1(\bar{x}, Y)\,, \\ X' = G_2(X, \bar{y})\,. \end{cases} \tag{3.73}$$

for any time-independent $\bar{x}$ and $\bar{y}$ for which G_i, $i = 1, 2$, are well defined. Further, it is assumed that the asymptotic solutions of (3.71)

$$\hat{x} = \lim_{t \to \infty} x(t)\,, \quad \text{and} \quad \hat{y} = \lim_{t \to \infty} y(t)\,,$$

are stationary

$$G_1(\hat{x}, \hat{y}) = G_2(\hat{x}, \hat{y}) = 0\,. \tag{3.74}$$

Clearly, $G_i(x, y)$, should be defined to allow the existence of these solutions. The change in size at time t is then defined as the change in size due to the small change in stimulatory activity around its stationary value and a small time increment

$$\Delta Y(t) = h_1\big(t + \Delta t, \hat{x} + \Delta X(t)\big) - h_1(t, \hat{x})\,, \tag{3.75}$$

where

$$\Delta X(t) = h_2\big(t + \Delta t, \hat{y} + \Delta Y(t)\big) - h_2(t, \hat{y})\,. \tag{3.76}$$

For sufficient smoothness of $G_1(x, y)$ and $G_1(x, y)$, the functions $h_1 = h_1(t, \hat{x})$ and $h_2 = h_2(t, \hat{x})$ are differentiable, so that

$$\Delta Y(t) = \frac{\partial h_1}{\partial t}(t, \hat{x})\Delta t + \frac{\partial h_1}{\partial \hat{x}}(t, \hat{x})\Delta X(t)\,, \tag{3.77}$$

$$\Delta X(t) = \frac{\partial h_2}{\partial t}(t, \hat{y})\Delta t + \frac{\partial h_2}{\partial \hat{y}}(t, \hat{y})\Delta Y(t)\,. \tag{3.78}$$

Equations (3.77–3.78) can be solved for $\Delta Y(t)$ to yield

$$\Delta Y(t) = \frac{\dfrac{\partial h_1}{\partial t}(t, \hat{x}) + \dfrac{\partial h_1}{\partial \hat{x}}(t, \hat{x})\dfrac{\partial h_2}{\partial t}(t, \hat{y})}{1 - \dfrac{\partial h_1}{\partial \hat{x}}(t, \hat{x})\dfrac{\partial h_2}{\partial \hat{y}}(t, \hat{y})}\,\Delta t\,. \tag{3.79}$$

In the hypothetical absence of the feedback, the function $h_1(t, \bar{x})$ should not depend on $\bar{x}$ explicitly and, therefore,

$$\frac{\partial h_1}{\partial \hat{x}}(t, \hat{x}) = 0 \,. \tag{3.80}$$

According to (3.77), the corresponding change in tumor size is then

$$\Delta \tilde{Y}(t) = \frac{\partial h_1}{\partial t}(t, \hat{x}) \, \Delta t \,. \tag{3.81}$$

In a formal sense, (3.79) and (3.81) complete the definition of the particular tumor size changes involved in (3.72). However, this definition is not very practical. Therefore, one can go a step further and express $\mathcal{M}$ in terms of partial derivatives of G_i. Again, we assume sufficient smoothness of G_i so that all formal operations below can be performed. From (3.73), and from the definition of h_i, $i = 1, 2$, together with $\hat{x}$, $\hat{y}$, it follows that

$$\hat{y} = \lim_{t \to \infty} h_1(t, \hat{x}) = f_1(\hat{x}) \,, \qquad \hat{x} = \lim_{t \to \infty} h_2(t, \hat{y}) = f_2(\hat{y}) \,. \tag{3.82}$$

The functions f_1 and f_2 represent the steady state characteristics of the dynamical system [DOa]. Taking the limes for $t \to \infty$ of (3.79) and making use of (3.81–3.82) and (3.73) yields

$$\Delta Y(\infty) = \frac{\Delta \tilde{Y}(\infty) + \dfrac{df_1}{d\hat{x}}(\hat{x}) \, G_2(\hat{x}, \hat{y})}{1 - \dfrac{df_1}{d\hat{x}}(\hat{x}) \, \dfrac{df_2}{d\hat{y}}(\hat{y})} \Delta t \,. \tag{3.83}$$

The very last term of (3.83) vanishes because of (3.74). Then, if the denominator in (3.83) differs from zero, from (3.83) and (3.72) one obtains

$$\mathcal{M} = \frac{1}{1 - \Omega} \,, \qquad \Omega = \frac{df_1}{d\hat{x}}(\hat{x}) \, \frac{df_2}{d\hat{y}}(\hat{y}) \,, \tag{3.84}$$

where Ω is the "open-loop gain" which represents the slope of the open-loop characteristic function $F = f_2 \circ f_1$ [DOa]. Taking into account (3.74) and (3.82), it follows

$$G_1\big(\hat{x}, f_1(\hat{x})\big) = 0 \,, \qquad G_2\big(f_2(\hat{y}), \hat{y}\big) = 0 \,, \tag{3.85}$$

and differentiation of implicit functions yields

$$\Omega = \frac{\dfrac{\partial G_1}{\partial \hat{x}}(\hat{x},\hat{y}) \, \dfrac{\partial G_2}{\partial \hat{y}}(\hat{x},\hat{y})}{\dfrac{\partial G_1}{\partial \hat{y}}(\hat{x},\hat{y}) \, \dfrac{\partial G_2}{\partial \hat{x}}(\hat{x},\hat{y})} . \tag{3.86}$$

Thus, the open-loop gain and the magnification factor can be calculated from the given model functions G_i. This makes it possible to characterize the positive feedback without even solving the system of equations (3.71), but only by finding its asymptotic critical points.

When $\mathcal{M} > 1$, the asymptotic change in size for growth with feedback is larger than for growth without feedback; this corresponds to the positive feedback, characterized also by $\Omega > 0$. For $\mathcal{M} = 1$, there is no feedback, and for $0 < \mathcal{M} < 1$, the feedback is negative ($\Omega < 0$). For the dynamical system (3.71), Doucet has shown that the stationary point $(\hat{x},\hat{y})$ is asymptotically stable if and only if $\Omega < 1$ [DOa].

For the autostimulation model (3.68–3.69), the magnification factor can be calculated in terms of model parameters exactly

$$\mathcal{M} = 1 + \left[1 + \frac{4b\,\beta\,\omega}{a\,\alpha_1}\left(1 - \frac{\omega}{\alpha_1}\right)\right]^{-1/2} . \tag{3.87}$$

For the asymptotically stable stationary point and for $\omega < \alpha_1$, it follows that $1 < \mathcal{M} < 2$; for $\omega > \alpha_1$ and other parameters set so that the term in brackets lies within the interval $(0, 1)$, the magnification factor is larger than 1.

In [BAa] we calculated the values of the magnification factor for 15 tumor growth curves of multicell tumor spheroids. We demonstrated that $\mathcal{M}$ can be estimated with a remarkably small error (less than 10% in 11 cases and less than 15% in four) in comparison to errors in model parameters which often exceeded 100 percent. The value of $\mathcal{M}$ ranged from 1.5 to 2. This implies that the model predicted a substantial reduction of tumor size when the positive feedback is blocked. The overall conclusion of the study [BAa] was that the magnification factor is a statistically sound parameter for characterization of the positive feedback mechanism.

3.7 Mathematical Models and Measured Growth Curves

The preceding discussion demonstrates a plethora of mathematical models proposed to describe and predict various aspects of tumor growth kinetics. Yet, only the Gompertz model has been *extensively* tested against measured tumor growth curves. Other models were tested more sporadically and on far fewer sets of growth data. We believe that further advancement in mathematical modeling of tumor growth kinetics critically depends on thorough testing of proposed models against data as they become more available with development of experimental techniques.

3.7.1 Growth data and Gompertz model

Many authors fitted the Gompertz function (3.14) to data by the least squares method and virtually all fits were adequate [LAa], [LAb], [LAd], [DUa], [SIa], [SUa], [NOa], [MAb], [MAe], [BSa], [BSb]. Often the Gompertz function was transformed into

$$\ln y = a + bu\,, \qquad u = \exp(-\alpha t)\,, \tag{3.88}$$

implying that for a given α the logarithms of tumor size should satisfy a linear dependence on u. The value of α was considered the best estimate when the linear regression yielded the least sum of squared errors. More recently, Bassukas and Maurer–Shultze [BSb] noticed that the Gompertz formula is equivalent to the recursion $\ln y(t_0+(n+1)\tau) = c + d\ln y(t_0+n\tau)$ where τ is a constant time interval. Thus, for the tumor size values measured regularly at times $n\tau$, $n = 1, 2, \ldots$, one can test the model by linear regression analysis. Another advantage of this approach is that it includes the pure exponential model ($d = 1$) and makes it possible to evaluate statistically the deviation from exponential growth, often observed at the initial stage. In a subsequent paper, Bassukas applied the recursion formula to the comparative analysis of tumor growth patterns in treated and untreated human renal cell carcinoma xenografts in nude mice [BSa]. It is interesting that the Gompertz recursion formula was derived earlier for tumor regression analysis [SUa], but was not used in actual fitting to data. Sullivan and Salmon demonstrated the almost universal applicability of the Gompertz model by fitting to the growth data of myeloma cells for the unperturbed growth and for the remission after treatment [SUa].

Norton et al. have found an interesting linear correlation between parameters k_+ and k_- of the Gompertz model (see (3.12)) for a given type of tumor, i.e., $\exp(k_+) = m\ln k_- + n$; here coefficients m and n characterize the type of tumor while k_+ and k_- vary for individual growth curves of the same tumor [NOb]. When m and n are determined, Norton et al. showed that only few initial points of a growth curve suffice for fits of the Gompertz model which then adequately describes the *entire* growth curve. This result suggests the high predictive potential of the Gompertz model. In other studies [VAa], [MAf], the prediction power of models of tumor growth was analyzed by the prediction error

$$E_k = \max_{i>k} \left| \frac{y(k,t_i) - y_i}{y_i} \right|, \tag{3.89}$$

where $y_i, i = 1, \ldots, n$, are data for tumor size at time t_i and $y(k, t_i)$, $k \leq n$, are the corresponding theoretical values obtained by fitting the model function to the first k data points. A comparison of the power of the Gompertz model, the generalized Gompertz model (Section 3.5), the Piantadosi model and the autostimulation model (Section 3.6.2) to predict the growth of multicell tumor spheroids showed that the Gompertz model was the most predictive [MAf]. However, in a study of induced sarcoma in mice and primary carcinoma of the human lung, Vaidya et al. found that the Gompertz model was not more predictive than the logistic model (Section 3.4) or the von Bertalanffy ("surface rule") model (Section 3.5) [VAa].

3.7.2 Comparative studies of deterministic tumor growth models

Few studies compare how different tumor growth models fit the same data, although such studies are essential for discrimination among models. In several instances it was possible to reject certain models by statistical analysis of fits.

Gratton et al. compared the Gompertz model, the logistic model, a three-parameter rational function, and the quadratic function by fitting to murine fibrosarcoma growth curves [GRa]. They concluded that all considered models described the data rather well, but that the Gompertz model was preferred. Michelson et al. reported similar results on the basis of the study of xenograft tumors in nude mice [MIa]. They showed that the Gompertz model fitted the data more adequately than the logistic model. The fits by the generalized logistic model (Section 3.4) yielded the value of exponent ν in (3.42) very close to 1 in four out of five different mixtures of two clones of tumor cells in xenografts. In other words, in these four cases the generalized logistic model was virtually equivalent to the Gompertz model.

Results quite different from Gratton et al. and Michelson et al. were obtained in the already mentioned study by Vaidya et al. [VAa]. Among the logistic, the von Bertalanffy ("surface rule"), and the Gompertz models, the authors found that the logistic model was preferred for human tumors *in situ* and the von Bertalanffy model for murine tumors *in situ*. In our recent study of models applied to multicell tumor spheroids [MAb], the logistic and the von Bertalanffy models could not fit any of the 15 growth curves considered, while the Gompertz model fitted all growth curves adequately (see Figure 3.1). This quite surprising result is an excellent example of clear-cut discrimination among mathematical models characterized by the same number of free parameters and all, to some extent, biologically founded. Vaidya et al. dealt with tumors in organisms with the immune system completely intact, so one can argue that the logistic and the von Bertalanffy models were adequate for tumors *in vivo*, but inadequate for multicell tumor spheroids or tumors in nude mice. Yet, the situation is not that simple.

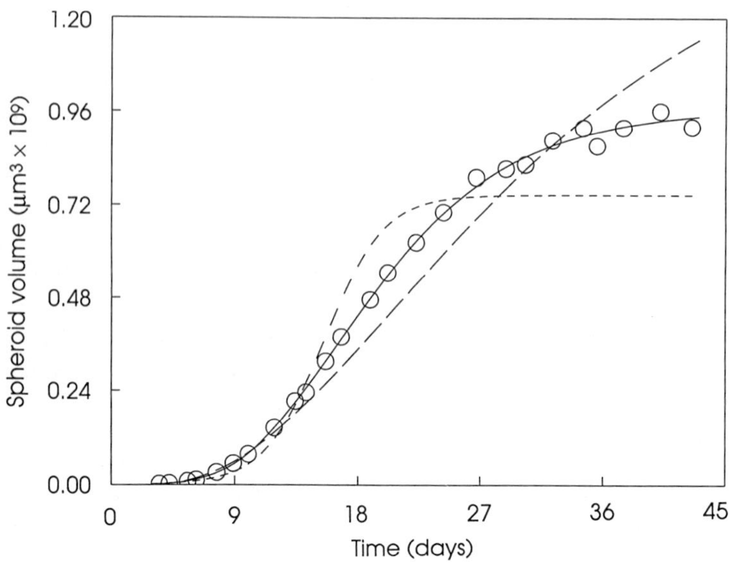

Figure 3.1 — Comparison of best-fit curves of the three "classical" tumor growth models fitted to the time-dependent volume of multicell tumor spheroids comprised of murine adenocarcinoma cells designated MAC2 (Data set No. 1 in [MAb]). Full line: Gompertz model; short-dashed line: logistic model; long-dashed line: von Bertalanffy model. Experimental and computational details as in [MAb].

Recently, we confirmed [MAe] the results of Michelson et al. [MIa] on two tumors in nude mice, i.e., we found that the logistic and the von Bertalanffy models were clearly inadequate in comparison to the Gompertz model. Then, we analyzed the same patient data (obtained by Schwartz [SCa]) studied by Vaidya et al. [VAa] and found that the Gompertz model yielded lower sums of squared errors than the logistic model in five out of seven growth curves. In contrast, it was found in [VAa] that the logistic model yielded lower sums of squared errors in four out of seven growth curves. We found that the difference between the fits resulted from the type of nonlinear regression applied. Vaidya et al. minimized the unweighted sum of squared errors (SSE) of tumor size, i.e.,

$$SSE = \sum_i \left[y_i - y(t_i)\right]^2, \tag{3.90}$$

and we minimized the unweighted sum of squared errors for the *logarithms* ($LSSE$) of tumor size

$$LSSE = \sum_i \left[\ln y_i - \ln y(t_i)\right]^2. \tag{3.91}$$

The minimum of SSE corresponds to the maximum likelihood for normally distributed volume measurements with standard deviation equal for all volumes. On the other hand, the minimum of $LSSE$ corresponds to the maximum likelihood of normally distributed volume measurements with standard deviations proportional to the volume, which is an assumption closer to observation. To further resolve the controversy in fitting the data by Schwartz, we assumed that the Gompertz model was the true model for description of the data and determined the best fit curve by the Gompertz model using (3.91). Then we computed tumor volumes predicted by the Gompertz model at times of true measurements and added normal noise to these values. The expectation of noise was zero and the standard deviation was proportional to volume and characterized by coefficient κ. A sufficient number (200) of such synthetic data sets was generated and used for fits of the Gompertz and logistic models by separate minimization of (3.90) and (3.91). For $\kappa = 0.2$, these fits showed that the logistic model yielded lower SSE in more than 80% of fits to the synthetic growth curves originally derived from the Gompertz curve. For $LSSE$, the logistic model was better in about 50% of fits. For smaller values of κ, i.e., for smaller measurement errors, the fits were more favorable for the Gompertz model, as expected; for the hardly attainable error of $\kappa = 0.05$, the Gompertz was still not favored in some 30% of fits for $LSSE$. These results show how difficult it is to discriminate the Gompertz model from the logistic model for the small number of data points measured beneath the growth plateau. This conclusion supports the previous experience that "*... when the data* *cover a wide range of sizes, the Gompertz equation usually gives better fit than either the logistic or the Bertalanffy equation"* [STa].

We scrutinized other models against data too, some models representing families of nested models, such as the generalized von Bertalanffy model with its special cases (Section 3.5), or the family of models based on the "generic model" [TUa], [PTa]. Similarly, we analyzed the model of Wheldon et al. and Cox et al. which is nested in both the Piantadosi model and the autostimulation model (Section 3.6.2). It is noteworthy that the Piantadosi model and the autostimulation model gave statistically indistinguishable fits to multicell tumor spheroid growth curves, but were clearly distinguishable by the predicted thickness of the rim of viable cells in spheroids; the Piantadosi model predicted a strongly time-dependent thickness, while predictions of the autostimulation model agreed with the observed thickness virtually independent in time.

From all comparative and other studies discussed here, we believe we can set some observations and guidelines for future studies:

1. Fitting the *families of nested models* of tumor growth curves makes it possible to discriminate among models more precisely than by fitting individual models.
2. The Gompertz model is the most parsimonious, still adequate, and almost universal description of tumor growth curves.
3. Some rather elaborate models, such as those by Wheldon et al. and Cox et al. describe data inadequately despite the "sufficient" number of free parameters. In other words, some models based on reasonable biological assumptions are not consistent with data although they include substantial freedom in parameters.
4. The autostimulation model fitted adequately all growth curves under study.
5. Comparative studies make discrimination possible between qualitative differences (different models) or just quantitative differences (different parameter values) for same tumors grown in different environments (e.g., as multicell spheroids and *in vivo*) [MAb].

3.8 Concluding Outlooks

In this review we focused on mathematical models for description and prediction of tumor growth curves — the primordial kinetic observations related to tumor growth. This is an old topic and we wished to condense decades of history and contribute towards a more coherent picture. However, the task turned out to be rather difficult as many isolated islands of developments have not been integrated by sufficiently abundant connections. We have tried to find mathematical or conceptual relations among different models and, indeed, in some instances such relations emerged (e.g., the relations among the Piantadosi model, the model of Gyllenberg and Webb, and the age-dependent model; Section 3.6.2). Admittedly, we are still far from any truly unified picture. The fruits of mathematical modeling that would significantly help understanding and curing cancer will have to come from more coherent efforts in the future. In this sense, here we list some directions:

1. The Gompertz model is deeply rooted in growth data, but is still lacking a truly fundamental explanation. Of the reviewed attempts towards such an explanation, most have merit, but none is convincing. We believe that the Gompertz model is more fundamental than, for example, the logistic model. Hence, let the quest for a deeper understanding of the empirical Gompertz law continue.
2. At this point, relations among different proposed models are vital for tumor growth modeling. Researchers in the field should make every attempt to find and elaborate such relations, and to compare their own models with models previously proposed but not rejected.
3. The time is ripe for extensive validation of various proposed deterministic models against data and for rejection of those which are inconsistent with observations. To bring coherence to the field, even models that have not been designed primarily for description and prediction of *tumor* growth curves should be examined. Most prerequisites for model validation are in place: more experimental data can be obtained with more precision, the software for model fitting has become more reliable and practical, and the computing power is not a problem anymore.

3.9 Acknowledgment

The authors thank Dr. Frank Prendergast for his steadfast support of mathematical modeling in biomedicine, and Mr. Ivo Penzar for his careful critical reading of the manuscript.

3.10 References

[ADa] Adam J.A. and Maggelakis S.A., Diffusion regulated growth characteristics of a spherical prevascular carcinoma, *Bull. Math. Biol.*, **52** (1990), 549–582.

[ADb] Adam J.A., General aspects of modeling tumor growth and immune response, in **A Survey of Models for Tumor-Immune System Dynamics**, Adam J.A. and Bellomo N. eds., Birkhäuser (1996).

[ARa] Aroesty J., Lincoln T., Shapiro N., and Boccia G., Tumor growth and chemotherapy: Mathematical methods, computer simulations, and experimental foundations, *Math. Biosci.*, **17** (1973), 243–300.

[BAa] Bajzer Ž., Marušić M., and Vuk-Pavlović S., Conceptual frameworks for mathematical modeling of tumor growth dynamics, *Math. Comput. Modeling*, **23** (1996), 31–46.

[BAb] Bajzer Ž., Marušić M., and Vuk-Pavlović S., Mathematical modeling of cellular interaction dynamics in multicellular tumor spheroids, in **Proc. First World Congress of Nonlinear Analysts**, Lakshmikantham V. ed., Vol. 4, Walter de Gruyter (1996), 3645–3654.

[BAc] Bajzer Ž., Pavelić K., and Vuk-Pavlović S., Growth self-incitement in murine melanoma B16, *Science*, **225** (1984), 930–932.

[BAd] Bajzer Ž. and Vuk-Pavlović S., Quantitative aspects of autocrine regulation in tumors, *CRC Crit. Rev. Oncogenesis*, **2** (1990), 53–73.

[BAe] Bajzer Ž. and Vuk-Pavlović S., Quantitation of autocrine regulation of tumor growth: A general phenomenological model. *Cancer Res.*, **47** (1987), 5330–5333.

[BEa] Beltrami E., **Mathematics for Dynamic Modeling**, Academic Press (1987).

[BLa] Bellomo N. ed., **Modelling and Simulation Problems on Tumor Immune System Dynamics**, *Math. Comp. Modelling – Special Issue*, **23** (1996).

[BLb] Bellomo N., Preziosi L., and Forni G., Tumor immune system interactions: The kinetic cellular theory, in **A Survey of Models for Tumor-Immune System Dynamics**, Adam J.A. and Bellomo N. eds., Birkhäuser (1996).

[BSa] Bassukas I.D., Comparative Gompertzian analysis of alterations of tumor growth patterns, *Cancer Res.*, **54** (1994), 4385–4392.

[BSb] Bassukas I.D. and Maurer–Schultze B., The recursion formula of the Gompertz function: A simple method for the estimation and comparison of tumor growth curves, *Growth, Development and Aging*, **52** (1988), 113–122.

[BTa] von Bertalanffy L., Quantitative laws in metabolism and growth, *Q. Rev. Biol.*, **32** (1957), 217–231.

[CAa] Calderón C.P. and Kwembe T.A., Modeling tumor growth, *Math. Biosci.*, **103** (1991), 97–114.

[CEa] Casey A.E., The experimental alteration of malignancy with an homologous mammalian tumor material I, *Am. J. Cancer*, **21** (1934), 760–775.

[COa] Cox E.B., Woodbury M.A., and Myers L.E., A new model for tumor growth analysis based on a postulated inhibitory substance, *Comp. Biomed. Res.*, **13** (1980), 437–445.

[DOa] Doucet P.G., On the static analysis of nonlinear feedback loops, *Math. Biosci.*, **78** (1986), 107–129.

[DUa] Durbin P.W., Jeung N., Williams M.H., and Arnold J.S., Construction of a growth curve for mammary tumors of the rat, *Cancer Res.*, **27** (1967), 1341–1347.

[EDa] Edelstein–Keshet L., **Mathematical Models in Biology**, Random (1988).

[FLa] Fletcher R.I., A general solution for the complete Richards function, *Math. Biosci.*, **27** (1975), 349–360.

[FRa] Frenzen C.L. and Murray J.D., A cell kinetics justification for Gompertz' equation, *SIAM J. Appl. Math.*, **46** (1986), 614–629.

[GOa] Gompertz B., On the nature of the function expressive of the law of human mortality, and on a new mode of determining the value of life contingencies, *Phil. Trans. Roy. Soc.*, **115** (1825), 513–585.

[GRa] Gratton R.J., Appleton D.R., and Alwiswasy M.K., The measurement of tumour growth rates, **Biomathematics and Cell Kinetics**, Elsevier/North-Holland Biomedical Press (1978), 325–332.

[GYa] Gyllenberg M. and Webb G.F., Quiescence as an explanation of Gompertzian tumor growth, *Growth, Development and Aging*, **53** (1989), 25–33.

[GYb] Gyllenberg M. and Webb G.F., A nonlinear structured population model of tumor growth with quiescence, *J. Math. Biol.*, **28** (1990), 671–694.

[HEa] Heppner G.H. and Miller C., Tumor heterogeneity: Biological implications and therapeutic consequences, *Cancer Metastasis Rev.*, **2** (1983), 5–23.

[HUa] Huxley J.S., **Problems in Relative Growth**, Dial (1932).

[IRa] Irvine D.H. and Savageau M.A., Efficient solution of nonlinear ordinary differential equations expressed in S-system canonical form, *SIAM J. Appl. Math.*, **27** (1990), 704–735.

[JAa] Jansson B. and Révész L., Analysis of growth of tumor cell populations, *Math. Biosci.*, **19** (1974), 131–154.

[JCa] Jackson E.A., **Prospectives of Nonlinear Dynamics**, Vols. 1 and 2, Cambridge University Press (1989).

[KEa] Kendal W.S., Gompertzian growth as a consequence of tumor heterogeneity, *Math. Biosci.*, **73** (1985), 103–107.

[KUa] Kuznetsov V.A., Makalkin I.A., Taylor M.A., and Perelson A.S., Nonlinear dynamics of immunogenic tumors: Parameter estimation and global bifurcation analysis, *Bull. Math. Biol.*, **56** (1994), 295–321.

[KUb] Kuznetsov V.A., Basic models of tumor-immune system interactions, in **A Survey of Models for Tumor-Immune System Dynamics**, Adam J.A. and Bellomo N. eds., Birkhäuser (1996).

[LAa] Laird A.K., Dynamics of tumor growth, *Brit. J. Cancer*, **18** (1964), 490–502.

[LAb] Laird A.K., Dynamics of tumor growth: Comparison of growth rates and extrapolation of growth curve to one cell, *Brit. J. Cancer*, **19** (1965), 278–291.

[LAc] Laird A.K., Tyler S.A., and Barton A.D., Dynamics of normal growth, *Growth*, **29** (1965), 233–248.

[LAd] Laird A.K., Dynamics of growth in tumors in normal organisms, *National Cancer Institute Monograph*, **30** (1969), 15–28.

[LIa] Ling Y. and He B., Entropic analysis of biological growth models, *IEEE Trans. Biomed. Eng.*, **40** (1993), 1193–1200.

[MAa] Marušić M. and Bajzer Ž., Generalized two-parameter equation of growth, *J. Math. Anal. Appl.*, **179** (1993), 446–461.

[MAb] Marušić M., Bajzer Ž., Freyer J.P., and Vuk-Pavlović S., Analysis of growth of multicellular tumour spheroids by mathematical models, *Cell Prolif.*, **27** (1994), 73–94.

[MAc] Marušić M., Bajzer Ž., Freyer J.P., and Vuk-Pavlović S., Modeling autostimulation of growth in multicellular tumor spheroids, *Int. J. Biomed. Comput.*, **29** (1991), 149–158.

[MAd] Marušić M., Bajzer Ž., and Vuk-Pavlović S., Modeling hormone-dependent cell-cell interactions in tumor growth: A simulation study, *Period. Biol. (Zagreb)*, **93** (1991), 649–656.

[MAe] Marušić M., Bajzer Ž., Vuk-Pavlović S., and Freyer J.P., Tumor growth in vivo and as multicellular spheroids compared by mathematical models, *Bull. Math. Biol.*, **56** (1994), 617–631.

[MAf] Marušić M. and Vuk-Pavlović S., Prediction power of mathematical models for tumor growth, *J. Biol. Systems*, **1** (1993), 69–78.

[MIa] Michelson S., Glicksman A.S., and Leith J.T., Growth in solid heterogeneous colon adenocarcinomas: comparison of simple logistical models, *Cell Tissue Kinet.*, **20** (1987), 343–355.

[MIb] Michelson S. and Leith J.T., Tumor Heterogeneity and Growth Control, in **A Survey of Models for Tumor-Immune System Dynamics**, Adam J.A. and Bellomo N. eds., Birkhäuser (1996).

[MUa] Murray J.D., **Mathematical Biology**, Springer (1989).

[NOa] Norton L., A Gompertzian model of human breast cancer growth, *Cancer Res.*, **48** (1988), 7067–7071.

[NOb] Norton L., Simon R., Brereton H.D., and Bogden A.E., Predicting the course of Gompertzian growth, *Nature*, **264** (1976), 542–545.

[PEa] Pearl R., **Studies in Human Biology**, Williams and Wilkins (1924).

[PIa] Piantadosi S., A model of growth with first-order birth and death rates, *Comp. Biomed. Res.*, **18** (1985), 220–232.

[PRa] Prescott D.M., Variations in the individual generation times of Tetrahymena geleii, *Exp. Cell Res.*, **16** (1959), 279–284.

[PTa] Pruitt K.M., DeMuth R.E., and Turner M.E. Jr., Practical application of generic growth theory and the significance of the growth curve parameters, *Growth*, **43** (1979), 19–35.

[QIa] Qi A.-S., Zheng X., Du C.-Y., and An B.-S., A cellular automaton model of cancerous growth, *J. Theor. Biol.*, **161** (1993), 1–12.

[RAa] Rashevsky N., Outline of a mathematical approach to the cancer problem, *Bull. Math. Biophys.*, **7** (1945), 69–81.

[RIa] Riggs D.S., **Control Theory and Physiological Feedback Mechanisms**, Williams and Wilkins (1970).

[RUa] Rubinow S.I., A maturity-time representation for cell populations, *Biophys. J.*, **8** (1968), 1055–1073.

[SAa] Savageau M.A., Allometric morphogenesis of complex systems: a derivation of the basic equations from first principles, *Proc. Natl. Acad. Sci. USA*, **76** (1979), 6023–6025.

[SAb] Savageau M.A., Growth of complex systems can be related to the properties of their underlying determinants, *Proc. Natl. Acad. Sci. USA*, **76** (1979), 5413–5417.

[SAc] Savageau M.A. and Voit E.O., Recasting nonlinear differential equations as S-systems: A canonical nonlinear form, *Math. Biosci.*, **87** (1987), 83–115.

[SCa] Schwartz M., A biomathematical approach to clinical tumor growth, *Cancer*, **14** (1961), 1272–1294.

[SHa] Sherratt J.A. and Nowak M.A., Oncogenes, antioncogenes and the immune response to cancer: a mathematical model, *Proc. R. Soc. Lond. B*, **248** (1992), 261–271.

[SIa] Simpson–Herren L. and Lloyd H.H., Kinetic parameters and growth curves for experimental tumor systems, *Cancer Chemotherapy Rep.*, **54** (1970), 143–174.

[SPa] Sporn M.B. and Roberts A.B., Autocrine growth factors and cancer, *Nature*, **313** (1985), 745–747.

[SPb] Sporn M.B. and Todaro G.J., Autocrine secretion and malignant transformation of cells, *N. Engl. J. Med.*, **303** (1980), 878–880.

[STa] Steel G.G., **Growth Kinetics of Tumors**, Clarendon Press (1977).

[SUa] Sullivan P.W. and Salmon S.E., Kinetics of tumor growth and regression in IgG multiple myeloma, *J. Clin. Invest.*, **51** (1972), 1697–1708.

[SWa] Swan G.W., **Some Current Mathematical Topics in Cancer Research**, Monograph Publishing on Demand, Sponsor Series, University Microfilms International, Ann Arbor (1977).

[SWb] Swan G.W., Role of optimal control theory in cancer chemotherapy, *Math. Biosci*, **101** (1990), 237–284.

[TUa] Turner M.E. Jr., Bradley E.L. Jr., Kirk K.A., and Pruitt K.M., A theory of growth, *Math. Biosci.*, **29** (1976), 367–373.

[VAa] Vaidya V.G. and Alexandro F.J. Jr., Evaluation of some mathematical models for tumor growth, *Int. J. Biomed. Comput.*, **13** (1982), 19–35.

[VAb] Vaidya V.G., Alexandro F.J. Jr., and Vaidya P.G., A bilinear control model for tumor growth and chemotherapy, *Int. J. Biomed. Comput.*, **17** (1985), 145–154.

[VAc] Vaidya P.G., Vaidya V.G., and Martin D.G., An application of the non-linear bifurcation theory to tumor growth modeling, *Int. J. Biomed. Comput.*, **27** (1991), 27–46.

[VEa] Verhulst P.F., Notice sur la loi que la population suit dans son accroissement, *Curr. Math. Phys.*, **10** (1838), 113–121.

[WHa] Wheldon T.E., Kirk J., and Grey W.M., Mitotic autoregulation, growth control and neoplasia, *J. Theor. Biol.*, **38** (1973), 627–639.

[WIa] Winsor C.P., The Gompertz curve as a growth curve, *Proc. Natl. Acad. Sci. USA*, **18** (1932), 1–8.

[WRa] Wright S., Book review, *J. Am. Stat. Assoc.*, **21** (1926), 493–497.

[WTa] Witten M., A return to time, cells, systems, and aging: III. Gompertzian models of biological aging and some possible roles for critical elements, *Mech. Ageing Develop.*, **32** (1985), 141–177.

[XUa] Xu X., The biological foundation of the Gompertz model, *Int. J. Biomed. Comput.*, **20** (1987), 35–39.

[XUb] Xu X. and Ling Y., A study on the expectational model for tumor growth, *Int. J. Biomed. Comput.*, **22** (1988), 135–141.

4

Tumor Immune System Interactions: The Kinetic Cellular Theory

N. Bellomo and L. Preziosi

Politecnico of Torino
Department of Mathematics
Torino, Italy

and
G. Forni

University of Torino
Department of Clinical and Biological Sciences
Orbassano, Italy

Abstract. The growth of a tumor and its relationships with the host environment are complex events that kinetically mutate during tumor progression. Several aspects of these interactions and their dynamical evolution can be modeled through equations that take into account a few key variables related to microscopic interacting populations: tumor, host, immune cells, cytokine signals.

This paper provides a review of the state of the art on the so called kinetic (cellular) theory. The development of the modeling starts from observation of the phenomenological behavior of the system and, in particular, of the cell populations and their cellular interactions. This analysis is followed by derivation of the evolution equations in the framework of nonequilibrium statistical mechanics. The following step is the development of simulation and validation techniques, which has to be related to the experimental activity in the field. The final part of the survey provides a critical analysis of this type of methodological approach and of its conceivable developments, which may hopefully contribute to medical research addressed to the competition against tumor aggression.

4.1 Introduction

The growth of a tumor and its relationships with the host environment are complex events that kinetically mutate during tumor progression [DOa], [GEa], [FOd]. Tumor growth is traditionally simulated by classical diffusion convection equations [CHe] in the framework of continuum mechanics. Although these models contribute to predict tumor behavior, they cannot take into account the tumor-host cell interactions. On the other hand, as usual in statistical mechanics, some aspects of these interactions and their dynamical evolution can be modeled through equations related to a few key variables related to microscopic interacting populations: tumor, host, immune cells, cytokine signals.

This methodological approach, which is typical of the kinetic theory of gases and of cellular mathematical biology, was first dealt with in [BEa], where a kinetic theory was proposed for the evolution of a system made up of by cells belonging to the tumor, growing in a host environment which feeds the tumor, and cells of the immune system competing with the tumor. In particular, the theory deals with the growth of the tumor and with the enhancing or inhibitory effects of its interactions with the immune system. The hope is that suitable elaborations of such a new approach will contribute to unravel the complexity of the system and allow realistic predictions and simulations. Here, we review the state of the art on this type of approach providing:

i) a phenomenological description of the system,
ii) modeling of the cellular interactions,
iii) derivation of the evolution equations,
iv) development of simulation and validation techniques.

The content is organized in ten sections. The first one is this introduction.
The second section provides a concise guide to the bibliography in the field.
The third section summarizes the guidelines that are followed in the development and application of the theory from observation of the system to simulation and application of the model.
The fourth section deals with the description of the phenomenological behavior of the system and, in particular, with the identification of the cell populations and activity.

The fifth section deals with the description of the cell populations and of their peculiar activity.
The sixth section refers to modeling and derivation of the evolution equations in the framework of nonequilibrium statistical mechanics.
The seventh section refers to the analysis of the experimental activity in the field and, in particular, to a survey of those experimental results that can be used in the analysis here developed.
The eighth section deals with some applications of the model, with simulation problems and validation.
The ninth section is addressed to applied mathematicians who may be interested to the mathematical problems (qualitative analysis) related to the analysis of the model.
The final section follows with a critical analysis of this type of methodological approach and of its conceivable developments.

The style of presentation of topics related to biological and immunological theory will be schematic. The treatment of this matter may not be sufficiently complete from the view point of experts in natural sciences. However, the pertinent bibliography will be indicated towards the reader who may be interested to a more complete insight into this field. The first survey of this book contributes to this purpose.

The reader must be aware that the program of deriving a mathematical model, in terms of a suitable system of evolution equations, and of developing a suitable simulation of the behavior of the real system, cannot be performed in oversimplified mathematical terms. Indeed, modeling requires to find a suitable balance between the extreme complexity of the real system and the need of reasonably simple and understandable mathematics. Such a balance is reached by means of the technical support that can be given by the scientific computation methods used to obtain quantitative results. The contents of Section 4.8 provide, in particular, a description of this link and support alongside the discussion on the simulation of the real system.

4.2 A Concise Guide to the Literature

This section aims to provide the reader with a guide to the pertinent literature. Although completeness is not claimed, an effort is made to select some titles among a vast literature that is dispersed in journals belonging to disparate research fields. The survey will also give some indications on the literature related to specific fields that are not strictly within the present subject, but are interesting as a scientific background, e.g. mathematical biology, modeling and mathematical methods, kinetic and continuum theories. With this in mind, we start with general fields progressing to more specialized ones.

Mathematical and Modeling Methods

The class of problems we are dealing with requires the use of mathematical techniques to solve problems related to ordinary and partial differential equations, generally in the nonlinear case. The analysis may refer either to evolution problems or to steady solutions. The selection of a bibliography in this field cannot avoid the personal biases.

With these premises we mention the books by Bellomo and Preziosi [BEb], that links modeling, mathematical methods and scientific computation, by Beltrami [BLa], that refers to modeling and qualitative analysis of dynamical systems modeled in terms of ordinary differential equations, and by Lin and Segel [LIa] mainly oriented to modeling methods in natural sciences. The book by Ash and Gardner [ASa] deals with probability theory and stochastic processes, mathematical fields strongly related to the models of this survey.

Kinetic Theory

This review refers to a kinetic (cellular) theory for distinct cell populations interacting *in vivo*. The methods used to derive the evolution equations of the models are the ones of the kinetic theory of gases. The book by Truesdell and Muncaster [TRa] is an excellent guide to this topic. Mathematical aspects are dealt with in the Lecture Notes [BEf].

In addition, we shall also mention the kinetic approach to population dynamics developed by various authors starting from the fundamental paper by Jager and Segel [JAa]. This paper proposes a model in which the individuals of a certain population are characterized by a physical state. The model defines the time evolution of the distribution of individuals over the range of definition of such a state. The evolution of this probability density is ruled by the interactions between individuals. Further developments of the model and the related mathematical analysis are proposed in [ARa] and [ARc].

The model proposed by Jager and Segel has several features of Boltzmann type kinetic models and will be a reference point for the kinetic approach to modeling the interactions between tumor and immune system.

Mathematical Biology

Although the subject of this survey is a specialized one, it is useful to cast the contents into the general framework of mathematical biology. As a matter of fact, the modeling technique used is based upon modeling population dynamics, which is one of the fundamental aspects of mathematical biology. The reader is then addressed to the book by Murray [MUa] and to the collection of papers by Levin [LEa]. The pertinent literature in the field can be recovered in the above cited books.

Modeling Cellular Phenomena

Cellular activities play crucial roles in the systems we are dealing with. A mathematical interpretation of these cell dynamics can contribute to the modeling of the interactions between tumors and the immune system. Considering the vast nature of this topic, only a few indications will be given with special attention to cellular features related to the immune system. In particular, we indicate the book edited by Herberman [HEa], the one written by Janeway and Travers [JNa], the papers by Perelson and coauthors [PEa,b], and the book by Segel [SEa], which is an excellent guide to modeling this type of phenomena. The general framework is the one of cellular and molecular immunology [ABa].

Modeling Tumor Dynamics

Modeling tumor dynamics when interacting with the immune system is the central topic of this survey. An attempt is made to cover at least the main subjects. The books by Steel [SLa] and Den Otter and Ruitenberg [DOa] deal with general aspects, the survey by Folkman and Klagsbrun [FLa] is devoted to the analysis of angiogenic factors, the collection of papers edited by Green, Cohen and McCluskey [GEa] deals with the mechanisms of tumor immunity, and the essay by Nossal [NOa] with a general description of the immune system referring to the competition with aggressive tumor cells.

Modeling tumor dynamics and interactions with the immune system requires a detailed analysis of cellular interactions; examples from this vast research field are the papers by Albert, Freedman and Perelson [AFa], De Boer and Högeweg [DEa,b], Grossman and Berke [GRa], Kuznetsov et al. [KUa,b], Inversen [IVa,b], Lefever et al. [LFa], Perelson et al. [PEa,b] and Prehn [PRa].

When tumor cells aggregate (or condense) in spheroidal shapes, see [LAa], models of continuum mechanics can be developed with a detailed analysis of the cellular interactions on the surface of the tumor. General descriptions can be found in the survey papers by Mueller [MEa] and by Sutherland [STa,b], while several other scientists are involved in the analysis and modeling of this type of physical systems and develop different aspects of the matter. We mention, among others, and starting from the pioneer paper by Greenspan [GSa], the papers by Adam [ADa–f], which develop models of tumor dynamics by partial differential equations and simple dynamical systems, see also [SWa].

The related stability and bifurcation analysis is referred to various aspects of tumor evolution. Chaplain [CHa–d] develops models and simulation in the framework of continuum mechanics with several types of interactions on the surface of quasi spheroidal tumors. The simulation is obtained by finite difference solutions of linear and nonlinear initial-boundary value problems for partial differential equations. The analysis developed by Michelson and Leith [MIa,b] and by the team organized by Bajzer [MRa–c], is referred to a detailed analysis and interpretation of experimental data, that gives relevance to the related analysis. Further studies are due to Maggelakis [MAa,b] and Markovitch [MKa]. The approach with the methods of kinetic theory has already been mentioned in the introduction. Predictions by solutions of the master equation are proposed by Yakovlev [YAa]. It is important to mention also the paper by Gyllenberg and Webb [GYa] that develops an analysis of quiescence and tumor growth by structured population dynamics.

In principle, to complete this guide to the literature, we should also cite papers concerning the experimental research in tumor immunology. However, being aware of the vastness of this field, the attention will be limited to the activity that is related to the kinetic description reviewed in this chapter. The interested reader is then addressed to Section 4.7, which is entirely devoted to this topic.

4.3 Guidelines: From Observation to Simulation

The modeling and simulation of the system we are dealing with is developed through a line that starts from the phenomenological observation of the system, goes through the modeling in the form of a set of evolution equations. The process is concluded by the design of the simulator for the behavior of the system as predicted by the model. The sequential steps are represented in the flow chart of Figure 4.1, where each block is developed in one of the sections that follow.

As it is shown, after the first block A that refers to the phenomenological observation of the system, one has to identify, as shown in Block B, the players of the game, i.e. cell populations and signals. This identification also refers to the activation state of cells. The role of cytokine signals is regulating the interactions between cells.

The step that follows — represented by Block C — is a crucial one, as it refers to modeling the interaction pairs: cell-cell and cell-signals. These interactions may either change the activation state of the cells or cause their destruction or proliferation. This type of representation is the output both of cellular theories and of experimental activity *in vivo*.

What follows is a technical treatment of the matter. Block D refers to the derivation of the evolution equations obtained by balance equations that are typical of the kinetic theory. The simulation is then organized

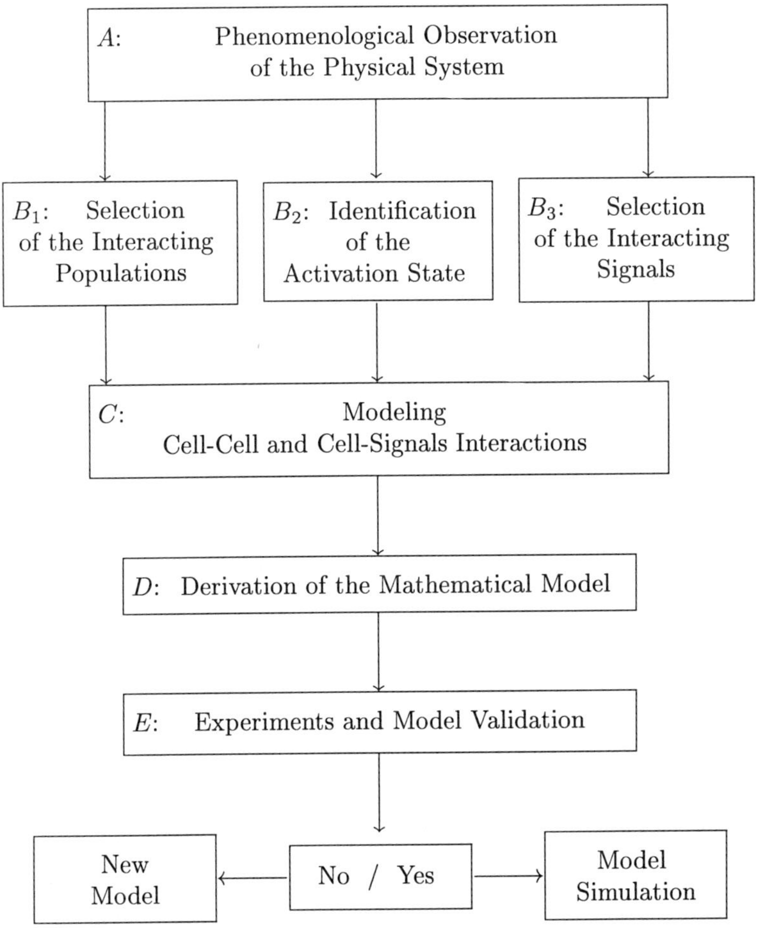

Figure 4.1 — Flow chart: From observation to modeling and simulation.

by the classical methods of applied mathematics. Model validation and a systematic simulation are the last steps of the whole process.

The contents of this survey follow the line of the flow chart. Therefore, we can re-examine the index referring to it. In particular, Section 4.4 is related to Block B, while Sections 4.5 and 4.6 to Blocks C and D. Block E is developed in Sections 4.7 and 4.8.

4.4 Cell Population and Activity

A vertebrate can be considered as a whole made by a huge number of interacting cells. In particular, in this type of modeling, we consider the interactions between tumor cells, environment and immune cells. Each cell is tagged by a variable, called **state**, either scalar or multi-dimensional, which functionally defines the cell activity.

The kinetic modeling approach is based upon the description of the statistical distribution over the state of the cells for each population and on the derivation of suitable evolution equations for the said probability distributions. The first step towards modeling is the phenomenological observation of the system and, in particular, the definition of the interacting cell populations. Then, for each population, it is necessary to identify the most important set of activities.

Each activity differs from population to population and is tagged by a suitable dimensionless variable u, that denotes the intensity with which the activities are performed. For the sake of simplicity, it will be assumed that u is a scalar variable with values in the range $[-1, 1]$. The value $u = 1$ corresponds to the highest value of the peculiar activities of the cell, while negative values correspond to their complete functional inhibition, or by the onset of new activities that are opposite to the positive ones. The largest negative activity occurs for $u = -1$.

In other words, we assume that the intensity by which peculiar activities of each cell of a given population are performed is randomly distributed over a certain range and that each cell can assume either positive or negative activities. The negative activities counteract the positive ones. In this way, we will attempt to model both the dormant and the proliferative behavior of the tumor on one side, and the tumor inhibitory or tumor stimulatory action of the immune and environmental cells on the other side.

In particular, a switch between activities of inverse effect is evident when the immune cells, that may inhibit the tumor aggression, degenerate into a cooperative action. On the other hand, during long phases of their natural history, tumor cells assume a dormant behavior (u approaching to 0), or can be pharmacologically induced to undergo towards programmed cell death (apoptosis corresponding to u tending to $u = -1$). In principle, one should operate to obtain a trend of the distribution of the tumor cells towards the range of negative values of the variable u.

Bearing this in mind, we identify the cell population and tumor-host relationships by means of the following assumptions:

Assumption 4.4.1. *Cells that actually take part to this process can be subdivided into three main populations:*

- *tumor cells, characterized by an anomalous proliferative activity and the difficulty to receiving inhibitory and apoptotic signals;*
- *environment cells characterized by promoting (feeding) influence over tumor cells;*
- *immune cells potentially able to either strongly hamper or favor tumor growth.*

Each population can be further subdivided. In general, we will deal with a number p of interacting populations. The activity of all these cell populations is regulated by soluble factors and cytokines and cell membrane signals.

Assumption 4.4.2. *The functional* **state** *of a each cell of a given population is described by the real number u with values in the interval $[-1, 1]$. Positive values of u denote:*

- *aggressive proliferation for tumor cells,*
- *adequate energy supply by the environment,*
- *strong anti-tumor activity by the immune cells*

Negative values correspond to opposite activities:

- *dormancy of tumor cells,*
- *tumor ischemic necrosis due to poor blood supply by the environment,*
- *tumor stimulating activity by the immune cells.*

Activation, or conversely inhibition, of the immune cells is regulated by cytokine and stimulatory signals, or by the lack of costimulation signals.

Assumption 4.4.3. *The statistical distribution within each population is defined by the density functions*

$$\mathbf{N} = \{N_i\}_{i=1}^{p}, \qquad N_i = N_i(t, u), \tag{4.1}$$

where $N_i(t, u)\,du$ defines the number of cells per unit volume at time t, with their state in the interval $[u, u + du]$ and where the number of interacting populations is generically indicated by p, although simulation will be developed for $p = 3$.

Admittedly, the definition of cell populations involved in this game for life and death, and the definition of their functions, is a gross simplification. Even if it is difficult to sketch the critical features that shape the process, one can consider that as a result of the accumulation of several gene mutations tumor cells proliferate without the usual restraints and respond no longer to the signals from the environment. Each tumor is characterized by a particular set of gene mutations that confers on it a more or less rapid expansion and independence from environmental signals that regulate normal proliferation or induce cells to die apoptotically. The accumulation of gene mutations and the intense proliferative activity also make the tumor different from the normal cells of the same tissue. The membrane expression of the altered proteins coded by the mutated genes and other membrane traits associated with the process whereby cells become neoplastic (collectively defined tumor associate antigens, TAA) allow tumor recognition by the immune cells, (see [BNa]).

Environment cells influence tumor growth. The first need for a growing tumor is to establish nutritional inter-relationships with the host. As has been mathematically modeled in a few recent papers [CHe,d], the microenvironment first provides nourishment to the tumor in the form of fluids that diffuse in the small initial tumor mass. When the mass becomes larger, it needs more energy: this major problem is solved by the tumor with the activation of endothelial cells that are induced to form new vessels to provide it. However, energy supply is a problem that is never satisfactorily solved by the tumor. The constant presence of ischemic necrotic areas inside the tumor shows the difficulty to provide nourishment to its inner part. Pharmacological inhibition of host endothelial cells, tumor vessel thrombosis or their mechanical legation leads to ischemic death of the tumor. The role of angiogenesis and blood supply in tumor development is discussed in other chapters of this book.

A growing tumor can also be perceived by environment cells as a foreign body. The signaling of **tumor foreigness** depends on the presence of a necrotic area or of the release of factors and cytokines that activate fibroblast and aspecific reactions. In several cases the tumor appears as a mass circumscribed by a reaction fibrotic capsule that clearly separates it by the host body. Very aggressive tumors, however, are not delimited by a capsule and directly contact normal tissues.

Long stages of a tumor's natural history are influenced by the microenvironment. The growth of incipient tumors can be inhibited by signals delivered by normal environmental cells. Indeed, traces of this environmental repression often persist even when a tumor has begun to expand and are responsible for the long dormancy that often characterizes tumor growth.

A particular case of interaction with the environment can be seen in the tumor's relationship with the immune system. This relationship depends on the membrane expression of TAA [BNa]. Leukocytes and natural killer lymphocytes are equipped with a rudimentary and broad spectrum recognition system, but are endowed with a very powerful antitumor activity [HEa]. Their antitumor reaction can be driven by antibodies and by cytokines secreted in the microenvironment by the tumor itself or by the immune cells, see [FOd]. Activation of T lymphocytes, on the other hand, follows the recognition of a fragment of the TAA presented by the glycoproteins of the major histocompatibility complex or by tumor cell surfaces of the host antigen-presenting cells. The activated T lymphocyte expands and produces clones of identical lymphocytes that assist in the activation of killer T lymphocytes. T lymphocytes also assist in the activation of B lymphocytes primed by a direct interaction with the TAA. B lymphocytes, too, expand clonally and secrete anti-TAA antibody [BNa], [JNa].

The effector arm of the immune system thus hampers tumor growth in four main ways:

a) Direct killing by lymphocytes;

b) Release of cytokines by T lymphocytes, which triggers and pilots the anti-tumor activity of several leukocytes;

c) Binding the antibodies to tumor cells, causing their death in the presence of serum factors. These antibodies also adhere to the membrane of leukocytes and guide their antitumor activity;

d) Induction of tumor ischemic necrosis by alteration of tumor vessels.

Bearing in mind that we have decided to operate in a simplified framework, we can now return to the kinetic model and we consider, in the case of scalar u, the problem of computing the result of the tumor-host relationship by knowing the densities N_i. In particular, the number of cells of the i-th population per unit volume at time t is

$$n_i(t) = \int_{-1}^{1} N_i(t,u)\, du\,. \tag{4.2}$$

Another important quantity is the mean value of u over the $i-$th population

$$E_i(u)(t) = \frac{\displaystyle\int_{-1}^{1} uN_i(t,u)\, du}{\displaystyle\int_{-1}^{1} N_i(t,u)\, du}\,. \tag{4.3}$$

The solution of mathematical problems related to the evolution equations for the densities N_i can give quantitative description of their time evolution. By means of moments, as the ones defined by Eqs. (4.2–4.3), the desired information on the behavior of the macroscopic observables of the system finally can be obtained.

4.5 Modeling Cell Interactions

Before dealing with the derivation of the evolution equation of the densities N_i, it is useful to identify, in a similar manner to kinetic theory [TRa], the cellular regimes that characterize the behavior of the system. Following [BEc], a classification can be proposed in order to distinguish the cellular regime from the condensed cell regime.

• **The free (dispersed) cells regime**, a situation where the cells move freely and homogeneously in space interacting by means of binary encounters.

• **The condensed (packed) cells regime**, a physical situation where the tumor cells are already packed in a quasi-spherical volume. In this case, the cells of the immune system and the feeding environment interact with the tumor surface only and interact among themselves as in the cellular regime.

The distinction between these two regimes is not, in physical reality, so simple as this and intermediate regimes should be taken into account. The contents of this chapter deal with the dispersed cell regime. This regime is particularly important as it refers to a physical situation for which medical action has still some possibility of being effective. This (conventional) classification will be critically discussed in the last section of this survey.

Cell interactions in **the free (dispersed) cells regime** will be modeled supposing that only binary encounters are significant.

The modeling of the cell interactions can be developed according to the following hypotheses:

Assumption 4.5.1. *Cell interactions can be divided into* **mass conservative encounters** *and* **interactions with cell proliferation or destruction** *(See Table 4.1).*
Cell interactions in the case of **mass conservative encounters** *will be defined by two physical quantities: the* **encounter rate** η *and the* **transition probability density** ψ. *Similarly,* **proliferative encounters** *will be described by two quantities: the* **proliferation rate** p *and the* **proliferation probability density** φ. **Destructive encounters** *will be described by the* **destruction rate** d.

Assumption 4.5.2. **Conservative encounters** *between the cell of the i-population (with state v) and the cell of the j-population (with state w), are quantitatively described by the* **transition rate**

$$T_{ij}(v, w; u) = \eta_{ij}(v, w)\psi_{ij}(v, w; u)\,, \tag{4.4}$$

where:

• $T_{ij}(v, w; u)$ *denotes the number of encounters, per unit volume and time, between cell pairs of the (i, j)-populations, respectively with states v and w, with transition of the i-cells into the state u;*

• $\eta_{ij}(v, w)$ *is the* **encounter rate**, *which denotes the number of encounters per unit volume and time between cell pairs of the (i, j)-populations with states v and w, respectively;*

• $\psi_{ij}(v, w; u)$ *is the* **transition probability density**, *which is the density of transition of the i-cell to the state u given its initial state v and the state w of the encountering cells belonging to the j-th population.*

Cell interactions	Encounter type	Parameters
Cell interactions	Mass conservative encounters	η encounter rate
		ψ transition probability density
	Proliferative destructive encounters	p proliferation rate
		d destruction rate
		φ proliferation probability density

Table 4.1 — Classification of cell interactions.

Assumption 4.5.3. Proliferative encounters *occur between cell pairs of the same or different populations, and cause generation of new cells in one or both populations. These interactions are quantitatively described by the* **proliferation rate**

$$P_{ij}(v,w;u) = p_{ij}(v,w)\varphi_{ij}(v,w;u)\,, \tag{4.5}$$

where:

• $P_{ij}(v,w;u)$ *denotes the number of the i-cells per unit volume and time which proliferate in the state u due to the encounter between cell pairs (with states v and w, respectively) of the (i,j)-populations;*

• $p_{ij}(v,w)$ *is the* **proliferation rate**, *which denotes the number of i-cells that are produced per unit volume and time due to the encounter of cell pairs (with states v and w, respectively) of the (i,j)-populations;*

• $\varphi_{ij}(v,w;u)$ *is the* **proliferation probability density**, *which is the density of the proliferation of the i-cell in the state u due to the encounter of two cells belonging, respectively, to the i-th population with state v and to the j-th population with state w.*

Assumption 4.5.4. Destructive encounters *occur between cell pairs* *of different populations, and cause death of one or both cells. These interactions are quantitatively described by the* **destruction rate**

- $d_{ij}(v, w)$, *that is the number of i-cells with state v that are suppressed in the interaction with the j-cells with state w.*

Note that the terms φ and ψ have the structure of a probability density

$$\int_{-1}^{1} \varphi_{ij}(v, w; u)\, du = \int_{-1}^{1} \psi_{ij}(v, w; u)\, du = 1\,, \tag{4.6}$$

$\forall\, i, j = 1, \ldots, p$.

4.6 Evolution Kinetic Equations

The evolution equations of the densities N_i, for $i = 1, \ldots, p$, can be derived by suitable balance equations which equate the total derivative of N_i to the **gain** term G_i minus the **loss** term L_i, where G_i and L_i are generated by the conservative interactions between cell pairs and their related change of state, plus the proliferation term S_i, minus the destruction term D_i. An additional term can be introduced in order to simulate the production g_i of cells of the i-th population due to the bone marrow or/and to any external source (e.g. injection)

$$\begin{aligned} \frac{\partial N_i}{\partial t}(t, u) = J_i[N](t, u) &= G_i[N](t, u) - L_i[N](t, u) \\ &\quad + S_i[N](t, u) - D_i[N](t, u) + g_i(t, u)\,, \end{aligned} \tag{4.7}$$

where all terms G_i, L_i, S_i, and D_i are assumed to depend on N in order to take into account relationship between the different cell-types.

In particular:

- G_i is obtained by summing (double integration over the variable v and w) all transitions, ruled by η and ψ, of the i-cells from the state v into u

$$G_i = \sum_{j=1}^{p} \int_{-1}^{1} \int_{-1}^{1} \eta_{ij}(v, w) \psi_{ij}(v, w; u) N_i(t, v) N_j(t, w)\, dv\, dw\,,$$

where the transitions occur after the encounter of the i-cell with all j-cells, which requires the sum over j. Furthermore, integration over

v refers to the original state distribution before the interaction, while integration over w refers to all possible states of the interacting j-cell.

- L_i is obtained by summing (simple integration over the variable v) all loss, ruled by η, from the state u due to the encounter with the cell with state v

$$L_i = N_i(t,u) \sum_{j=1}^{p} \int_{-1}^{1} \eta_{ij}(u,v) N_j(t,v)\, dv\,,$$

where the loss occurs after the encounter of the i-cell with all j-cells having all possible states, which requires the sum over j and the integration over v, respectively.

- S_i is obtained by summing (double integration over the variable v and w) all proliferation rates, ruled by p and φ, into u

$$S_i = \sum_{j=1}^{p} \int_{-1}^{1} \int_{-1}^{1} p_{ij}(v,w) \varphi_{ij}(v,w;u) N_i(t,v) N_j(t,w)\, dv\, dw\,,$$

where proliferations occur after the encounter of the i-cell with all j-cells, which requires the sum over j and the integration over v and w, respectively.

- D_i is obtained summing (simple integration over the variable v) all destructions, ruled by d, of the cells with state u due to the encounter with cells with state v

$$D_i = N_i(t,u) \sum_{j=1}^{p} \int_{-1}^{1} d_{ij}(u,v) N_j(t,v)\, dv\,,$$

where the destruction can occur after the encounter of the i-cell with all j-cells, which requires the sum over j and the integration over v, respectively.

- g_i is a source term due to inner (for instance, from bone marrow) or outer inlets.

Remark 4.6.1. *The computation implies a statistical independence of the distributions N_i and N_j. This hypothesis is generally used in phenomenological kinetic theory, but is not genuinely true. It can be accepted as an approximation of physical reality for bounded times.*

Then the following evolution equation is obtained

$$\frac{\partial N_i}{\partial t}(t,u) = \sum_{j=1}^{p} \int_{-1}^{1} \int_{-1}^{1} \eta_{ij}(v,w) \psi_{ij}(v,w;u) N_i(t,v) N_j(t,w)\, dv\, dw$$

$$- N_i(t,u) \sum_{j=1}^{p} \int_{-1}^{1} \eta_{ij}(u,v) N_j(t,v)\, dv$$

$$+ \sum_{j=1}^{p} \int_{-1}^{1} \int_{-1}^{1} p_{ij}(v,w) \varphi_{ij}(v,w;u) N_i(t,v) N_j(t,w)\, dv\, dw$$

$$- N_i(t,u) \sum_{j=1}^{p} \int_{-1}^{1} d_{ij}(u,v) N_j(t,v)\, dv + g_i(t,u)\,. \tag{4.8}$$

Or, in a more compact form

$$\frac{\partial N_i}{\partial t}(t,u) = \sum_{j=1}^{p} \int_{-1}^{1} \int_{-1}^{1} A_{ij}(v,w;u) N_i(t,v) N_j(t,w)\, dv\, dw$$

$$- N_i(t,u) \sum_{j=1}^{p} \int_{-1}^{1} B_{ij}(u,v) N_j(t,v)\, dv + g_i(t,u)\,, \tag{4.9}$$

where

$$A_{ij}(v,w;u) = \eta_{ij}(v,w) \psi_{ij}(v,w;u) + p_{ij}(v,w) \varphi_{ij}(v,w;u) \tag{4.10}$$

and

$$B_{ij}(u,v) = \eta_{ij}(u,v) + d_{ij}(u,v)\,. \tag{4.11}$$

We point out that the model that we have just built can be regarded as a superposition of a kinetic and a population dynamics model. It retains some features of both classes of models. As a matter of fact, the model refers to both the phenomenological behaviors of the system: population dynamics with competition and kinetic interactions with stochastic state transition. In particular, one can have either totally **conservative models**

$$\frac{\partial N_i}{\partial t}(t,u) = \sum_{j=1}^{p} \int_{-1}^{1} \int_{-1}^{1} \eta_{ij}(v,w) \psi_{ij}(v,w;u) N_i(t,v) N_j(t,w)\, dv\, dw$$

$$- N_i(t,u) \sum_{j=1}^{p} \int_{-1}^{1} \eta_{ij}(u,v) N_j(t,v)\, dv\,, \tag{4.12}$$

or totally **competitive models**

$$\frac{\partial N_i}{\partial t}(t,u) = \sum_{j=1}^{p} \int_{-1}^{1} \int_{-1}^{1} p_{ij}(v,w)\varphi_{ij}(v,w;u) N_i(t,v) N_j(t,w)\, dv\, dw$$

$$- N_i(t,u) \sum_{j=1}^{p} \int_{-1}^{1} d_{ij}(u,v) N_j(t,v)\, dv + g_i(t,u)\,. \tag{4.13}$$

We remark that integration of Eq. (4.8) over u yields

$$\frac{\partial n_i}{\partial t} = G_i(t) + \sum_{j=1}^{p} \int_{-1}^{1} \int_{-1}^{1} \Big[p_{ij}(v,w) - d_{ij}(v,w) \Big] N_i(t,v) N_j(t,w)\, dv\, dw\,, \tag{4.14}$$

where $n_i = n_i(t)$ is the density of i-cells, and

$$G_i(t) = \int_{-1}^{1} g_i(t,u)\, du\,. \tag{4.15}$$

Equation (4.14) defines the rate of growth of the number of cells for each population. The absence of the term ψ in the equation is due to the fact that it only changes the status of the cells, but not their number. In other words, this term was involved in the so-called conservative equation. Note that Eq. (4.14) cannot be integrated independently from Eq. (4.13) as it also involves the N_i terms. In particular, this means that conservative encounters influence the density of the i-cells only because changing the state of the cells influence proliferation and destruction.

It is plain that the model reported in (4.8) or (4.9) is only a general framework that cannot be immediately used for the applications. Specific applicable models involve the identification of the matrices

$$[\eta] = [\eta_{ij}]\,, \quad [p] = [p_{ij}]\,, \quad [d] = [d_{ij}]\,, \quad [\psi] = [\psi_{ij}]\,, \quad [\varphi] = [\varphi_{ij}]\,. \tag{4.16}$$

The identification may require assumptions on the analytic structure of the above-mentioned terms. In general, a simple structure can contribute to the design of the experiments addressed to the identification itself.

The evolution of the densities N_i is then obtained by solving Eqs. (4.7) with suitable initial conditions. Methods and results of simulations will be reported in Section 4.8.

As we shall see in Section 4.8, the identification of the matrices indicated in Eq. (4.16) needs to assume suitable analytic expressions for the densities ψ and φ. Particular assumptions are the ones proposed in [BEc] and [BEe], that seem useful for the identification of parameters.

An immediate simplification is obtained assuming, as is reasonable, that new-born cells retain the same activation state as the generating cells, independently on the states of the encountered cells, that is

$$\varphi_{ij}(v, w; u) = \delta(u - v)\,, \tag{4.17}$$

for all pairs i, j.

In this case, it is convenient to write the evolution equation after having separated the contributions to the evolution due to conservative and nonconservative terms

$$\begin{aligned}\frac{\partial N_i}{\partial t}(t, u) = &\sum_{j=1}^{p} \int_{-1}^{1} \eta_{ij}(v, w)\psi_{ij}(v, w; u) N_i(t, v)) N_j(t, w)\, dv\, dw \\ &- N_i(t, u) \sum_{j=1}^{p} \int_{-1}^{1} \eta_{ij}(u, v) N_j(t, v)\, dv \\ &+ N_i(t, u) \sum_{j=1}^{p} \int_{-1}^{1} \mu_{ij}(u, v) N_j(t, v)\, dv + g_i(t, u)\,,\end{aligned} \tag{4.18}$$

where the term μ corresponds both to proliferative and destructive encounters

$$\mu_{ij}(u, v) = p_{ij}(u, v) - d_{ij}(u, v)\,, \tag{4.19}$$

that consequently can assume negative and positive values.

Furthermore, following Assumption 4.4.1, the number of populations can be reduced by considering a system constituted by three interacting populations:

- Tumor cells, corresponding to $i = 1$;
- Cells of the immune system, corresponding to $i = 2$;
- Environmental cells, corresponding to $i = 3$.

In addition, it will be assumed that $N_3 = N_{30}(u)$ is constant in time and with a given distribution over the state u. This simplification, and letting $g_i = 0$, yields a system of two population dynamics

$$\begin{aligned}\frac{\partial N_1}{\partial t}(t, u) = &\int_{-1}^{1}\int_{-1}^{1} \eta_{11}(v, w)\psi_{11}(v, w; u) N_1(t, v) N_1(t, w)\, dv\, dw \\ &+ \int_{-1}^{1}\int_{-1}^{1} \eta_{12}(v, w)\psi_{12}(v, w; u) N_1(t, v) N_2(t, w)\, dv\, dw\end{aligned}$$

$$
\begin{aligned}
&+ \int_{-1}^{1} \eta_{13}(v,w)\psi_{13}(v,w;u)N_1(t,v)N_{30}(w)\,dv\,dw \\
&- N_1(t,u)\int_{-1}^{1}\Big[\eta_{11}(u,v)N_1(t,v) \\
&+ \eta_{12}(u,v)N_2(t,v) + \eta_{13}(u,v)N_{30}(v)\Big]\,dv \\
&+ N_1(t,u)\int_{-1}^{1}\Big[\mu_{11}(u,v)N_1(t,v) \\
&+ \mu_{12}(u,v)N_2(t,v) + \mu_{13}(u,v)N_{30}(v)\Big]\,dv\,, \qquad (4.20a)
\end{aligned}
$$

and

$$
\begin{aligned}
\frac{\partial N_2}{\partial t}(t,u) = &\int_{-1}^{1}\int_{-1}^{1} \eta_{21}(v,w)\psi_{21}(v,w;u)N_2(t,v)N_1(t,w)\,dv\,dw \\
&+ \int_{-1}^{1}\int_{-1}^{1} \eta_{22}(v,w)\psi_{22}(v,w;u)N_2(t,v)N_2(t,w)\,dv\,dw \\
&+ \int_{-1}^{1} \eta_{23}(v,w)\psi_{23}(v,w;u)N_2(t,v)N_{30}(w)\,dv\,dw \\
&- N_2(t,u)\int_{-1}^{1}\Big[\eta_{21}(u,v)N_1(t,v) \\
&+ \eta_{22}(u,v)N_2(t,v) + \eta_{23}(u,v)N_{30}(v)\Big]\,dv \\
&+ N_2(t,u)\int_{-1}^{1}\Big[\mu_{21}(u,v)N_1(t,v) \\
&+ \mu_{22}(u,v)N_2(t,v) + \mu_{23}(u,v)N_{30}(v)\Big]\,dv\,. \qquad (4.20b)
\end{aligned}
$$

Further, the characterization of the terms ψ can be developed identifying, as in [BEd], these terms by most probable value and variance. This can even be done, according to [BEe], by delta functions over the output of the variable v

$$
\psi(v,w;u) = \delta\big(u - m(v,w)\big)\,. \qquad (4.21)
$$

These relatively simple equations will be used for the discussion and simulation problems dealt with in Section 4.8. In particular, the system can be further specialized according to the assumptions reported in Eqs. (4.17–4.21). Moreover, the construction of specific model will take into account only interaction terms, that are significant to the evolution of the system. This point will be further clarified in Section 4.8.

On the other hand, the bridge between the contents of this section, that only provide a general framework, and a detailed modeling of well defined physical systems, is found in the next section. There, a phenomenological description of the interactions among the various cell populations is given, and some particular behaviors of the system are reported. The goal of mathematical models is to describe these behaviors.

4.7 Experimental Activity

This section provides a report of some representative experimental conditions that could be interpreted on the basis of the approach based on the kinetic (cellular) theory. This topic is documented in papers [BOa], [FOa–c], [LOa] and bibliography therein cited.

4.7.1 Transition to neoplastic behavior and tumor proliferation

In natural conditions, a cell becomes neoplastic as the result of the accumulation of multiple gene mutations. This accumulation requires a long time period. Then, the neoplastic cell may expand. Small initial and clinically imperceptible tumors may persist throughout the body life and develop very slowly, with stages of expansion alternating with stages of dormancy, or even a long dormancy until a final stage of tumultuous, uncontrollable growth. This behavior is represented in Figure 4.2.

The neoplastic growth may be contrasted by the competition with the active cells of the immune system. This competition is visualized in Figure 4.3.

Because of the accumulation of mutations, it is quite probable that tumor cells display on their cell membrane altered glycoproteins acting as tumor associate antigens TAA or TAA peptides presented by MHC glycoproteins on tumor cell surfaces. However, these TAAs are, in general, unable to activate a significant immune reaction because both the immune suppressive factors released by tumor cells and the their poor presentation in the absence of costimulatory molecules by tumor cells expressing scanty MHC glycoproteins on their surface.

By using the code of the proposed model, when tumor cells in the condensed (packed) cell regime start to proliferate progressively, most of them

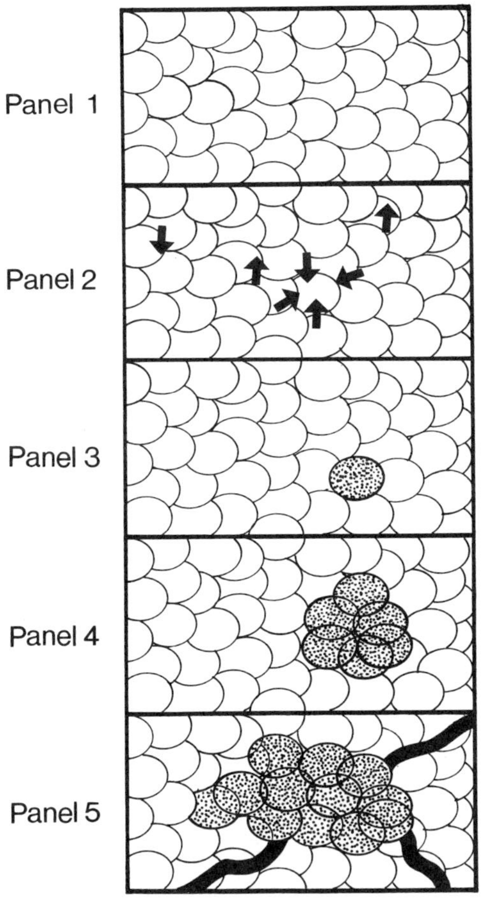

Figure 4.2 — When several gene alterations (**mutations**) involving cell reproductive activity accumulate, a normal cell (Panel 1) may become fully neoplastic (Panel 2) even if its growth is still inhibited for long period by signals delivered by neighboring normal cells (Panel 3). Suddenly, neoplastic cells grow without the usual restraints (Panel 4) and give rise to a tumor and induce blood vessel formation (Panel 5).

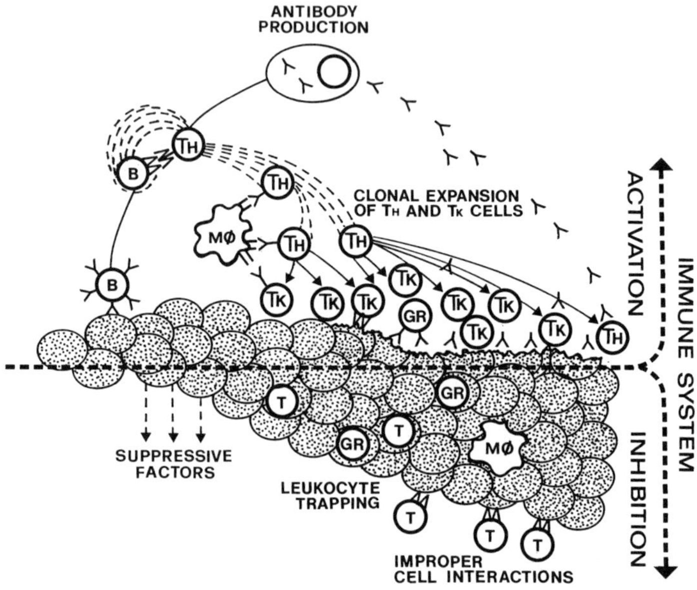

Figure 4.3 — Competition between immune system and neoplastic cells.

acquire a state with u values approaching to 1, and interact and proliferate with a rate that can be assumed to be constant. Proliferating tumor cells are surrounded by environment cells in a state characterized by u approaching to 1, since they are induced by tumor released factors to provide an adequate blood supply. By contrast, tumor-borne suppressor factors, along with the absence of correct costimulation signals, impede immune activation and elicit first a local response. Then systemic immunosuppression occurs, thus conferring to the immune cells a state characterized by u approaching to -1. The rate of immune-tumor cell encounters is low. Following these interactions, immune cells are unable to recognize TAA and to react against the tumor, and thus destructive encounters do not take place.

Instead, following these interactions, immune cells can be induced to release various factors that act on the environment cells promoting angiogenesis or act on immune cells providing tumor rejection, see Figure 4.3.

4.7.2 Preimmunization and recognition of antigens

Both antitumor preimmunization through *optimally presented* tumor antigens and the recognition of foreign histocompatibility antigens and tumor

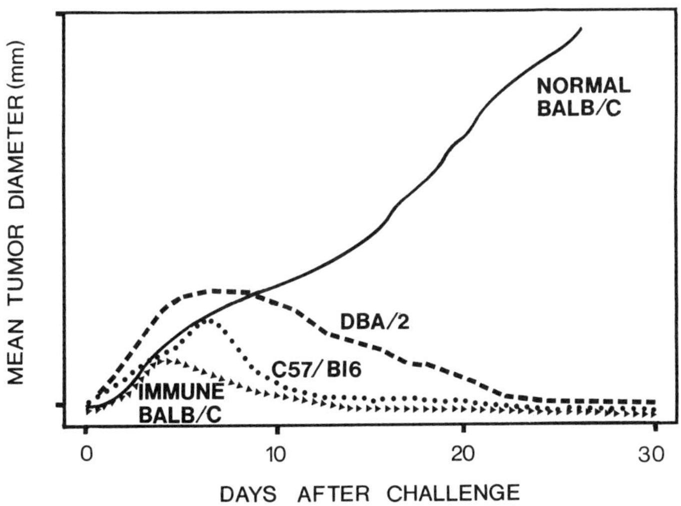

Figure 4.4 — Pattern of tumor growth in different host environment. Normal or preimmunized BALB/c(H-2^d, Mls^b), C57/Bl6 (H-2^d, Mls^b), and DBA/2 (H-2^d, Mls^b) mice were challenged subcutaneously in the left groin with $2.5 \cdot 10^4$ cells of an highly aggressive and moderately differentiated mammary adenocarcinoma (TSA), see [NAa]. The incidence and growth of TSA tumors were evaluated by measuring neoplastic masses with calipers in the two perpendicular diameters. All mice bearing neoplastic masses with a diameter larger than 10 millimeters were killed for humane reasons. TSA cells grow progressively in normal syngeneic BALB/c mice, whereas they are rejected by histocompatible DBA/2 and C57/Bl6 mice. TSA tumor is also rejected in syngeneic BALB/c mice preimmunized with TSA cells inactivated with mitomycin-C, see [ALa].

associated antigens put immune cells in a state characterized by u approaching to 1 and allow to destroy the tumor as documented in Figure 4.4.

Following tumor or foreign histocompatibility antigen recognition, poised immune cells encounter tumor cells and undergo proliferation and differentiation into killer cells. The state of immune cells becomes progressively characterized by u approaching to 1. The ensuing encounter between tumor and immune cells are of destructive type and are often characterized by a high tumor destruction rate. The acquisition of an activation state by poised immune cells is a rapid event taking place before proliferating tumor cells (again characterized by a state of activation characterized by u approaching to 1) expand and release enough suppressive factors to impair immune reactivity. Under these conditions it can be assumed that tumor microenvironment has a neutral influence, its state being characterized by u approaching to 1 available both to the destructive action of the immune cells and to tumor expansion, see Figure 4.4.

4.7.3 Cytokine genes

Another case of tumor-host immune relationship takes place when tumor cells are genetically engineered by the transduction of genes that normally are not expressed by the tumor cells, namely cytokine genes. Following the transfection of a particular cytokine gene, tumor cells begin to pump the specific cytokine into the tumor microenvironment. These tumor cells can be regarded as actively self-replicating minipumps that, by expanding, secrete increasing amounts of a given cytokine. Engineered tumor cells proliferate with the same rate of untreated parental tumor cells with an activation state also characterized by u-values approaching to -1.

However, when the cytokines that is released by the expanding tumor cells, reaches a pharmacological threshold in the tumor microenvironment, it elicits a strong immune reaction that places various populations of the immune system in an activation state characterized by u-values approaching to 1, see Figure 4.5.

Moreover, the released cytokines can markedly enhance their local recruitment, thus increasing the encounter rate between immune cells and tumor cells. Because of the action of the secreted cytokine, these encounters are of the proliferative type, leading to an expansion and differentiation of the immune cells. The ensuing encounters between tumor and immune cells are of the destructive type and are characterized by a high destruction rate of tumor cells. In addition, the tumor-secreted cytokines, acting both on the microenvironment cells and through secondary cytokines released by activated immune cells, negatively influence the environment vessel cells that acquire an activation state characterized by u-values approaching to -1.

Fibrosis, collagen production and vessel obliteration (thrombosis), inhibition or destruction provoke a major deficit in the tumor mass. This lack of energy supply by the microenvironment causes the tumor to collapse by ischemic necrosis. Direct cell lysis and ischemic necrosis hamper tumor expansion and often leads to the complete tumor eradication, see Figure 4.5.

These situations represented in the above figures show the importance of a immune system and environment manipulation and the necessity to be able to predict the final results.

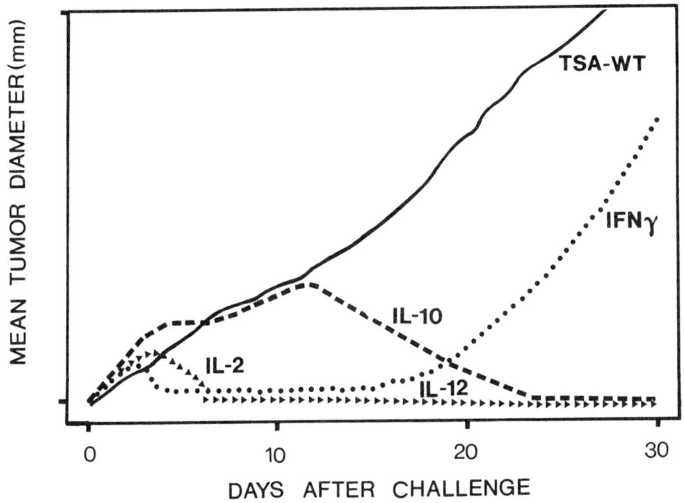

Figure 4.5 — Growth and rejection in syngenic mice of wild-type TSA cells or of TSA cells engineered to release interleukin-2, interleukin-10 or interferon-gamma. Gene transfection has been previously described in [ALa] and [CAa]. Each cytokine activates an anti-tumor reaction of different efficacy. Interleukin-10 slowly activates host killer activity and necrosis due to vessel obliteration. Interferon-γ activating macrophages induces tumor dormancy, but their reaction is not enough to eradicate the tumor that eventually grows progressively and kills the mice.

4.8 Simulation and Validation Problems

This section is divided in three parts. The first one deals with a survey of the mathematical (computational) methods to obtain the simulation of the behavior of the system. The second part develops an approach to the identification of the parameters of the model. This enables us to make some comparisons between theory and experimental results. Finally, the third paragraph describes some simplified models and deals with some related identification problems. Obviously, these problems will be relatively simple with respect to the ones involved by the full model.

4.8.1 Simulation methods

The simulation of the model essentially consists in the solution of the initial value problem related to Eqs. (4.7), that can be rewritten as

$$\begin{cases} \dfrac{\partial N_i}{\partial t}(t,u) = J_i[N](t,u) \\ N_{i0} = N_i(t=0,u)\,, \end{cases} \tag{4.22}$$

for $i = 1, \dots, n$, where $N = \{N_i\}_{i=1}^n$.

This problem can be regarded as an initial value problem for an ordinary differential equation depending on a parameter. Mathematical aspects related to the qualitative analysis of the solutions to Problem (4.22) are discussed in Section 4.9. Here we simply report, with reference to the specialized literature, e.g. Chapter 4 and Appendix 2 of [BEb], the technical methods to obtain the numerical solution to such a problem.

In particular, the solution can be obtained by a suitable discretization of the variable u

$$I_u = \{u_1, \dots, u_h, \dots, u_m\}\,, \tag{4.23}$$

followed by interpolation of the densities $N_i(t,u)$ over u

$$N_i(t,u) \cong \sum_{h=1}^{m} L_h(u) N_{ih}(t)\,, \qquad N_{ih}(t) = N_i(t,u_h)\,, \tag{4.24}$$

where $L_h = L_h(u)$, (which denotes the generic element of a set of fundamental interpolants corresponding to the collocation (4.23)), is characterized by the property

$$L_h(u_k) = \delta_{hk}\,, \tag{4.25}$$

where δ_{hk} is the Kronecker delta. Fundamental splines, Lagrange polynomials and Sinc functions satisfy such a property, for instance see [BEb].

Using this property allows the transformation of the integro-differential system into a suitable system of $n \times m$ ordinary differential equations

$$\begin{aligned} \frac{dN_{ih}}{dt}(t) = J_{ih}[N](t) &= \sum_{j=1}^{n} \sum_{p,q=1}^{m} w_{ijhpq} N_{ip}(t) N_{jq}(t) \\ &\quad - N_{ih}(t) \sum_{j=1}^{n} \sum_{p=1}^{m} w^*_{ijhp} N_{jp}(t) + g_{ih}(t)\,, \end{aligned} \tag{4.26}$$

where

$$w_{ijhpq} = \int_{-1}^{1}\int_{-1}^{1} \Big[\eta_{ij}(v,w)\psi_{ij}(v,w;u_h) + s_{ij}(v,w;u_h)\Big] L_p(v) L_q(w)\, dv\, dw$$

and

$$w^*_{ijhp} = \int_{-1}^{1} [\eta_{ij}(u_h, v) + d_{ij}(u_h, v)]\, L_p(v)\, dv$$

can be computed once and for all before starting computing the actual evolution of the system.

Therefore, Problem (4.22) is now reformulated in terms of a system of nonlinear ordinary differential equations

$$\begin{cases} \dfrac{dN_{ih}}{dt}(t) = J_{ih}[N] \\ N_{ih0} = N_{ih}(t=0)\,, \end{cases} \tag{4.27}$$

for $i = 1, \ldots, n$ and $h = 1, \ldots, m$.

The solution of Problem (4.27) can be obtained by well known methods for the integration of ordinary differential equations. Considering that a large number of sums has to be computed in J_{ih}, predictor-corrector methods may be suggested, while Chebyshev collocations appear to be more convenient because of their spectral accuracy. In this case, the quadrature rule described above is known as Cleanshaw–Curtis rule. The same rule can be used to compute the moments (4.2) and (4.3) which provide interesting information. Examples of simulations will be reported in the next sub-section.

4.8.2 Some identification and validation problems

The central problem is the identification of the parameters of the model and, consequently, its validation by suitable comparisons with experimental data, in the framework of the kinetic cellular theory reported in this essay.

As we have seen, cellular interactions are identified by the matrices $[\eta]$, $[\psi]$, $[p]$, $[\varphi]$, and $[d]$. In principle, their identification should be based upon a detailed analysis of the properties and modeling of the cell behavior including their characterization at a sub-cellular level. Unfortunately, this topic is only partially understood. Indeed, it is a research perspective, and we have therefore to rely on a purely phenomenological identification.

The identification procedure proposed in [BEc] is based on assumptions of a suitable analytic structure for the various terms of the above matrices, so that the identification is reduced to a limited number of constants. This is the case, for instance, when the densities $\psi = \psi(v, w; u)$ and $\varphi = \varphi(v, w; u)$ are assumed to have a continuous distribution over the range $[-1, 1]$ of the variable u, and are characterized by two parameters only, that may depend on v and w, $m = m(v, w)$ and $\sigma = \sigma(v, w)$. Here, m is the mean value, alternatively the most probable value, and σ is the standard variation. An additional simplification consists in assuming that the standard deviation tends to zero and that the probability densities ψ and φ tend to delta functions.

The reader can refer to [BEc] and [BEe] for specific calculations of this type. Here we will show some simulation results based on a suitable modeling of the parameters that gives an interesting description of the behavior of the system. In particular, it is important to show that the model can describe the two conflicting situations: fast activation of the immune system and depletion of the tumor cells, or fast growth of the tumor cells and inhibition of the immune system. Both behaviors can be observed after a dormancy period that may be surprisingly long. Indeed, in the framework of this theory, the dormancy time interval corresponds to a slow activation of tumor cells that move from negative values to positive values of the activation state.

Still remaining at a survey level, we rely on papers [BEc] and [BEe] to characterize a specific model and show the qualitative behavior mentioned above. To be more specific, we limit our attention to the physical system represented in Eqs. (4.20). The system is then constituted by three interacting populations: tumor cells corresponding to $i = 1$, cells of the immune system corresponding to $i = 2$, environment cells for $i = 3$, while, as a further simplification, the number of environment cells remains constant during the observation time of the phenomenon. It appears however that this crude simplification, that compresses the action of the immune system into one population only, is still sufficient to enable a careful description of the relevant features of the behavior of the system.

The interactions among the various cells are visualized in Figure 4.6, where wavy lines refer to conservative encounters (in the figure only between tumor and immune cells), continuous straight lines refer to feeding activity or any other cause generating tumor growth (between environment and tumor cells as well as suppressed immune system and tumor cells), double continuous lines refer to destructive interactions (active immune system and tumor cells). Straight dashed lines refer to production of immune cells due to interaction with tumor cells, while cytokine actions are indicated by wavy dashed lines and affect the conservative interactions.

Referring to Figure 4.6, we have to model interactions among three populations and describe the influence of cytokine signals over these interactions. In particular, it will be assumed that the signals modify conservative interactions only, while destructive proliferative encounters are ruled by the activation state reached by the cells through the mediation of the signals.

Referring now to **conservative encounters**, the following two assumptions are stated:

Assumption 4.8.1. *The temperature of the environment remains constant during the observation time, so that the encounter rates η_{ij} are also constant. The interactions that generate change of state (nontrivial in-*

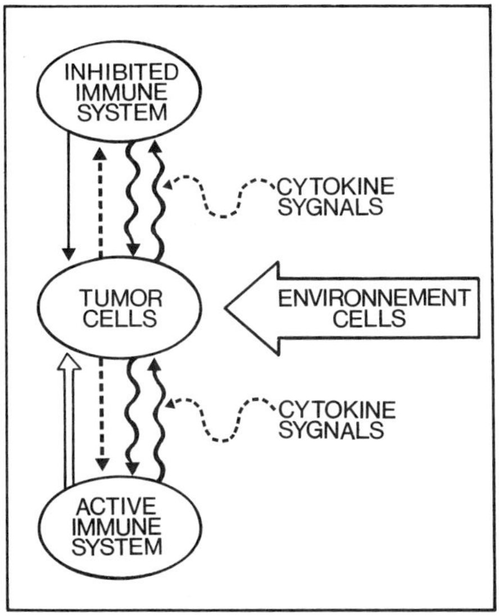

Figure 4.6 — Interaction schemes.

teractions) are significant only for interactions between cells of tumor and immune system

$$\eta_{12} = \eta_{21} = \alpha\,, \tag{4.28a}$$

where α is constant in time. The assumption that the other encounters do not generate change of state yields

$$\psi_{11} = \psi_{13} = \psi_{22} = \psi_{23} = \delta(v - u)\,, \tag{4.28b}$$

which means that the contributions to the gain and loss terms $G_i[N]$ and $L_i[N]$ are equal and cancel out.

Assumption 4.8.2. *The transition probability densities are probability densities with two parameters: variance σ and most probable output value defined by*

$$m_{12}(v,w) = \begin{cases} v & \text{if } w > 0 \text{ and } v \leq 0 \\ v - \beta_{12}^{+} w v & \text{if } w > 0 \text{ and } v > 0 \\ v - \beta_{12}^{-} w(1-v) & \text{if } w \leq 0\,, \end{cases} \tag{4.29}$$

and

$$m_{21}(v,w) = \begin{cases} v - \beta_{21} w(1+v) & \text{if } w > 0 \\ v & \text{if } w \leq 0\,, \end{cases} \tag{4.30}$$

where $\beta_{12}^{+}, \beta_{12}^{-}, \beta_{21} \in [0,1]$.

Remark 4.8.1. *The above assumptions correspond to the following physical behavior:*

i) If the interacting immune cell is inactive, i.e. $w = 0$, or if the tumor cell is dormant, i.e. $v \leq 0$, then its state does not change

$$m_{12}(v, w = 0) = v\,,$$
$$m_{12}(v \leq 0, w \geq 0) = v\,.$$

ii) If the interacting immune cell is active, i.e. $w > 0$, then the state of the active tumor cell decreases, being always above the limiting dormant state $v = 0$,

$$0 \leq m_{12}(v > 0, w > 0) \leq v\,.$$

The higher the activity w of the immune cell, the stronger the disactivation of the tumor cell. In particular, β_{12}^{+} can be measured as the decrease of activation of a fully active ($v = 1$) tumor cell due to its encounter with a fully active ($w = 1$) immune cell.

iii) If the interacting immune cell is suppressed, i.e. $w < 0$, then the state of the tumor cell increases, being always below the limiting activation state $v = 1$

$$v \leq m_{12}(v, w < 0) \leq 1\,.$$

If the tumor cell has already reached its maximum activity $v = 1$, it cannot increase further

$$m_{12}(v = 1, w < 0) = 1\,.$$

The higher the suppression of the immune cell, the stronger the activation of the tumor cell. In particular, if a dormant cell encounters an immune cell with suppressed state

$$w < -\frac{1}{\beta_{12}^{-}\left(1 - \frac{1}{v}\right)},$$

then it will probably activate. β_{12}^{-} *can be measured as the activation of an inactive* ($v = 0$) *tumor cell due to its encounter with a fully suppressed* ($w = -1$) *immune cell.*

iv) *If the interacting tumor cell is dormant, i.e.* $w \leq 0$, *then the state of the immune cell does not change*

$$m_{21}(v, w \leq 0) = v\,.$$

v) *If the interacting tumor cell is active, i.e.* $w > 0$, *then the state of the immune cell decreases, being always above the maximum state* $v = -1$

$$-1 \leq m_{21}(v, w > 0) \leq v\,.$$

If the immune cell has already reached its maximum suppression state $v = -1$, *it cannot decrease further*

$$m_{21}(v = -1, w > 0) = -1\,.$$

The higher the activity w *of the tumor cell, the stronger the disactivation of the immune cell. In particular,* β_{21} *can be measured as the suppression of an inactive* ($v = 0$) *immune cell due to its encounter with a fully active* ($w = 1$) *tumor cell.*

Assumptions with a similar mathematical structure can now be made referring to proliferative and destructive encounters.

Assumption 4.8.3. *Proliferative and destructive encounters are ruled by the following phenomenological assumptions*

- *Both production and destruction are localized in the state* v *independently of the value of* w

$$\varphi_{ij}(v, w; u) = \delta(v - u)\,. \tag{4.31}$$

- *Proliferation of tumor cells is significant only for interactions with the suppressed immune cells, i.e.* $w < 0$, *and with the environmental cells. Proliferation only occurs for aggressive states* $u > 0$, *and is directly* *proportional to the aggressivity power of the tumor u and to the negative activation of the suppressed immune cells $-w$ and to the activation of the environmental cells.*

- *Proliferation of immune cells only occurs in the interaction with active tumor cells and is independent on the activation state of the pair.*
- *Destruction of immune cells only occurs in the interaction with the host environment (or, equivalently, by natural death) and is independent of the activation state of the cells.*
- *Destruction of aggressive tumor cells only occurs in the interaction with active immune cells and is directly proportional to the activation state of the immune cells.*

This means that

$$\mu_{11} = p_{11} - d_{11} = 0\,, \tag{4.32a}$$

$$\mu_{12} = p_{12} - d_{12} = \begin{cases} -\delta_{12} w & \text{if } w \geq 0 \text{ and } u > 0 \\ -\gamma_{12} u w & \text{if } w < 0 \text{ and } u > 0 \\ 0 & \text{if } u \leq 0\,, \end{cases} \tag{4.32b}$$

$$\mu_{13} = p_{13} - d_{13} = \begin{cases} \gamma_{13} u w & \text{if } u > 0 \\ 0 & \text{if } u \leq 0\,, \end{cases} \tag{4.32c}$$

$$\mu_{21} = p_{21} - d_{21} = \begin{cases} \gamma_{21} & \text{if } w \geq 0 \\ 0 & \text{if } w < 0\,, \end{cases} \tag{4.33a}$$

$$\mu_{22} = p_{22} - d_{22} = 0\,, \tag{4.33b}$$

$$\mu_{23} = p_{23} - d_{23} = -\delta_{23}\,. \tag{4.33c}$$

Assumption 4.8.4. *The bone marrow constantly produces active immune cells uniformly distributed over the (positive) activation state*

$$g_2(t,u) = \begin{cases} g_2 & \text{if } u \geq 0, \\ 0 & \text{if } u < 0. \end{cases} \tag{4.34}$$

The evolution equations are obtained by Eqs. (4.20) with the specialization due to the above assumptions

$$\frac{\partial N_1}{\partial t}(t,u) = \alpha \int_{-1}^{1}\int_{-1}^{1} \psi_{12}(u, m_{12}(v,w)) N_1(t,v) N_2(t,w)\, dv\, dw$$

$$- N_1(t,u)\Big\{ \alpha \int_{-1}^{1} N_2(t,v)\, dv + \Big[\gamma_{12} u \int_{-1}^{0} v N_2(t,v)\, dv$$

$$+ \delta_{12} \int_{0}^{1} v N_2(t,v)\, dv - \gamma_{13} u \int_{0}^{1} v N_{30}(v)\, dv \Big] H(u) \Big\} \quad (4.35a)$$

$$\frac{\partial N_2}{\partial t}(t,u) = \alpha \int_{-1}^{1}\int_{-1}^{1} \psi_{21}(u, m_{21}(v,w)) N_2(t,v) N_1(t,w)\, dv\, dw$$

$$+ N_2(t,u) \Big[\gamma_{21} \int_{0}^{1} N_1(t,v)\, dv - \alpha \int_{-1}^{1} N_1(t,v)\, dv$$

$$- \delta_{23} \int_{0}^{1} N_{30}(v)\, dv \Big] + g_2 H(u)\,, \quad (4.35b)$$

where the terms

$$\psi_{ij}(v,w;u) = \psi_{ij}(u, m_{ij}(v,w))$$

are modeled as indicated in Assumption 4.8.2 and

$$H(u) = \begin{cases} 1 & \text{if } u \geq 0 \\ 0 & \text{if } u < 0 \end{cases}$$

is the Heaviside function.

The simulation consists in the solution of the initial value problem related to such an evolution model. With this in mind, we can focus on the role of the parameters characterizing the model

- α is related to the speed of evolution of the system and can be included in the time-scale.
- β_{12}^{+} characterizes the ability of the active immune system to disactivate the aggressive tumor cells.
- β_{12}^{-} characterizes the negative action of the suppressed immune system to activate the aggressive tumor cells.
- β_{21} characterizes the ability of the tumor cells to inhibit the immune system.

- γ_{12} characterizes the proliferative behavior of the tumor cells in their encounter with the suppressed immune system.
- γ_{13} characterizes the proliferative behavior of the tumor cells in their encounter with the host environment.
- γ_{21} characterizes the proliferative behavior of the immune cells in their encounter with tumor cells.
- δ_{12} characterizes the suppression of the tumor cells in their encounter with the active immune system.
- δ_{23} characterizes the suppression of the immune cells in their encounter with the host environment, or, equivalently, their natural extinction.
- g_2 characterizes the input of active immune cells from the bone marrow.

Therefore, in this simplified model, parameters β are related to transitions in conservative encounters, parameters γ are related to proliferative activity, while parameters δ are related to destructive activity. Practical simulations have shown that the variance σ holds a secondary role.

Such a specialization of the parameters is useful for their identification. For instance, in [BEe] it is discussed how cytokine signals can be related to the parameters β. The reader is referred to [BEe] for detailed comparisons between theory and experiments.

The solution technique is the one summarized in the preceding paragraph. The figures that follow show some aspects of the behavior of the system. They are all obtained assuming that the host environment is always fully active

$$N_{30}(u) = \delta(u-1)\,,$$

where δ is the Dirac delta, and setting

$$\begin{aligned} &\beta_{12}^{+} = \beta_{12}^{-} = \beta_{21} = 0.1\,, \\ &\gamma_{13} = 1\,, \\ &g_2 = \delta_{23} = 0.2\,. \end{aligned} \tag{4.36}$$

All simulations start from a uniform distribution over the state with density normalized to one, i.e.

$$N_{10}(u) = N_{20}(u) = 0.5\,.$$

The following example give an indication of the possible scenarios that might present:

- Figure 4.7 shows the fast growth of the number of tumor cells. This behavior is obtained for the following values of the parameters

$$\alpha = 0.3\,, \quad \gamma_{12} = \gamma_{21} = 0.5\,, \quad \delta_{12} = 0.2\,,$$

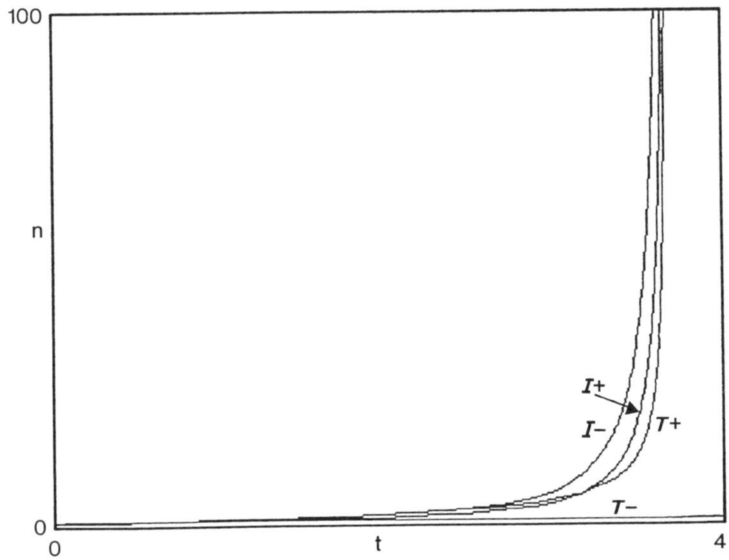

Figure 4.7 — Blow up of both tumor and immune cells. I^- and I^+ indicate, respectively, the number of suppressed and active immune cells, while T^- and T^+ indicate, respectively, the number of dormant and active tumor cells.

besides those already set in Eq. (4.36). In this case, the aggressivity of the immune system is not sufficient to control tumor growth. On the contrary, its cells, due to the action of the tumor, enhance its growth.

- Figure 4.8 shows the persistence of a small tumor over a long period with stages of expansions alternated with stages of depletion with final sudden blow up of the tumor. This behavior is obtained for the following values of the parameters

$$\alpha = 0.3 \,, \quad \gamma_{12} = \gamma_{21} = 0.5 \,, \quad \delta_{12} = 1 \,,$$

besides those already set in Eq. (4.36). With respect to the previous case, the immune system is more aggressive, leading to a temporary control of tumor growth. The decrease of tumor cells generate a decrease in the proliferation of immune cells. This favors a new growth of the tumor, which cause an immune response. This cycle may repeat several times. In the meantime, however, the tumor succeeds in suppressing a

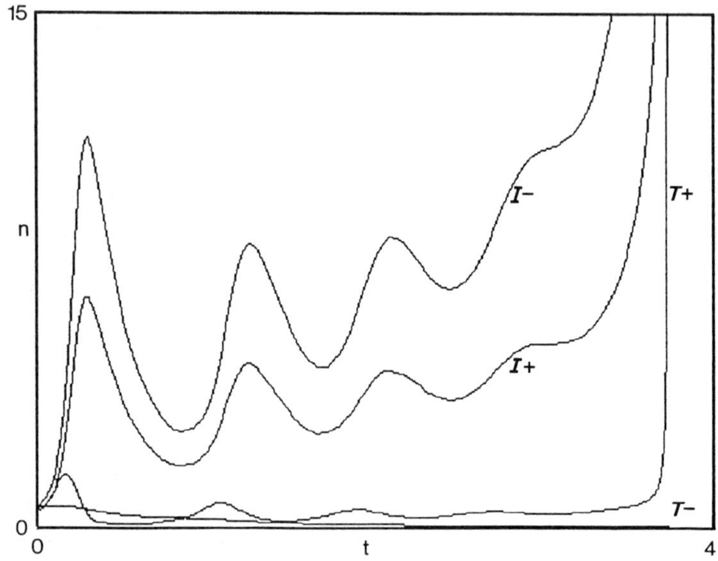

Figure 4.8 — Persistence of a small tumor over a long period with stages of expansions alternated with stages of depletion with final sudden blow up of the tumor. I^- and I^+ indicate, respectively, the number of suppressed and active immune cells, while T^- and T^+ indicate, respectively, the number of dormant and active tumor cells.

sufficient number of immune cells to enhance its final blow up.

- Figure 4.9 shows the persistence of a small tumor throughout the body life with an initial sequence of stages of expansions alternated with stages of depletion and the trend toward an asymptotic coexisting configuration. This behavior is obtained for the following values of the parameters

$$\alpha = 0.2\,, \quad \gamma_{12} = \gamma_{21} = 0.5\,, \quad \delta_{12} = 1\,,$$

besides those already set in Eq. (4.36). With respect to the previous case, conservative encounters leading, among other things, to degeneracy of the immune system are less frequent and this leads to an insufficient degeneration of the immune system to generate tumor blow up as in the previous case.

- Figure 4.10 shows total suppression of the tumor due to prompt response of the immune system. This behavior is obtained for the following values

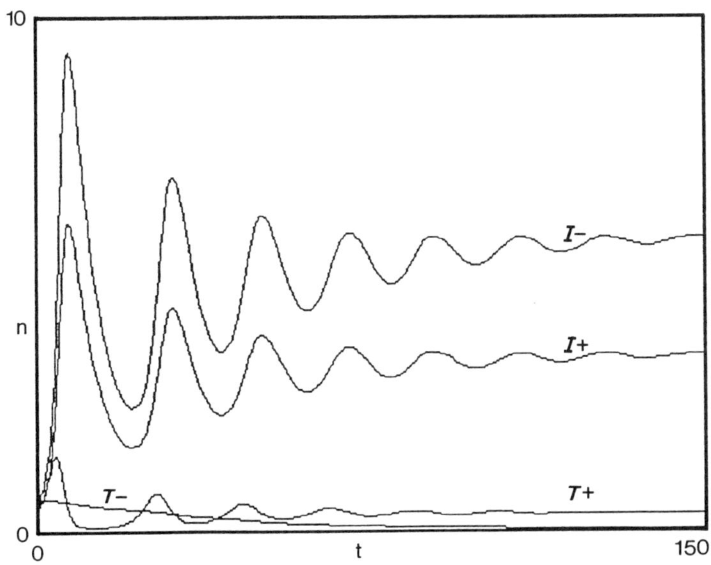

Figure 4.9 — Equilibrium between tumor and immune cells with an initial sequence of stages of expansions alternated with stages of depletion and final trend toward an asymptotic coexisting configuration. I^- and I^+ indicate, respectively, the number of suppressed and active immune cells, while T^- and T^+ indicate, respectively, the number of dormant and active tumor cells.

of the parameters

$$\alpha = 0.3 \,, \quad \gamma_{12} = 0.5 \,, \quad \gamma_{21} = 2 \,, \quad \delta_{12} = 1 \,,$$

besides those already set in Eq. (4.36). With respect to Figure 4.8, immune cells proliferate faster in the presence of the tumor. This leads to an initial alternation of stages of expansion and depletion with final destruction of the tumor.

These figures reproduce the behavior experimentally observed as reported in Section 4.6.

As we have seen above, the different behaviors have been obtained for different values of the parameters characterizing the model. The simulation was obtained using two parameter distribution functions with small variance. The results that are obtained when the variance tends to zero are

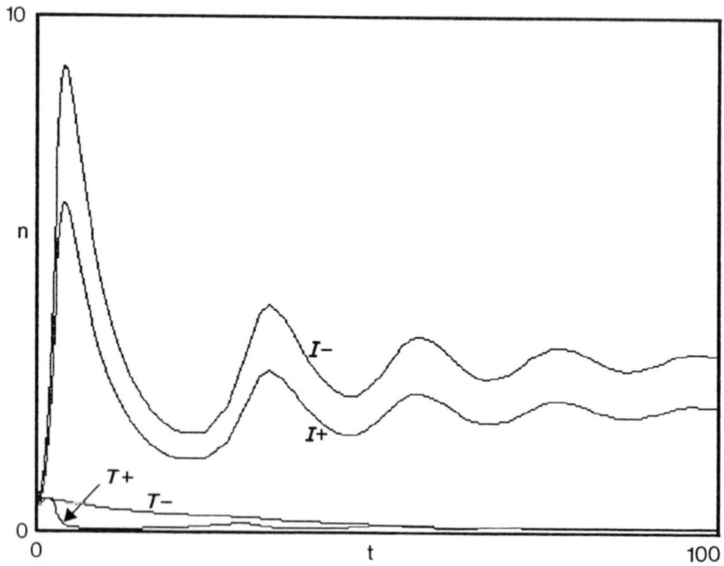

Figure 4.10 — Suppression of tumor due to prompt response of the immune system. I^- and I^+ indicate, respectively, the number of suppressed and active immune cells, while T^- and T^+ indicate, respectively, the number of dormant and active tumor cells.

very close, so that the parametric identification can be effectively restricted to the most probable output.

It is plain that the simulation can provide information not only to describe the dynamics of the system, but also to improve the model and move some way towards understanding of the complex system we are examining. One of the crucial points is to understand more deeply the role of the parameters β that are related to the activity of cytokine signals. The analysis has to be developed for fixed values of γ and δ that characterize the proliferative and destructive actions of the tumor and immune cells. An example of this type of simulation is given in the above figures. Indeed, the objective is to evaluate the possibility of modifying the evolution of a neoplastic system within the environment of a vertebrate characterized by a certain immune system.

The role of the parameters γ and δ can be further understood by dealing with the simulation and organization of suitable experiments corresponding to some extreme physical situations. The analysis of these situations may even be useful for a direct measurements of the parameters γ and δ.

For instance, one can consider the physical situation, that can be artificially created, of a vertebrate with totally suppressed immune system. In this case, if the states of tumor and environment cells are concentrated in the most active state, then Eq. (4.35a) yields a very simple evolution equation for the number density n_1 of the tumor cells

$$\frac{dx_1}{dt} = \gamma_{13} n_{30} x_1 \,, \qquad x = \frac{n_1}{n_{10}} \,, \tag{4.37}$$

that can be solved as follows

$$x_1 = e^{\lambda t} \,, \qquad \lambda = \gamma_{13} n_{30} \,. \tag{4.38}$$

This solution shows that the tumor grows exponentially in a vertebrate with a totally suppressed immune system. The rate of growth is proportional to the aggressive power of the tumor and to the feeding capacity of the environmental cells. As known [BEa], this situation can be experimentally created and observed as documented in Figures 4.11 and 4.12 that show the exponential growth of CE-2 and TS/A tumors in BALB mice. This experiment is useful to identify and classify the aggressive power of different tumor cells, by means of the parameter λ.

On the other hand, if the vertebrate is not deprived of its immune reaction, then the early growth is contrasted by it. Such a behavior is experimentally observed and shown, still in Figures 4.11 and 4.12, that shows the initial growth of the same tumors in BALB mice with fully active immune systems.

When the immune system is active, then its behavior is described by the full integro-differential system. Nevertheless, one can simplify and idealize the description to obtain again a very simple dynamical system. For instance, the use of cytokine signals can prevent the inhibition activity of the tumor cells against the immune system. Then, the immune system is totally active against the the tumor cells. This behavior is described by the simple system

$$\begin{cases} \dfrac{dx}{dt} = \lambda x - \delta^* xy \\[2em] \dfrac{dy}{dt} = \gamma^* xy \,, \end{cases} \tag{4.39}$$

where x was already defined in Eq. (4.37) and y refers to immune cells.

This simple dynamical system can be regarded as one of the several phenomenological models that can be proposed based on observation of the

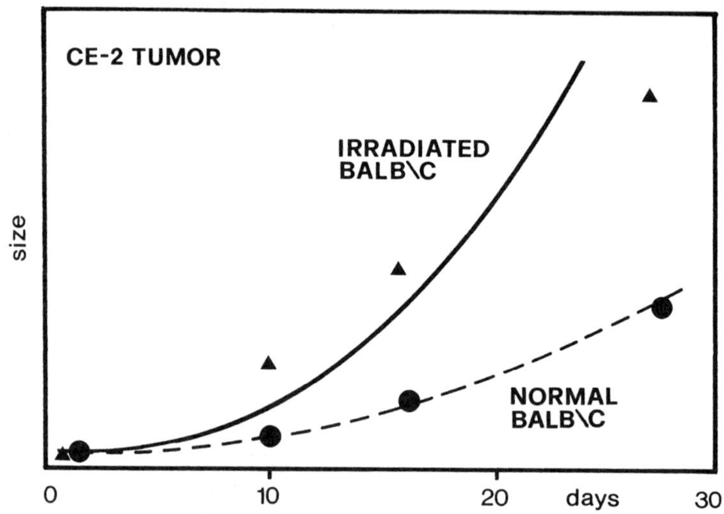

Figure 4.11 — Growth of CE-2 tumor cells in an irradiated BALB mice (continuous line) and with active immune system (dashed line).

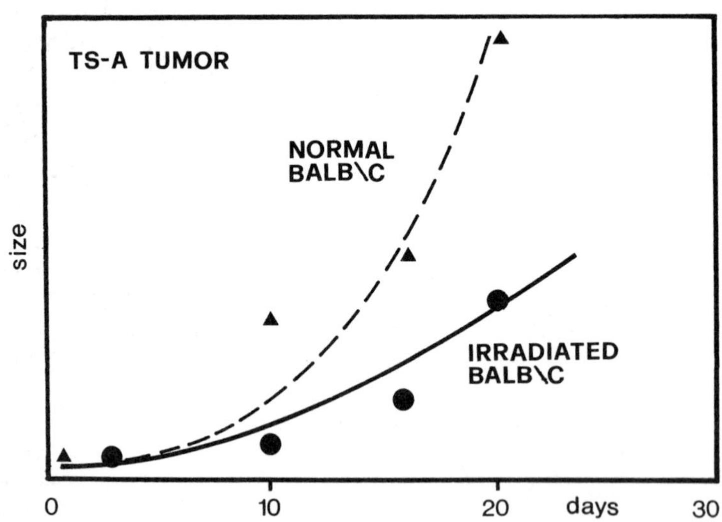

Figure 4.12 — Growth of TS/A tumor cells in an irradiated BALB mice (continuous line) and with active immune system (dashed line).

system. Examples of these models can be found in the chapters of this book and, in particular in the one by Michelson and Leith. On the other hand, the correct link between the cellular kinetic theory and dynamical systems described by ordinary differential equations is given by the discrete models that are presented in the subsection that follows.

4.8.3 Discrete models

Discrete models are often proposed in the literature in order to provide simple and immediate modeling. On the other hand, these models are generally too simple to be able to cover the real behavior of the system. In particular, classical population dynamics models can describe proliferative and destructive encounters, but not the change of activity due to conservative encounters.

An interesting description, that is developed by Lo Schiavo [LSa], is given by discretized models, namely models for which the state u is discretized over a certain number of fixed states as in (4.28), such that the corresponding densities are denoted by

$$N_i^\ell = N_i^\ell(t)\,, \qquad i = 1, \dots, p\,, \qquad \ell = 1, \dots, m\,. \tag{4.40}$$

This approach is useful, and differs from the discretization described in Section 4.8.3, if one can select a small number of states. Typically, one can select two states $u = -1$ and $u = 1$.

A discrete model can be obtained by the general continuous model (4.8), corresponding to the above stated discretization under the assumption

$$N_i(t, u) = \sum_{\ell=1}^{n} N_i^\ell(t)\delta(u - u_\ell)\,, \qquad i = 1, \dots, p\,, \qquad \ell = 1, \dots, m\,. \tag{4.41}$$

Models obtained in this way, although relatively simpler than the continuous ones, will retain the essential features of the original model: the modification of activation state and the competition among the various cell populations. In particular, let

- $G_{ij}^{hk}(\ell)$ be the transition rate into the state u_ℓ due to the encounters between the cell of the i-population, with state v_h, with the cell of the j-population, with state v_k,
- $P_{ij}^{hk}(\ell)$ be the proliferation rate into the state u_ℓ due to the encounters between the cell of the i-population, with state v_h, with the cell of the j-population, with state v_k,

and

- $L_{ij}^{\ell k}$ be the loss of i-cells with state u_ℓ due to the conservative encounters with the cell of the j-population, with state v_k.

- $D_{ij}^{\ell k}$ be the destruction i-cells with state u_ℓ due to destructive encounters with the cell of the j-population, with state v_k.

The discrete model is obtained replacing the integrals by finite sums

$$\frac{dN_i^\ell}{dt} = \sum_{j=1}^{p} \sum_{h,k=1}^{m} \left[G_{ij}^{hk}(\ell) + P_{ij}^{hk}(\ell) \right] N_i^h N_j^k$$

$$- N_i^\ell \sum_{j=1}^{p} \sum_{h,k=1}^{m} \left(L_{ij}^{\ell k} + D_{ij}^{\ell k} \right) N_j^k \,. \tag{4.42}$$

The rate G can be obtained as product of the encounter rates and a suitable **transition probability density**. For instance,

$$G_{ij}^{hk}(\ell) = \eta_{ij}^{hk} \psi_{ij}^{hk}(\ell) \,, \tag{4.43}$$

where

$$\sum_{\ell=1}^{m} \psi_{ij}^{hk}(\ell) = 1 \,, \quad \forall i, j, h, k \,. \tag{4.44}$$

Similar calculations can be developed for the interactions ruled by the terms P, L, and D.

The models proposed in [LSa] appear to be very interesting for applications. Therefore, it is worth developing this research line that may provide interesting models with a structure much simpler than the one of the models which are reported in this survey.

4.9 Remarks Addressed to Applied Mathematicians

Although this survey is almost totally devoted to modeling and simulation, the evolution equations of the model originate some interesting problems that are worth of the attention of applied mathematicians. Non specialists can avoid going through this section, which is devoted to the description of the mathematical problems and to a brief review of the solved and open problems related to the equations reported in Section 4.6.

The aim is to address the mathematical research, e.g. qualitative analysis of the solutions to the initial value problem, towards a deeper understanding of the properties of the integro-differential system reported in Section 4.6.

In particular, consider the initial value problem for the autonomous case, i.e. $g_i = 0$,

$$\frac{\partial N}{\partial t}(t,u) = \mathcal{J}(N)(t,u)\,, \quad \mathcal{J} = \{J_i\}_{i=1}^p\,,\ N = \{N_i\}_{i=1}^p\,,\ N(0,u) = N_0(u)\,. \tag{4.45}$$

The analysis follows the usual line

i) Definition of a suitable Banach space;

ii) Statement of solution to the initial value problem;

iii) Proof of existence, uniqueness, regularity and asymptotic behavior of the solutions.

Referring to the papers already published on this topic, the analysis is generally developed in the Banach space $\left(L^1[-1,1]\right)^p$, such that on its elements $N = \{N_i\}_1^p$ the norm

$$\|N\| = \sum_{k=1}^{p} \|N_k\| = \sum_{k=1}^{p} \int_{-1}^{1} |N_k|\, du \tag{4.46}$$

is defined. Solutions are sought in the positive cone X^+ of X defined by the functions $N \in X$, such that $N_i \geq 0$, for $i = 1, \ldots, p$.

The analysis can be related to the mild form

$$\begin{aligned} N_i(t,u) =& N_{i0}(u) \exp\left(-\int_0^t \mathcal{L}_i[N](s,u)\, ds\right) \\ &+ \int_0^t \mathcal{Q}_i[N](s,u) \exp\left(\int_s^t \mathcal{L}_i[N](r,u)\, dr\right) ds\,, \end{aligned} \tag{4.47}$$

that corresponds, with obvious meaning of notations related to Eq. (4.7), to the initial value problem

$$\begin{cases} \dfrac{\partial N_i}{\partial t} + N_i \mathcal{L}_i[N] = \mathcal{Q}_i[N] \\ \\ N_i(t=0,u) = N_{i0}(u)\,. \end{cases} \tag{4.48}$$

A set of functions N is defined **solution to the initial value problem** with $N \in X^+$ if it is a map from $[0,T]$ into X^+, if it is continuously differentiable in $[0,T]$, and satisfies both the differential evolution equation and the initial conditions N_0.

The qualitative analysis is developed, in the literature, mainly for conservative models (4.12). Mathematical results are given in [ARa] and [ARc]. The first paper proves existence and uniqueness of solutions to the initial value problem. The analysis is further developed in the second paper where the existence theory is generalized to models with multiple interactions. The same paper shows the existence of equilibrium points. The problem of the stability of equilibrium points still remains open, although the computational experiments developed by Preziosi [PZa] have shown that two populations, interacting according to well specified terms η and ψ generally have an asymptotic trend to stable equilibrium distributions.

Conservative models have not a direct impact on the contents of this essay. However, they are of interest in the analysis of population dynamics and, in particular, to describe a dynamics in absence of destructive proliferative activities. Nevertheless, one can look at the analysis developed in [ARa] and [ARc] as the first step towards the qualitative analysis of the full model. In particular, the analysis of the full equation is a problem of great mathematical interest, and has a relevant impact with immunological problems we are dealing with. The presence of proliferative and competitive terms either activates a fast growth, in norm, of the solutions, or produces their asymptotic trend.

The analysis of [ARb] refers to an early edition of the model (4.11), that is characterized by some technical differences with respect to the one reported in this survey. In particular, it develops an analysis of existence of solutions locally in time for general mathematical models. Then, it develops an analysis of the asymptotic behavior of the solutions for particular choices of the parameters characterizing the model. Indeed, it is shown that under a suitable choice of the parameters, the model predicts qualitative behaviors that are experimentally observed.

Paper [ARb] proposes some interesting and useful results; however a systematic analysis has still to be developed and certainly is a challenging problem for those applied mathematicians interested in the qualitative analysis of the solutions to nonlinear differential problems.

4.10 Perspectives

A survey of the kinetic (cellular) modeling of the interactions between the immune system and tumor cells was proposed. The reader should realize that the analysis refers to early stages of the competition, that is when interactions occur at a cellular level. Once tumor cells have condensed in a compact block, approximately a sphere, then the system has to be modeled by equations of continuum mechanics. The mathematical problem can then be stated as a moving boundary problem with interactions, between the tumor and the outer system, on the surface of the tumor itself. The modeling discussed by Chaplain [CHa–e], also reviewed in this book, proceeds in that direction.

Referring to the modeling of cellular interactions and evolution, we have seen that the core of the modeling is the identification of the terms η, ψ, p, d, and φ. Indeed, once these quantities have been evaluated, the derivation of the evolution equations can be obtained by straightforward calculations. Moreover, the simulation of the behavior of the system can be developed by efficient methods such as the ones reviewed in Section 4.8.

Up to now, the identification of the terms η, ψ, p, φ, and d was reached by means of a suitable comparison between predictions of the model and experimental results. In this approach, we assume a simple analytic expression of the above mentioned terms, so that the few parameters involved in these expressions can be identified using experimental information. The analysis of the phenomenological behavior of the system can identify the terms that have an influence upon the evolution of the system.

Although this approach has given some promising results, such as the ones reported in [BEc], it cannot be regarded as totally satisfactory. Indeed, it would be important to obtain a theory, or at least a model, suitable to describe the behavior of the cells directly from the modeling of the dynamics of the cell interaction itself. The relevance of an analysis of this type does not need to be emphasized. If achieved, it would provide a fully self-consistent theory and would open new perspectives in the modeling of cellular phenomena in physical contexts, that may be characterized by some differences with respect to the ones dealt with in this survey.

Some work in this area has already been carried out. For instance, we mention the modeling and simulation of the immune network with special attention to reconstruction of the interaction among cells of the immune system and recognition of the state shape. In particular, we refer to the research activity developed by De Boer, Högeweg, Segel and Perelson, see [DEa,b], [SEb], [PEc]. The problem is to discover and formalize the link between cellular activities and the kinetic (cellular) theory of tumor immune system interactions. This topic is posed by immunologists. An example is given in [TOa] where a detailed description of the phenomenon and some modeling is proposed.

The above mentioned topic appears to be a relevant research perspective. However, the interest of researchers should also be directed towards condensation mechanisms [SMa] that lead to spheroid forms, and towards modeling the link between equations of continuum mechanics, related to the dynamics of solid tumors, with the outer cellular systems. The interest in this matter is also clearly motivated by medicine. Indeed, the struggle against tumors is initiated also when the tumor is condensed. This is documented in the research activity by Mulè [MLa], Rosenberg and coworkers

[ROa], and, in general, on methods based by activation of the immune system against the aggressive power of the tumor cells fighting their ability to inhibit the immune system [FOd]. In this physical situation, one has to study a mathematical problem with moving boundaries as documented in [CHe]. The boundaries divide the inner necrotic zone from the middle zone of the vascularized carcinoma and the outer zone of the environment.

In all cases, that is for both cellular and continuum theories, the analysis of control problems, or solution of inverse problems related to identification of parameters by experimental data, is relevant to the development of this branch of mathematical biology. It is also necessary developing molecular aggregation models such as the one described in [ACa], [SMa], and [SRb,c]. The mathematical analysis of this type of equations is well documented in the literature [SRa].

We conclude noting again the relevance of the contribution that simulation devices can give to research activity in medicine and immunology. Indeed, a parallel support to experiments *in vivo* may hopefully reduce the amounts of experiments and direct them, if necessary, in more successful directions. Indeed, considering that it is necessary to develop experiments *in vivo*, then any effort has to be made to reduce their number. This matter is well emphasized in the article by Taubes [TAa], which stimulates scientific activity towards simulation of the various phenomena, interaction and competition, of cells.

In addition, simulation can also provide relevant quantitative information on the behavior of the system, and will hopefully address medical research into the competition against aggressive tumors.

4.11 References

[ABa] Abbas A.K., Lichtmann A.H., and Pober J.S., **Cellular and Molecular Immunology**, Saunders (1991).

[ACa] Ackleh A.S., Fitzpatrick B.G., and Hallam T.G., Approximation and parameter estimation problems for algal aggregation models, *Math. Models Meth. Appl. Sci.*, **4** (1994), 291–312.

[ADa] Adam J.A., A simplified mathematical model of tumor growth, *Math. Biosci.*, **81** (1986), 229–244.

[ADb] Adam J.A., A mathematical model of tumor growth II: Effects of geometry and spatial nonuniformity on stability, *Math. Biosci.*, **86** (1987), 183–211.

[ADc] Adam J.A., A mathematical model of tumor growth III: Comparison with experiment, *Math. Biosci.*, **86** (1987), 213–227.

[ADd] Adam J.A., Diffusion models of prevascular and vascular tumor growth – A review, in **Mathematical Population Dynamics**, Arino O. et al. eds., Dekker (1991).

[ADe] Adam J.A. and Noren R., Equilibrium model of a vascularized spherical carcinoma with central necrosis – Some properties of the solution, *J. Math. Biol.*, **81** (1993), 735–745.

[ADf] Adam J.A., Effects of vascularization on lymphocyte/tumor cell dynamics: Qualitative features, *Math. Comp. Modelling - Special Issue on Modelling and Simulation Problems on Tumor-immune System Dynamics*, Bellomo N. ed., **23** (1996), 1–10.

[AFa] Albert A., Freedman M., and Perelson A.S., Tumors and the immune system: The effects of a tumor growth modulator, *Math. Biosci.*, **50** (1980), 25–58.

[ALa] Allione A., Consalvo M., Nanni P., Lollini P.L., Cavallo F., Giovarelli M., Forni M., Gulino A., Colombo M.P., Dellabona P., Hock H., Blanckstain T., Rosenthal F., Gansbacher B., Colombo M.C., Musso T., Gusella L., and Forni G., Immunizing and curative potential of replicating and nonreplicating murine mammary adenocarcinoma cells engineered with IL2, IL4, IL6, IL7, IL10, TNFα, GM-CSF and IFNγ gene or admixed with conventional adjuvants, *Cancer Res.*, **54** (1994), 6022–6026.

[ARa] Arlotti L. and Bellomo N., On a new model of population dynamics with stochastic interaction, *Transp. Theory Statist. Phys.*, **24** (1995), 431–443.

[ARb] Arlotti L. and Lachowicz M., Qualitative analysis of a nonlinear integro-differential equation modelling tumor-host dynamics, *Math. Comp. Modelling - Special Issue on Modelling and Simulation Problems on Tumor-immune System Dynamics*, Bellomo N. ed., **23** (1996), 11–30.

[ARc] Arlotti L. and Bellomo N., On the Cauchy problem for a nonlinear integral differential equation in population dynamics, *Appl. Math. Letters*, **9** (1996), 65–70.

[ASa] Ash R. and Gardner M., **Topics in Stochastic Processes**, Academic Press (1975).

[BEa] Bellomo N. and Forni G., Dynamics of tumor interaction with the host immune system, *Math. Comp. Modelling*, **20** (1994), 107–122.

[BEb] Bellomo N. and Preziosi L., **Modelling, Mathematical Methods and Scientific Computation**, CRC Press (1995).

[BEc] Bellomo N., Forni G., and Preziosi L., On a kinetic (cellular) theory for the competition between tumors and host-immune system, *J. Biol. Systems*, to appear.

[BEd] Bellomo N. ed., **Modelling and Simulation Problems on Tumor Immune System Dynamics**, *Special Issue Math. Comp. Modelling*, **23** (1996).

[BEe] Bellomo N., Firmani B., Guerri G., and Preziosi L., On the kinetic (cellular) theory of tumor-immune system dynamics: Citokine mediated interaction between tumors and immune system, work in progress.

[BEf] Bellomo N. ed., **Lecture Notes on the Mathematical Theory of the Boltzmann Equation**, World Sci. (1995).

[BLa] Beltrami E., **Mathematics for Dynamic Modelling**, Academic Press (1987).

[BNa] Boon T., Gajewski T., and Coulie G., From defined human tumor antigens to effective immunization, *Immunol. Today*, **16** (1955), 334–335.

[BOa] Bosco M., Giovarelli M., Forni M., Scarpa S., Masuelli L., and Forni G., Low doses of IL-4 injected perilymphatically in tumor-bearing mice inhibit the growth of poorly and apparently nonimmunogenic tumors and induce a tumor specific immune memory, *J. Immunol.*, **145** (1990), 3136–3143.

[CAa] Cavallo F., Giovarelli M., Gulino A., Vacca A., Stoppacciaro A., Modesti A., and Forni G., Role of Neutrophils and $CD4^{+}T$ lymphocytes in the primary and memory response to nonimmunogenic mammary adenocarcinoma made immunogenic by IL-2 gene transfection, *J. Immunol.*, **149** (1992), 3627–3635.

[CHa] Chaplain M. and Stuart A.M., A model mechanism for the chemotactic response of endothelial cells to tumor angiogenesis factor, *IMA J. Math. Appl. Med. Biol.*, **8** (1991), 191–220.

[CHb] Chaplain M. and Britton N.F., On the concentration profile of a growth inhibitory factor in multicell spheroids, *Math. Biosci.*, **115** (1993), 233–245.

[CHc] Chaplain M. and Sleeman B.D., Modelling the growth of solid tumors and incorporating a method for their classification using nonlinear elasticity theory, *J. Math. Biol.*, **31** (1993), 431–479.

[CHd] Chaplain M., Benson D.L., and Maini P.K., Nonlinear diffusion of a growth inhibitory factor in multicell spheroids, *Math. Biosci.*, **121** (1994), 1–13.

[CHe] Chaplain M., A vascular growth, angiogenesis, and vascular growth in solid tumors: The mathematical modelling of stages of tumor developments, *Math. Comp. Modelling - Special Issue on Modelling and Simulation Problems on Tumor-immune System Dynamics*, Bellomo N. ed., **23** (1996), 47–88.

[DEa] De Boer R.J. and Högeweg P., Tumor escape from immune elimination: Simplified precursor bound cytotoxicity models, *J. Theor. Biol.*, **113** (1985), 719–736.

[DEb] De Boer R.J. and Högeweg P., Interactions between macrophages and T-lymphocytes, *J. Theor. Biol.*, **120** (1986), 331–354.

[DOa] Den Otter W. and Ruitenberg E.J. eds., **Tumor Immunology. Mechanisms, Diagnosis, Therapy**, Elsevier (1987).

[FLa] Folkman J. and Klagsbrun M., Angiogenic factors, *Science*, **235** (1987), 442–447.

[FOa] Forni G. and Comoglio P.M., Growth of syngenetic tumors in unimmunized newborn and adult hosts, *Brit. J. Cancer*, **27** (1973), 120–127.

[FOb] Forni G., Giovarelli M., Santoni A., Modesti A., and Forni M., Interleukin-2 activated tumor inhibition in vivo depends on the systemic involvement of host immunoreactivity, *J. Immunol.*, **138** (1987), 4031–4033.

[FOc] Forni G., Varesio L., Giovarelli M., and Cavallo G., Dynamic state of a spontaneous immune reactivity towards a mammary adenocarcinoma, in **Tumor Associate Antigens and Their Specific Immune Response**, Spreafico F. and Arnon R. eds., Academic Press (1979), 167–192.

[FOd] Forni G., Foa R., Santoni A., and Frati L. eds., **Cytokine Induced Tumor Immunogeneticity**, Academic Press (1994).

[GEa] Green I., Cohen S., and McCluskey R. eds., **Mechanisms of Tumor Immunity**, Wiley (1977).

[GRa] Grossman Z. and Berke G., Tumor escape from immune elimination, *J. Theor. Biol.*, **83** (1980), 276–296.

[GSa] Greenspan H., On the growth and stability of cell cultures and solid tumors, *J. Theor. Biol.*, **56** (1976), 229–242.

[GYa] Gyllenberg M. and Webb G., A nonlinear structured population model of tumor growth with quiescence, *J. Math. Biol.*, **28** (1990), 671–694.

[HEa] Herberman R.B., **NK Cells and Other Natural Effector Cells**, Academic Press (1982).

[IVa] Iversen O., What's new in endogenous growth stimulators and inhibitors (chalones), *Path. Res. Pract.*, **180** (1985), 77–80.

[IVb] Iversen O., The hunt for endogenous growth-inhibitory and tumor suppression factors - Their role in physiological and pathological growth-regulation, *Adv. Cancer Res.*, **57** (1991), 413–453.

[JAa] Jager E. and Segel L., On the distribution of dominance in a population of interacting anonymous organisms, *SIAM J. Appl. Math.*, **52** (1992), 1442–1468.

[JNa] Janeway C.A. and Travers P., **Immunobiology**, Current Biology (1994).

[KUa] Kuznetsov V.A., **Dynamics of Immune Processes During Tumor Growth**, Nauka (1992), in Russian.

[KUb] Kuznetsov V.A., Malakin A.M., Taylor M.A., and Perelson A.S., Nonlinear dynamics of immunogenic tumors: Parameter estimation and global bifurcation analysis, *Bull. Math. Biol.*, **56** (1994), 295–321.

[LAa] Landry J., Freyer J.P., and Sutherland R.M., A model for the growth of multicell spheroids, *Cell Tissue Kinet.*, **15** (1982), 585–594.

[LEa] Levin S., **Frontiers in Mathematical Biology**, Springer (1994).

[LFa] Lefever R.J., Hiernaux J., Urbain J., and Meyers P., On the kinetics and optimal specificity of cytotoxic reactions mediated by T-lymphocytes clones, *Bull. Math. Biol.*, **54** (1992), 839–873.

[LIa] Lin C.C. and Segel L.A., **Mathematics Applied to Deterministic Problems in Applied Sciences**, SIAM Publ. (1988).

[LOa] Lollini P., Bosco M., Cavallo F., De`Giovanni C., Giovarelli M., Landuzzi L., Musiani P., Modesti A., Nicoletti G., Palmieri G., Santoni A., Young H., Forni G., and Nanni P., Inhibition of tumor growth and enhancement of metastasis after transfection of the γ-Interferon gene, *Int. J. Cancer*, **55** (1993), 320–329.

[LSa] Lo Schiavo M., Discrete kinetic cellular models of tumors immune system interactions, *Math. Models Meth. Appl. Sci.*, **6** (1996), to appear.

[MAa] Maggelakis S. and Adam J.A., Mathematical model for prevascular growth of a spherical carcinoma, *Math. Comp. Modelling*, **13** (1990), 23–38.

[MAb] Maggelakis S., Type α and type β transforming growth factors as regulators of cancer cellular growth: A mathematical model, *Math. Comp. Modelling*, **18** (1993), 9–16.

[MEa] Mueller-Klieser W., Multicellular spheroids: A review on cellular aggregates in cancer research, *J. Cancer Res. Clin. Oncol.*, **113** (1987), 101–122.

[MIa] Michelson S. and Leith J., Growth factors and growth control of heterogeneous cell populations, *Bull. Math. Biol.*, **55** (1993), 993–1011.

[MIb] Michelson S. and Leith J., Autocrine and paracrine growth factors in tumor growth: A mathematical model, *Bull. Math. Biol.*, **53** (1991), 639–656.

[MKa] Markovitch S., The particular role of cell loss in tumor growth, *Math. Comp. Modelling*, **18** (1993), 83–89.

[MLa] Mulè J., Shu S., Schwarz S., and Rosenberg S., Successful adoptive immunotherapy of established pulmonary metastases with LAK cells and recombinant IL-2, *Science*, **255** (1993), 1487–1489.

[MRa] Marusic M., Bajzer Z., Freyer J.P., and Vuk-Pavlovic S., Modelling autostimulation of growth in multicellular tumor spheroids, *Int. J. Biomed. Comp.*, **149** (1991), 149–158.

[MRb] Marusic M. and Vuk-Pavlovic S., Prediction power of mathematical models for tumor growth, *J. Biological Systems*, **1** (1993), 69–78.

[MRc] Marusic M., Bajzer Z., Freyer J.P., and Vuk-Pavlovic S., Tumor growth *in vivo* and as multicellular spheroids compared by mathematical models, *Bull. Math. Biol.*, **56** (1994), 617–631.

[MUa] Murray J., **Mathematical Biology**, Springer (1994).

[NAa] Nanni P., De Giovanni C., Lollini P., Nicoletti G., and Prodi G., TS/A: A new metastasiging cell line originated from a BALB/c spontaneous mammary adenocarcinoma, *Clin. Exp. Med.*, **1** (1983), 373–380.

[NOa] Nossal G.J.V., Life, death and the immune system, *Scientific American*, **269** (1993), 53–72.

[PEa] Perelson A.S. and Bell G.I., Delivery of lethal hits by cytotoxic T lymphocytes in multicellular conjugates occurs sequentially but randomly, *J. Immunol.*, **129** (1982), 2796–2801.

[PEb] Perelson A.S. and MacKean C.A., Kinetics of cell-mediated cytotoxicity: Stochastic and deterministic multistage models, *J. Math. Biol.*, **170** (1984), 161–194.

[PEc] Perelson A.S. ed., **Theoretical Immunology**, Addison-Wesley (1988).

[PRa] Prehn R.T, Stimulatory effects of immune reactions upon the growth of transplanted tumors, *Cancer Res.*, **55** (1994), 908–914.

[PZa] Preziosi L., From population dynamics to the competition between tumors and immune system, *Math. Comp. Modelling - Special Issue on Modelling and Simulation Problems on Tumor-immune System Dynamics*, Bellomo N. ed., **23** (1996), 135–152.

[ROa] Rosenberg S., Lotze M., Yang J., Aebersold P., Linehan W., Seipp C., and White D., Experience with the use of high-dose interleukin-2 in the treatment of 652 cancer patients, *Ann. Surg.*, **210** (1989), 474–484.

[SEa] Segel L., **Modelling Dynamic Phenomena in Molecular and Cellular Biology**, Cambridge University Press (1984).

[SEb] Segel L. and Perelson A.S., Computations in phase space. A new approach to immune network theory, in **Theoretical Immunology II**, Addison-Wesley (1988), 321–342.

[SLa] Steel G.G., **Growth Kinetics of Tumors**, Clarendon (1977).

[SMa] Smoluchowski M.V., Versuch einer mathematischen theorie der koagulationskinetik, *Z. Phys. Chem.*, **92** (1917), 129–168.

[SRa] Stewart I.W., Global existence theorem for the general coagulation fragmentation equation with unbounded kernels, *Math. Meth. Appl. Sci.*, **11** (1989), 627–648.

[SRb] Stewart I.W., On the coagulation-fragmentation equation, *J. Appl. Math. Phys.*, **41** (1990), 746–756.

[SRc] Stewart I.W., Density conservation for a coagulation equation, *J. Appl. Math. Phys.*, **42** (1991), 746–756.

[STa] Sutherland R.M. and Durand R.E., Growth and cellular characteristics of multicell spheroids, *Recent Results in Cancer Research*, **95** (1984), 24–49.

[STb] Sutherland R.M., Cell and environment interactions in tumor microregions: The multicell spheroid model, *Science*, **240** (1988), 177–184.

[SWa] Swan G.W., The diffusion of an inhibitor in a spherical tumor, *Math. Biosci.*, **108** (1992), 75–79.

[TAa] Taubes G., Do immunologists dream of electric mice?, *Science*, **265** (1994), 886–888.

[TOa] Tomlison I.P. and Bodmer W.F., Failure of programmed cell death and differentiation as causes of tumors: Some simple mathematical models, *Proc. Natl. Acad. Sci. USA*, **92** (1995), 11130–11134.

[TRa] Truesdell C. and Muncaster R., **Fundamentals of Maxwell Kinetic Theory of a Simple Monoatomic Gas**, Academic Press (1980).

[YAa] Yakovlev A.Yu., Tsodikov A., and Asselain B., **Stochastic Models of Tumor Latency and their Applications**, World Sci. (1995).

5

From Mutation to Metastasis: The Mathematical Modelling of the Stages of Tumour Development

M.A.J. Chaplain

University of Bath
School of Mathematical Sciences
Bath, UK

ABSTRACT. Cancer is a complicated multi-stage process beginning at the intra-cellular level of genetic mutation processing to the inter-cellular level and then in some cases the inter-organ level (metastasis). There are three well-recognised carcinogenic agents which are known to directly cause tumour growth in animals or induce cell transformation and purposeless proliferation *in vitro*-viruses, chemical carcinogens and radiation. The genetic mutations occurring at the single cell level lead among other things to the transformed cells escaping the normal growth control mechanisms. This in turn, coupled with a favourable local environment and adequate nutrient supply, leads to the formation of a rapidly growing mass of tissue — a solid tumour. In the case of a malignant tumour, such as a carcinoma, this early growth remains avascular and limited in size to a few millimeters in diameter (cf. multicellular spheroids). The tumour cells may then secrete certain chemicals (angiogenic factors) which induce neighbouring blood vessels to form a well-organised capillary network which grows toward and connects with the primary tumour. Once supplied with its own micro-circulation invasive growth of the tumour is possible and the tumour cells may then spread to distant parts of the body via the lymph or blood systems. This chapter presents some mathematical models describing avascular tumour growth, angiogenesis and pre-invasive growth.

5.1 Introduction

The growth and development of solid tumours occurs in two distinct stages — the avascular growth phase and the vascular growth phase. During the former growth phase the tumour remains in a diffusion-limited, dormant state of a few millimeters in diameter (cf. multicell spheroids, carcinoma *in situ*) while during the latter growth phase, invasion and metastasis may take place. In order to accomplish the transition from avascular to vascular growth, solid tumours may secrete diffusible substances known as tumour angiogenesis factors (TAF) into the surrounding tissue. Endothelial cells which form the lining of neighbouring blood vessels respond to this chemotactic stimulus in a well-ordered sequence of events. Capillary sprouts are formed which migrate towards the tumour eventually penetrating it and permitting vascular growth to take place. It is during this stage of growth that the insidious process of invasion takes place. This paper will present several mathematical models (partial differential equations models, nonlinear elasticity models) which deal with the various stages of growth and development of solid tumours.

In vivo cancer growth, and as a particular example in this paper, solid tumour growth, is a complicated phenomenon involving many interrelated processes and as such presents the mathematical modeller with a correspondingly complex set of problems to solve. Even deciding which simplifying assumptions to make is a non-trivial task. In this paper we present a variety of mathematical models describing the various phases of solid tumour growth.

Solid tumours are known to progress through two distinct phases of growth — the avascular phase and the vascular phase [FOb], [FOc]. The initial avascular growth phase can be studied in the laboratory by culturing cancer cells in the form of three-dimensional *multicell spheroids* [DUb], [SUc], [MUE]. It is well known that these spheroids, whether grown from established tumour cell lines or actual *in vivo* tumour specimens, possess growth kinetics which are very similar to *in vivo* tumours. Typically, these avascular nodules grow to a few millimeters in diameter. Cells towards the centre, being deprived of vital nutrients, die and give rise to a necrotic core. Proliferating cells can be found in the outer three to five cell layers. Lying between these two regions is a layer of quiescent cells, a proportion of which can be recruited into the outer layer of proliferating cells. Much experimental data has been gathered on the internal architecture of spheroids, and studies regarding the distribution of vital nutrients (e.g. oxygen) and metabolites within the spheroids have been carried out [DUb], [BRUM], [DER], [ADG], [DUc], [FRa], [BG]. Indeed, recent research into the phenomenon of hypoxia [BRO] has meant that such studies are enjoying a new lease of life.

The transition from the dormant avascular state to the vascular state, wherein the tumour possesses the ability to invade surrounding tissue and metastasise to distant parts of the body, depends upon its ability to induce new blood vessels from the surrounding tissue to sprout towards and then gradually penetrate the tumour, thus providing it with an adequate blood supply and microcirculation. In order to accomplish this neovascularization, it is now a well-established fact that tumours secrete a number of diffusible chemical substances into the surrounding tissues and extracellular matrix. Much work has been carried out into the nature of such substances and their effect on endothelial cells since initial research began in the early 1970's with Folkman, culminating in the purification of several angiogenic factors, the cloning of their genes from libraries of complementary DNA (cDNA) and the determination of their amino acid sequences [FOd]. The extensive current literature on the subject is testimony to its importance in our understanding of the mechanisms by which solid tumours develop and grow (see, for example, the reviews of [FOd] and [PAW]).

The first events of angiogenesis are rearrangements and migration of EC situated in nearby vessels [PAK]. The main function of EC is in the lining of the different types of vessels such as venules and veins, arterioles and arteries, small lymphatic vessels and the thoracic duct. They form a single layer of flattened and extended cells and the intercellular contacts are very tight. Large intercellular spaces are not visible and any easy penetration of the established layer of cells is impossible. Special processes must take place for the intra- and extravasation of different cellular elements of the blood or the lymphatic fluids and tumour cells. Even intravascular tumour cells have to induce the formation of gaps in the single layer of EC in order to leave the respective vessels. These cells are the principal characters in the drama of angiogenesis and are always centre stage [PAW].

In response to the angiogenic stimulus, EC in the neighbouring normal capillaries which do not possess a muscular sheath are activated to stimulate proteases and collagenases. The endothelial cells destroy their own basal lamina and start to migrate into the extracellular matrix. Small capillary sprouts are formed by accumulation of EC which are recruited from the parent vessel. The sprouts grow in length by migration of the endothelial cells [SHO]. The experimental results of [SHO] demonstrated that EC are continually redistributed among sprouts, moving from one sprout to another. This permits the significant outgrowth of a network of sprouts even when cell proliferation is prevented [SHO]. At some distance from the tip of the sprout the EC divide and proliferate to contribute to the number of migrating EC. The mitotic figures are only observed once the sprout is already growing out and cell division is largely confined to a region just behind the sprout tip. Solid strands of EC are formed in the extracellular matrix. Lumina develop within these strands and mitosis continues.

Initially the sprouts arising from the parent vessel grow in a more or less parallel way to each other. They tend to incline toward each other at a definite distance from the origin when neighbouring sprouts run into one another and fuse to form loops or *anastomoses.* Both tip-tip and tip-branch anastomosis occur and the first signs of circulation can be recognised. From the primary loops, new buds and sprouts emerge and the process continues until the tumour is eventually penetrated.

Once vascularized the tumours grow rapidly as exophytic masses. In certain types of cancer, e.g. carcinoma arising within an organ, this process typically consists of columns of cells projecting from the central mass of cells and extending into the surrounding tissue area. The local spread of these carcinoma often assume an irregular jagged shape. By the time a tumour has grown to a size whereby it can be detected by clinical means, there is a strong likelihood that it has already reached the vascular growth phase.

In this chapter we present a review of some recent mathematical models which attempt to describe the various stages and processes involved in solid tumour growth — the avascular growth phase, tumour angiogenesis (capillary sprout formation) and vascular growth — while also presenting some new developments. In the following section we begin with a simple but general model for the growth of an avascular tumour nodule or multicell spheroid which focusses on the potential role played by one or more growth inhibitory factors and the effect of the spatial distribution of this factor on cell mitosis. In Section 5.3 we present a model for the growth and development of capillary sprouts during tumour angiogenesis. The model focusses on the roles of endothelial cell proliferation and migration during angiogenesis. New results concerning 2-dimensional simulations are presented. Section 5.4 develops and extends the model of Section 5.2 by introducing a growth promoting factor into the mathematical model and assesses the potential implications this may have for vascular tumour growth and invasion using reaction-diffusion theory. In Section 5.5 the relative merits and demerits of each model are discussed and various concluding remarks are made.

5.2 Avascular Tumour Growth: The Multicell Spheroid Model

The first mathematical model for the growth of a solid tumour which we present in this section focusses on the initial avascular stage of growth, wherein the tumour, or from an experimental point of view, the multicell spheroid, grows to a diffusion-limited size of a few millimeters in diameter.

To incorporate all of the known and observed experimental results into a mathematical model, even for an avascular tumour (multicell spheroid), would be a very formidable task indeed. Furthermore, from such a complicated model it would be difficult to focus on the roles of individual processes. Even deciding upon simplifying assumptions can be difficult. However, at minimum a realistic model of spheroid growth should include certain nonuniformities in the central processes of inhibition of mitosis, consumption of nutrients, cell proliferation; as well as the dependence of cell mitotic rate on growth inhibitor concentration, geometrical constraints and central necrosis.

Several papers ([ADJa], [DEG]) have focussed attention on the chemical inhibition of mitosis within multicell spheroids, the main assumption of the modelling being that a growth inhibitory factor (GIF) is produced within the spheroid in some prescribed spatially-dependent manner to reflect the observed cellular heterogeneity within spheroids.

The existence and properties of chemicals which inhibit mitosis are very well documented in [BRU] and [MAR]. Indeed there is experimental evidence concerning the specific effects of extracts from necrotic areas in tumours. It has been demonstrated that these extracts possess the ability to reduce the proliferation of cultured cells [LE] and also of monolayer tumour cells [FRe], [FRf] and the same effects have been proposed to occur in tumours *in vivo* [HA]. Initially we focus attention on the *diffusion* of a growth inhibitory factor within a multicell spheroid and its possible effect on cell mitosis and proliferation. To this end, instead of a nonlinear production term, we consider the effects of introducing a nonlinear, spatially-dependent diffusion coefficient. It is known that in spheroids normal structural associations (e.g. cell-cell junctions) are disrupted and hence the possibility arises of normal intercellular signals being disrupted also. Nonlinear diffusion of the GIF within the spheroid is one possible and simple way to take account of this. The results of this approach are then be compared and contrasted with those produced when a nonlinear production term is assumed.

The control of mitosis in tissues can be modelled as a schematic mechanism in which self-regulating growth is achieved as a result of negative feedback from the growing tissue [SHY]. In this approach mitosis is assumed to be controlled by a discontinuous switch-like mechanism, such that if the concentration of the (GIF) is less than some threshold level θ, say, in any region within the tissue, mitosis occurs in this region, whereas if the concentration is greater than θ, mitosis is completely inhibited. The differential equation describing the diffusion, production and degradation of the GIF within a spheroid can be written

$$\frac{\partial C}{\partial t} = D\nabla^2 C + f(C) + \lambda S(\mathbf{r}), \qquad \mathbf{r} \in \Omega, \tag{5.1}$$

where $C = C(\mathbf{r}, t)$ is the concentration of GIF within the spheroid occupying the region $\Omega \in \mathcal{R}^3$ and λ is the inhibitor production rate (molecules per unit volume per second).

A more detailed description of the background biology and the derivation of the above equation can be found in [ADJa] and [SHY]. Previous papers make the assumptions that the GIF is produced throughout the tissue by the individual cells, modelled by a source function $S(\mathbf{r})$, diffuses with a *constant* diffusion coefficient D and is depleted everywhere at a prescribed rate $f(C)$. [ADJa–c] and [SHY] use the function $f(C) = -\gamma C$, where γ is the decay or loss constant. Various forms for the source function $S(\mathbf{r})$ have been used. In the original model of [SHY], the GIF is assumed to be produced at a constant rate throughout the tissue yielding the *uniform* source function

$$\begin{cases} S(r) = 1\,, & 0 \le r \le R\,, \\ S(r) = 0\,, & r > R\,, \end{cases} \tag{5.2}$$

In an attempt to model more accurately the heterogeneity of cells within tumours, the models of [ADJa-c] consider a *non-uniform* source function of the form

$$\begin{cases} S(r) = 1 - r/R\,, & 0 \le r \le R\,, \\ S(r) = 0\,, & r > R\,, \end{cases} \tag{5.3}$$

where r is the distance from the origin. However, as shown by [BRI], the non-uniform source term of [ADJa–c] is unrealistic from a biological point of view since $S'(0) \neq 0$ and they suggest a smooth source function of the form

$$S(r) = \begin{cases} 1 - r^2/R^2\,, & 0 \le r \le R, \\ 0\,, & r > R. \end{cases} \tag{5.4}$$

If the above system is studied in a spherical geometry, with radial symmetry, that is a sphere of radius R, where the GIF concentration depends only on the radial distance from the centre of the sphere ($C \equiv C(r)$) then it may be used to model mitotic inhibition within multicell spheroids. As stated in the introduction, there is a large body of experimental data available for multicell spheroids which can be used to study tumour microregions, the results of which can be applied to *in vivo* tumours [SUc] [SUa]. Small spheroidal nodules of tumour cells can be grown in the laboratory, the growth kinetics of which closely follow the first avascular stage of *in vivo* tumour growth such as carcinomas. These grow to a diffusion-limited steady-state size a few millimeters in diameter. Cells at the centre of the avascular nodule are starved of vital nutrients and die [GREc], forming a central necrotic core. A thin layer of live, proliferating cells three to five cell layers thick forms at the periphery of the nodule while sandwiched between these two regions is a layer of quiescent cells. A proportion of the quiescent cells is reproductively viable and may be recruited into the proliferating compartment. One feature of spheroid growth which has hitherto not been treated in detail by mathematical models is the importance of cell-cell contacts. It is known that spheroids are held together by various surface membrane microprojections, extracellular matrix and a variety of cell-cell junctions including spot desmosomes, tight junctions, junctional complexes and gap junctions. It is possible that the loss of coupling between cells may play a critical role in the uncontrolled proliferation in cancer [LO]. In addition to this, whether through gap junctions or by other structures, intercellular permeability may not be constant between cells at different stages of spheroid growth [DER], [ADG], [HUL]. These observations suggest that diffusion of chemicals between cells may not be constant [FRa]. In this paper therefore, we examine the effect of spatial nonuniformity not on the production term but on the diffusion coefficient and to this end the model we consider is

$$\frac{\partial C}{\partial t} = \nabla . \left(D(\mathbf{r}) \nabla C \right) + f(C) + \lambda S(\mathbf{r}) \,, \qquad \mathbf{r} \in \Omega \,, \tag{5.5}$$

$$\frac{\partial C}{\partial r} = 0 \,, \qquad \mathbf{r} = \mathbf{0} \,, \tag{5.6}$$

$$D(\mathbf{r}) \frac{\partial C}{\partial n} + PC = 0 \,, \qquad \text{on} \quad \partial\Omega \,, \qquad P \geq 0 \,, \tag{5.7}$$

where we assume (initially) that production of GIF is via the uniform source function given in (5.2); P is the permeability of the tissue surface and the diffusion coefficient $D(\mathbf{r})$ in the above equation is now assumed to be spatially dependent i.e. it varies throughout the interior of the spheroid, for which there is experimental evidence [KAR]. Thus the observed cellular heterogeneity within spheroids, the heterogeneous intercellular permeability and the composition of the extracellular matrix is accounted for via nonlinear diffusion. The boundary conditions (5.6) and (5.7) have been dealt with at length elsewhere ([ADJa-c], [SHY]) and we will not discuss their derivation here.

Considering the spherical geometry described in the introduction and assuming radial symmetry, the above system reduces to

$$\frac{\partial C}{\partial t} = \frac{1}{r^2} \frac{\partial}{\partial r} \left(r^2 D(r) \frac{\partial C}{\partial r} \right) - \gamma C + \lambda \,, \qquad r \leq R \,, \tag{5.8}$$

$$\frac{\partial C}{\partial r} = 0 \,, \qquad r = 0 \,, \tag{5.9}$$

$$D(r)\frac{\partial C}{\partial r} + PC = 0\,, \qquad r = R\,. \tag{5.10}$$

In order to facilitate analysis of the above system it is convenient to nondimensionalise and hence we choose appropriate reference variables. The obvious variables to choose [CHAd] are, as the reference length R, the radius of the spheroid under consideration, as a reference GIF concentration, θ the critical threshold level of C and as a reference time R^2/D. Thus we define new variables

$$\tilde{r} = \frac{r}{R}\,, \qquad \tilde{C} = \frac{C}{\theta}\,, \qquad \tilde{t} = \frac{Dt}{R^2}\,.$$

We also assume that we can write

$$D(r) = Dd(r)\,,$$

where D is a constant. The system now becomes, upon dropping the tildes for notational convenience,

$$\frac{\partial C}{\partial t} = \frac{1}{r^2}\frac{\partial}{\partial r}\left(r^2 d(r)\frac{\partial C}{\partial r}\right) - L^2 C + aL^2\,, \tag{5.11}$$

$$\frac{\partial C}{\partial r} = 0\,, \qquad r = 0\,, \tag{5.12}$$

$$d(r)\frac{\partial C}{\partial r} + \frac{L}{\eta}C = 0\,, \qquad r = 1\,, \tag{5.13}$$

where

$$\kappa^2 = \frac{\gamma}{D}\,, \qquad L = \kappa R\,, \qquad a = \frac{\lambda}{\gamma\theta}\,, \qquad \eta = \frac{\sqrt{\gamma D}}{P}\,.$$

With this nondimensionalisation we see that once the parameters for a particular spheroid are determined, the only undetermined parameter is the radius R. The solutions to the above equation can therefore be monitored for different sized spheroids. Thus we can analyse the system using different values for the spheroid radius R while holding constant the various observable parameters associated with the system i.e. D, γ, P and λ/θ [SHY]. It is our intention to discover if a concentration profile of GIF inside the spheroid can be found corresponding to the observed pattern of necrosis seen experimentally.

Since it is known that rapidly growing tumours enlarge at a rate of the order 0.4–0.7 mm/day [BUL], while diffusing chemical substances, with diffusion coefficients of order $10^{-6}\text{cm}^2\text{s}^{-1}$, reach steady-state on a time-scale of the order of a few minutes, then it is sufficient to consider the corresponding steady-state equation given by

$$0 = \frac{1}{r^2}\frac{\partial}{\partial r}\left(r^2 d(r)\frac{\partial C}{\partial r}\right) - L^2 C + aL^2\,, \tag{5.14}$$

together with the boundary conditions (5.12) and (5.13). In order to accomplish this, (5.11) was solved using the NAG routine D03PGF, with zero initial conditions $C(r,0) = 0$. The steady-state solutions evolved on a time scale of $O(1)$. Different forms for the function $d(r)$ were considered, which we assume is some monotonic function of r. Both monotonically increasing functions of $d(r)$ ($d(0) < d(1)$) and monotonically decreasing functions ($d(0) > d(1)$) were investigated. For our purposes we chose $d(r) = 0.8 + 0.2r^2$ as an example of the former and $d(r) = 1.0 - 0.2r^2$ as an example of the latter (variability in diffusion constants between spheroids grown from different cell lines has been verified experimentally [FRa]). As stated above, once the observable parameters have been fixed, the concentration profile for different sized spheroids can be easily obtained from the steady-state solutions of (5.11) simply by varying one parameter, namely the spheroid radius R. Mathematical models for this stage of spheroid growth involving the dynamic evolution of the radius $R(t)$ can be found in, for example, [BUR] and [MAG]. In these models, since the initial growth of the spheroids is avascular, they grow to a *finite*, diffusion-limited size a few millimeters in diameter. Mathematically, as $t \to \infty$, $R(t) \to R^*$. Thus by varying (i.e. increasing) the value for R in (5.11) from an initial value $R(0)$, say, up to R^*, we can effectively follow the development of the GIF concentration profile within the spheroid as the spheroid grows. This seems intuitively more appropriate rather than letting $R \to \infty$ which does not happen in practice. We also note that a consequence of the nondimensionalisation is that in each case the critical threshold level for mitosis occurs at $C = 1$.

5.2.1 Results

The results presented in this section are compared with the experimental data of [FOa]. In order to compare and contrast our results with previous mathematical models, following [CHAd] and [SHY] we choose $D = 5 \times 10^{-7}\text{cm}^2\text{s}^{-1}$, $P = 10^{-4}\text{cms}^{-1}$ and $\gamma = 5 \times 10^{-5}\text{s}^{-1}$. Correspondingly, $\kappa = 10\text{cm}^{-1}$ and $\eta = 0.05$. We note that in accordance with our assumption of a spatially varying diffusion coefficient the value of D given above will hold only at $r = 1$, i.e. the tumour edge. The value of the diffusion coefficient in the interior of the spheroid will vary according to the prescribed function $d(r)$. In order to find a value for the parameter a, we follow the procedure of [CHAd] and use the experimental observation of [FOa] that when the

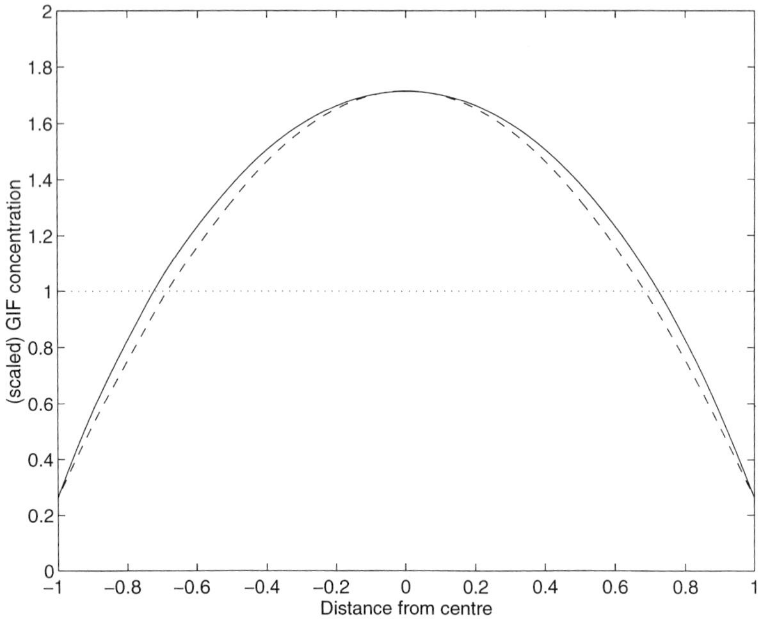

Figure 5.1 — Plot of GIF concentration profile within multicell spheroid of size $R = 0.05$cm; $D = 5 \times 10^{-7}$cm^{2}s^{-1}, $P = 10^{-4}$cms^{-1}; $\gamma = 5 \times 10^{-5}$s^{-1}; $a = 32.5$; $L = 0.5$; $\eta = 0.05$; (i) $d(r) = 0.8 + 0.2r^2$ (monotonically increasing), hatched line; (ii) $d(r) = 1.0 - 0.2r^2$ (monotonically decreasing), full line; constant source term.

spheroids are approximately 0.05cm in radius, the volume of the active mitotic zone is 0.6 of the total volume of the tissue. A simple calculation then shows that the size of the inner radius of the necrotic core must be 0.037cm. In terms of the nondimensionalized variables we therefore require that $C = 1$ when $r = 0.74$, $L = 0.5$, $\eta = 0.05$. Equation (5.11) was solved numerically with various values of the parameter a and allowed to evolve to steady-state. Figure 5.1 shows the steady-state profiles achieved with a value of

$$a = 32.5 \qquad \text{i.e.} \quad \frac{\lambda}{\theta} = 1.625 \times 10^{-3}\text{s}^{-1}$$

for (i) a monotonically increasing and (ii) a monotonically decreasing diffusion coefficient respectively. It can be seen from Figure 5.1 that this value of a (approximately) satisfies the above experimental constraint. Exact agreement could not be easily obtained since the analytic solution of (5.11) is not known. Figure 5.2 shows the steady-state GIF profiles within a spheroid of size 4mm in diameter i.e. the diffusion limited size. Once again the two curves correspond to (i) a monotonically increasing and (ii) a monotonically decreasing diffusion coefficient respectively. The horizontal line drawn at $C = 1$ in all figures is the threshold value for the GIF. Hence in any region of the spheroid where the GIF concentration is greater than 1 then mitosis will be inhibited here. This enables regions within the spheroid where mitosis is taking place and where mitosis is inhibited (necrotic core) to be easily distinguished. As can be clearly seen from Figure 5.2 the final steady-state GIF profile achieved is in good agreement with the experimental data of [FOa] where at the stable, diffusion-limited size there was a narrow layer of one or two cells which was mitotically active surrounding the necrotic core. These results also parallel those of [CHAd].

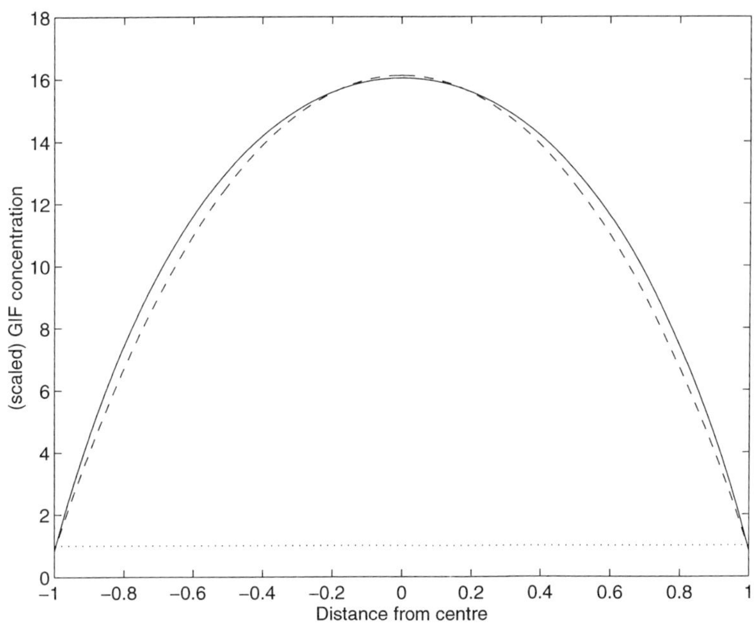

Figure 5.2 — Plot of GIF concentration profile within multicell spheroid of ultimate size $R = 0.2$cm; $D = 5 \times 10^{-7}\text{cm}^2\text{s}^{-1}$, $P = 10^{-4}\text{cms}^{-1}$; $\gamma = 5 \times 10^{-5}\text{s}^{-1}$; $a = 32.5$; $L = 2$; $\eta = 0.05$; (i) $d(r) = 0.8 + 0.2r^2$ (monotonically increasing), hatched line; (ii) $d(r) = 1.0 - 0.2r^2$ (monotonically decreasing), full line; constant source term.

We now also consider solving the above system with the constant source term being replaced by a spatially nonuniform source function of the type

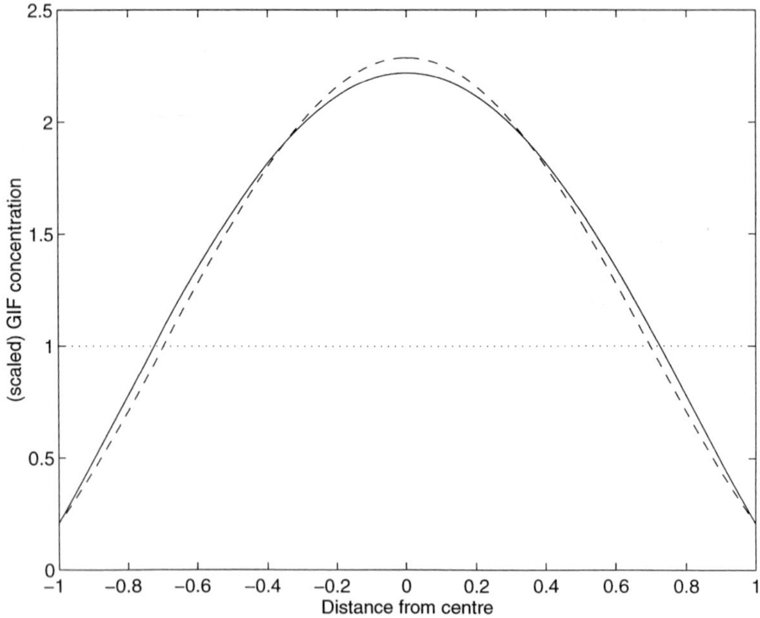

Figure 5.3 — Plot of GIF concentration profile within multicell spheroid of size $R = 0.05$cm; $D = 5 \times 10^{-7}\text{cm}^2\text{s}^{-1}$, $P = 10^{-4}\text{cms}^{-1}$; $\gamma = 5 \times 10^{-5}\text{s}^{-1}$; $a = 65$; $L = 0.5$; $\eta = 0.05$; (i) $d(r) = 0.8 + 0.2r^2$ (monotonically increasing), hatched line; (ii) $d(r) = 1.0 - 0.2r^2$ (monotonically decreasing), full line; nonlinear source term.

suggested by [CHAd] and [BRI] i.e.

$$S(r) = \begin{cases} 1 - r^2/R^2\,, & 0 \leq r \leq R, \\ 0\,, & r > R. \end{cases} \tag{5.15}$$

After nondimensionalization, the model equation now becomes

$$\frac{\partial C}{\partial t} = \frac{1}{r^2}\frac{\partial}{\partial r}\left(r^2 d(r)\frac{\partial C}{\partial r}\right) - L^2 C + aL^2(1 - r^2)\,. \tag{5.16}$$

Figure 5.3 shows the steady-state GIF concentration profiles obtained with a value of $a = 65$ for (i) a monotonically increasing and (ii) a monotonically decreasing nonlinear diffusion term respectively. Once again this value for a enables the experimental observation of [FOa] concerning the ratio of the volume of the active mitotic zone to the total tissue volume to be satisfied.

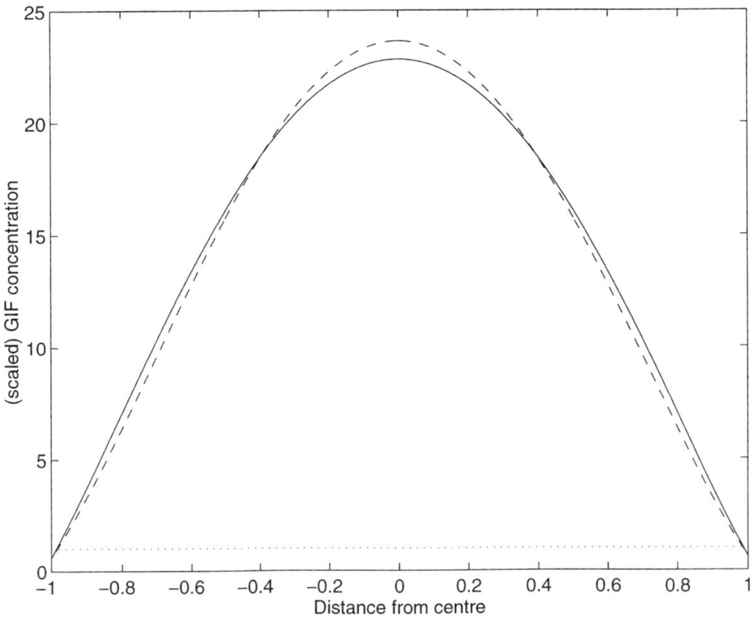

Figure 5.4 — Plot of GIF concentration profile within multicell spheroid of ultimate size $R = 0.2$cm; $D = 5 \times 10^{-7}\text{cm}^2\text{s}^{-1}$, $P = 10^{-4}\text{cms}^{-1}$; $\gamma = 5 \times 10^{-5}\text{s}^{-1}$; $a = 65$; $L = 2$; $\eta = 0.05$; (i) $d(r) = 0.8 + 0.2r^2$ (monotonically increasing), hatched line; (ii) $d(r) = 1.0 - 0.2r^2$ (monotonically decreasing), full line; nonlinear source term.

Figure 5.4 shows the corresponding steady-state GIF concentration profiles for a spheroid of ultimate size 0.4cm diameter. Again these show good agreement with the experimental observations.

We note for completeness that similar results to those of [BRI] can be obtained upon straightforward application of the maximum principle to (5.11–5.13) and (5.16). Using these techniques it is easily shown that, qualitatively, the final GIF concentration profile depends only on the qualitative form of the function $d(r)$ which can be chosen to model the interior heterogeneity of the spheroids.

5.3 Tumour Angiogenesis. Capillary Sprout Formation and Growth

In this section and throughout the rest of the paper wherever angiogenesis is mentioned, we choose to focus on the model system of [GI] [MUT] wherein a fragment of tumour is implanted into the cornea of a test animal and an angiogenic response is elicited from blood vessels situated in the nearby limbus region of the cornea. The mathematical model presented here is a development and extension of that of [CHAc].

Tumour angiogenesis factor having concentration $c(\mathbf{x}, t)$ is secreted by the solid tumour and diffuses into the surrounding tissue. Upon reaching neighbouring endothelial cells situated in, for example, the limbal vessels, the TAF stimulates the release of enzymes by the endothelial cells which degrade their basement membrane. As described in the introduction, after degradation of the basement membrane has taken place, the initial response of the endothelial cells is to begin to migrate towards the source of angiogenic stimulus. Capillary sprouts are formed and cells subsequently begin to proliferate at a later stage. Once the capillary sprouts have formed, mitosis is largely confined to a region a short distance behind the sprout tips [PAW], [SHO], [AUS], [STOb]. In [AUS] it was hypothesised that the reason for this proliferation was that these cells or vessels at the sprout tips were *acting as sinks* for the TAF. [BAL] also suggested that a sink term could be included in their model of capillary growth. Following [CHAc] and [CHAb], we thus incorporate a sink term for the TAF *in addition to* a natural decay term for the TAF. The conservation equation for the TAF concentration is thus given by

$$\boxed{\begin{array}{l}\text{rate of increase}\\ \text{of concentration}\\ \text{of moiety}\end{array}} = \boxed{\begin{array}{l}\text{diffusion}\\ \text{of moiety}\end{array}} + \boxed{\begin{array}{l}\text{production}\\ \text{of moiety}\end{array}} - \boxed{\begin{array}{l}\text{decay}\\ \text{of moiety}\end{array}}$$

which, under the assumption of linear Fickian diffusion, can be written mathematically as

$$\frac{\partial c}{\partial t} = D_c \nabla^2 c - f(c)g(n) - h(c)\,, \tag{5.17}$$

where D_c is the TAF diffusion coefficient. We assume that the local rate of uptake of TAF by the endothelial cells (modelled by the function $f(c)$) is governed by Michaelis–Menten kinetics (cf. [CHAb,c]) and that it also depends on the cell density, hence the inclusion of the function $g(n)$ i.e. the greater the density of endothelial cells, the more TAF will be removed by the cells acting as sinks (cf. [AUS] and [CHAb]). In general, the function $g(n)$ can therefore be chosen to be some strictly increasing function to account for this. For simplicity the actual function used in the model is given by $g(n) = n/n_0$, a simple linear function. More complicated choices are also possible however and do not affect the model qualitatively. We also assume that the decay of TAF with time is governed by first-order kinetics, a standard assumption cf. [SHE]. This leads to the following equation for the TAF in the external tissue

$$\frac{\partial c}{\partial t} = D_c \nabla^2 c - \frac{Qcn}{(K_m + c)n_0} - dc\,. \tag{5.18}$$

The initial condition is

$$c(\mathbf{x}, 0) = c_0(\mathbf{x})\,, \tag{5.19}$$

where $c_0(\mathbf{x})$ is a prescribed function chosen to describe qualitatively the profile of TAF in the external tissue when it reaches the limbal vessels cf. [CHAb]. The TAF is assumed to have a constant value c_b on the boundary of the tumour and to have decayed to zero at the limbus [CHAb] giving the boundary conditions as

$$c(0, t) = c_b\,, \qquad c(L, t) = 0\,. \tag{5.20}$$

Endothelial Cell Population Balance Equation

The endothelial cells are the principal characters in the drama of angiogenesis and are always centre stage [PAW]. It is therefore highly desirable and logical to include in our model an equation modelling the endothelial cells. The cascade of events which goes to make up the complex process of angiogenesis is essentially driven by the endothelial cells. We will thus follow the route of the endothelial cells from their origin in their parent vessel (e.g. the limbus), their crossing of the extracellular matrix and other material in the surrounding host tissue, to their destination within the tumour.

The first events of angiogenesis are rearrangements and migration of endothelial cells rather than induction of cell division [PAW], [PAK]. In response to the angiogenic stimulus, endothelial cells in the neighbouring normal capillaries which do not possess a muscular sheath are activated to stimulate proteases and collagenases. The endothelial cells destroy their own basal lamina and start to migrate into the extracellular matrix. Small capillary sprouts are formed by accumulation of endothelial cells which are recruited from the parent vessel. The sprouts grow in length by migration of the endothelial cells [SHO], [CLI], [SCH], [WAR]. The experimental evidence of [SHO] demonstrated that endothelial cells are continually redistributed among sprouts, moving from one sprout to another. This permits the significant outgrowth of a network of sprouts even when cell proliferation is prevented [SHO]. At some distance from the tip of the sprout the endothelial cells divide and proliferate to contribute to the number of migrating endothelial cells. The mitotic figures are only observed once the sprout is already growing out and cell division is largely confined to a region just behind the sprout tip. Solid strands of endothelial cells are formed in the extracellular matrix. Lumina develop within these strands and mitosis continues.

Initially the sprouts arising from the parent vessel grow in a more or less parallel way to each other. They tend to incline toward each other at a definite distance from the origin when neighbouring sprouts run into one another and fuse to form loops or *anastomoses.* Both tip-tip and tip-branch anastomosis occur and the first signs of circulation can be recognised. From the primary loops, new buds and sprouts emerge and the process continues until the tumour is eventually penetrated.

We now attempt to account for the above sequence of events using a population balance equation for the endothelial cells and to interpret the processes described above by analysing the endothelial cell density profile. The main events we model are the *migration* and the *proliferation* of the endothelial cells (the processes of anastomosis and budding will be accounted for implicitly in the model). We note that the migration and replication of endothelial cells are not linked together. Different types of stimuli are necessary for these two processes and we take this important fact into account in our model. We begin then with a general conservation equation for the endothelial cell density $n(\mathbf{x}, t)$ which is of the form [CHAc]

$$\frac{\partial n}{\partial t} + \nabla.\mathbf{J} = F(n)G(c) + H(n)\,, \tag{5.21}$$

where $\mathbf{J}$ is the cell flux, $F(n)$ and $H(n)$ are functions representing a normalised growth term and a loss term respectively for the endothelial cells. We assume that mitosis is governed by logistic type growth and that cell loss is a first order process [SHO], [CHAc]. Thus

$$F(n) = rn\left(1 - \frac{n}{n_0}\right)\,, \tag{5.22}$$

$$H(n) = -k_p n\,, \tag{5.23}$$

where r is a positive constant related to the maximum mitotic rate and k_p is the proliferation rate constant which is taken to be the reciprocal of the endothelial cell doubling time [STOb], [SHE]. We note that (5.22) contains a second order loss term while (5.23) is a first order loss term. [BAL] considered cell loss due to anastomosis (both tip-tip and tip-branch) as essentially a second order process, while [STOb] modelled endothelial cell loss due to budding as a first order loss term. Moreover they assumed that the probability of budding was uniform in all sprouts for all positions and all times. Thus these two terms implicitly account for endothelial cell loss due to anastomosis and budding respectively. Further we assume that the endothelial cell proliferation is controlled in some way by the TAF ([PAW], [PAK]) and this is reflected by the inclusion of the function $G(c)$ which is assumed to be nondecreasing. As stated previously, the initial response of endothelial cells to the angiogenic stimulus is one of migration [PAW], [PAK]. Proliferation is a crucial but secondary response. In order to account for this through the function $G(c)$ we assume that there is a threshold concentration level of TAF below which proliferation does not occur. Thus in the present model we chose $G(c)$ to be of the form

$$G(c) = \begin{cases} 0\,, & c \le c^*, \\ \dfrac{c - c^*}{c_b}\,, & c^* < c\,, \end{cases} \tag{5.24}$$

where $c^* \le c_b$. We note that a similar approach was used by [SHE] in modelling the chemical control of epithelial cells during wound healing.

There is substantial evidence that the response of the endothelial cells to the presence of the TAF is a chemotactic one ([AUS], [STOb]) and following [CHAc] we assume that the flux $\mathbf{J}$ of endothelial cells consists of two parts, one representing random motion and the other chemotactic motion of the cells. Thus

$$\mathbf{J} = \mathbf{J}_{\text{diffusion}} + \mathbf{J}_{\text{chemotaxis}}\,.$$

Once again we assume linear diffusion so that

$$\mathbf{J}_{\text{diffusion}} = -D_n \nabla n\,,$$

where D_n is the diffusion coefficient of the endothelial cells and

$$\mathbf{J}_{\text{chemotaxis}} = n\chi(c)\nabla c\,,$$

the well-known form for the chemotactic flux. Various functional forms have been proposed for $\chi(c)$ including a logarithmic law

$$\chi(c) = \frac{\chi_0}{c}\,,$$

a receptor kinetic law

$$\chi(c) = \frac{\chi_0 k}{(k+c)^2},$$

and a constant law

$$\chi(c) = \chi_0 \quad \text{(a constant)}.$$

For mathematical simplicity, throughout this paper we adopt the latter i.e. we take $\chi(c) = \chi_0$, a constant. We note however that the present model could easily be adapted to incorporate either the logarithmic law or the receptor kinetic law. The cell conservation equation can be written

rate of increase of cell density	=	cell migration	+	mitotic generation	−	cell loss

With the above assumptions we thus have the following population diffusion-chemotaxis equation for the endothelial cells

$$\frac{\partial n}{\partial t} = D_n \nabla^2 n - \chi_0 \nabla.(n\nabla c) + rn\left(1 - \frac{n}{n_0}\right) G(c) - k_p n, \tag{5.25}$$

where $G(c)$ is given by (5.24). We assume that initially the endothelial cell density at the limbus is a constant n_0 and zero elsewhere, giving initial condition

$$n(\mathbf{x}, 0) = \begin{cases} n_0, & x = L \\ 0, & x < L. \end{cases} \tag{5.26}$$

We assume that throughout the subsequent motion, the cell density remains constant at the limbus and hence the boundary condition here becomes

$$n(L, t) = n_0. \tag{5.27}$$

As stated previously, the main aim of the model is to monitor the progress of the endothelial cells (in particular those at the sprout tips) as they cross the ECM and eventually reach the tumour. Once they reach the tumour and penetrate it interactions with the tumour cells become important [PAW] and the assumptions of the present model no longer hold. The modelling of this stage of the process is considered by [LIO] and [CHAa]. Thus within the assumptions and limitations of the present model we consider the following boundary condition at $\mathbf{x} = \mathbf{0}$:

$$n = 0 \quad \text{at} \quad \mathbf{x} = \mathbf{0}. \tag{5.28}$$

Under the assumptions of the model this boundary condition will remain valid up to the time when the endothelial cells at the sprout tips first reach the tumour.

Following [CHAb,c] we normalize the equations using the following reference variables

- reference TAF concentration: c_b, the value of the TAF concentration at the tumour boundary;
- reference cell density: n_0, the value of the endothelial cell density at the limbus;
- reference length: L, the distance from the tumour boundary to the limbal vessels;
- reference time unit: $\tau = L^2/D$.

We thus define new variables:

$$\tilde{c} = c/c_b\,, \qquad \tilde{n} = n/n_0\,, \qquad \tilde{x} = x/L\,, \qquad \tilde{t} = t/\tau\,.$$

Dropping the tildes and specialising to a one dimensional geometry the equations now become

$$\frac{\partial c}{\partial t} = \frac{\partial^2 c}{\partial x^2} - \frac{\alpha n c}{\gamma + c} - \lambda c\,, \tag{5.29}$$

$$\frac{\partial n}{\partial t} = D\frac{\partial^2 n}{\partial x^2} - \kappa \frac{\partial}{\partial x}\left(n\frac{\partial c}{\partial x}\right) + \mu n(1-n)G(c) - \beta n\,, \tag{5.30}$$

where

$$\begin{aligned} G(c) &= \begin{cases} 0\,, & c \le c^* \\ c - c^*\,, & c^* < c\,, \end{cases} \\ \alpha &= \frac{L^2 Q}{D_c c_b}\,, \quad \gamma = \frac{K_m}{c_b}\,, \quad \lambda = \frac{L^2 d}{D_c}\,, \\ D &= \frac{D_n}{D_c}\,, \quad \kappa = \frac{c_b \chi_0}{D_c}\,, \quad \mu = \frac{L^2 r}{D_c}\,, \\ \beta &= \frac{L^2 k_p}{D_c}\,. \end{aligned} \tag{5.31}$$

The initial and boundary conditions become respectively

$$c(x,0) = c_0(x)\,, \tag{5.32}$$

$$n(x,0) = \begin{cases} 1\,, & x = 1 \\ 0\,, & x < 1\,, \end{cases} \tag{5.33}$$

$$c(0,t) = 1\,, \qquad c(1,t) = 0\,, \tag{5.34}$$

$$n(1,t) = 1\,, \tag{5.35}$$

$$n = 0 \quad \text{at} \quad x = 0\,. \tag{5.36}$$

As we have mentioned previously, angiogenic factors must be able to provoke three main activities of the endothelial cells, namely

i) production and secretion of enzymes capable of digesting extracellular matrix,

ii) the initiation of *migration*, and

iii) cell *proliferation*. It is clear from experimental evidence ([SHO], [WRI], [REI]) that *different* types of stimuli are necessary for ii) and iii) and we note that this is accounted for in the model i.e. migration is governed by chemotaxis while proliferation is governed by the function $G(c)$ which essentially only depends on the TAF concentration. As stated previously the processes of anastomosis and budding are also (implicitly) accounted for through the second and first order loss terms respectively in Eq. (5.30). Moreover, the form of the function $G(c)$ ensures that the second order loss term implicitly modelling anastomosis will only take effect after the sprouts have reached a certain distance into the extracellular matrix which is precisely what is observed experimentally [PAW], [PAK].

We now present the results from the numerical simulation of Eqs. (5.29–5.30) with appropriate boundary and initial conditions. As far as possible parameter values are chosen to correspond to available experimental data.

For a reference length we choose L = 2mm, an average distance between a tumour implant and the limbal vessels, and the value for τ is taken to be 14 days, an average time for neovascularization to occur [STOb], [BAL]. According to the nondimensionalisation in Eq. (5.31), this gives a value for D_c of $3.3 \times 10^{-8}\text{cm}^2\text{s}^{-1}$. [SHE] found values of $3.1 \times 10^{-7}\text{cm}^2\text{s}^{-1}$ and $5.9 \times 10^{-6}\text{cm}^2\text{s}^{-1}$ as estimates for diffusion coefficients of chemicals. Correspondingly, they estimated the diffusion coefficients D_n of the epithelial cells under consideration in their model as $3.5 \times 10^{-10}\text{cm}^2\text{s}^{-1}$ and $6.9 \times 10^{-11}\text{cm}^2\text{s}^{-1}$. Using these values the ratio D_n/D_c thus varies between 1.1×10^{-3} and 1.2×10^{-5}. In accordance with this range we choose D to be 10^{-3}.

[STOd] have measured the value for the chemotaxis coefficient χ_0 of endothelial cells migrating in a medium containing unpurified acidic fibroblast growth factor (aFGF) as $2600\text{cm}^2\text{s}^{-1}\text{M}^{-1}$. As above, the value for D_c is estimated at $3.3 \times 10^{-8}\text{cm}^2\text{s}^{-1}$. In the numerical simulations carried out the (nonzero) values for κ varied between 0.3 and 1.0 which from Eq. (5.31) gives a value of c_b of approximately 10^{-11}M which is not unreasonable.

From equation (5.25) we assume that the parameter r is a positive constant related to the maximum mitotic rate. Using data based on epidermal wound healing ([WIN], [SHE]) estimated that the maximum value $r_{\max}$ for this parameter was 10 times the proliferation rate constant. Based on *in vitro* experiments on endothelial cell proliferation [WIL] and [STOb] estimated the proliferation rate constant k_p of endothelial cells to be 0.056hr^{-1} under the assumption that all cells proliferate. However cell mitosis in the sprouts is mainly confined to a region close to the tips. To compensate for this, in most of their simulations Stokes and Lauffenburger reduced the value of k_p to 0.02hr^{-1} and assumed that all cells in a sprout may proliferate. Thus in the following numerical simulations we assume a range for $r_{\max}$ of $0.2\text{hr}^{-1} - 0.56\text{hr}^{-1}$. Under this assumption this gives a range of values for the cell proliferation parameter μ of approximately $70 - 190$.

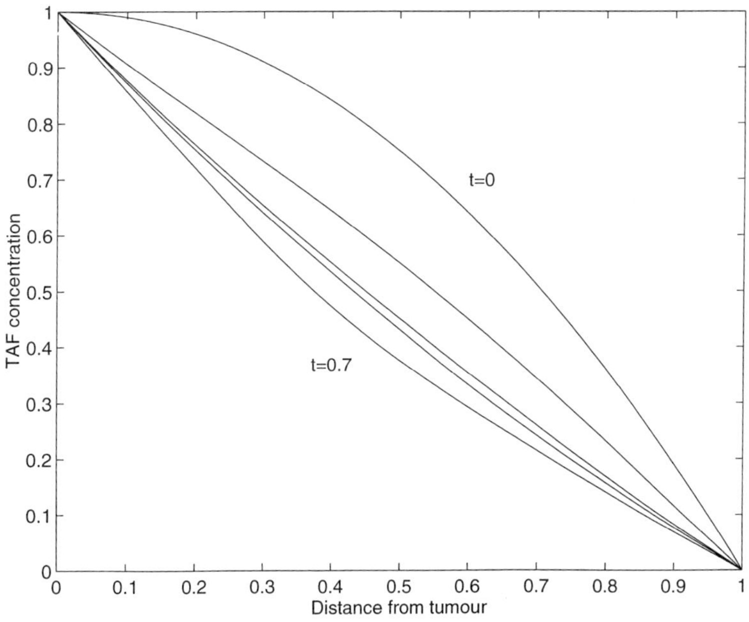

Figure 5.5 — Profile of the TAF concentration in the external host tissue at times $t = 0, 0.1, 0.3, 0.5, 0.7$ showing changing gradient profile. Parameter values: $\alpha = 10$, $\gamma = 1$, $\delta = 1$, $D = 0.001$, $\kappa = 0.7$, $\mu = 100$, $\beta = 4$, $c^* = 0.2$.

The parameter k_p is the reciprocal of the endothelial cell doubling time (cf. [SHE]). As seen above [SHE] estimated this to lie within the range $0.02\text{hr}^{-1} - 0.056\text{hr}^{-1}$. Also, from experimental data on epidermal cells [WRI], [SHE] estimated this to be 0.01hr^{-1}. This gives a range of values for the cell loss parameter β of approximately $3 - 18$.

The initial condition (5.19) was taken to be $c(x, 0) = c_0(x) = 1 - x^2$ which is of the correct qualitative shape for the TAF profile in the external tissue i.e. a constant value of 1 at the tumour edge decaying away to 0 at the limbus.

Figures 5.5 and 5.6 show the profiles of the TAF concentration and the endothelial cell density respectively in the external host tissue at various different times. As can be seen from Figure 5.2, shortly after $t = 0.7$ the model loses its validity since the endothelial cells reach the tumour and interactions between tumour cells and endothelial cells become important. The time taken for the endothelial cells to first reach the tumour corresponds to a real time of approximately 11 days which is within the experimentally observed timescale cf. [BAL]. By varying the parameters μ and κ the time taken for the endothelial cells (and hence the capillary sprouts) to reach the tumour can also be varied.

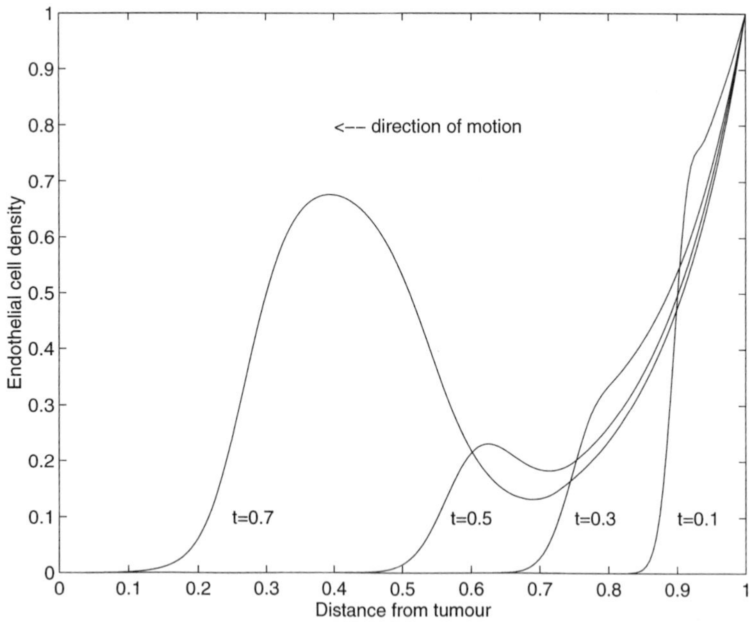

Figure 5.6 — Profile of the endothelial cell density in the external host tissue at times $t = 0, 0.1, 0.3, 0.5, 0.7$. Shortly after $t = 0.7$ the endothelial cell reach the tumour and the assumptions of the model no longer hold. Parameter values as per Figure 5.5.

Figure 5.7 shows the endothelial cell density profile when the chemo-

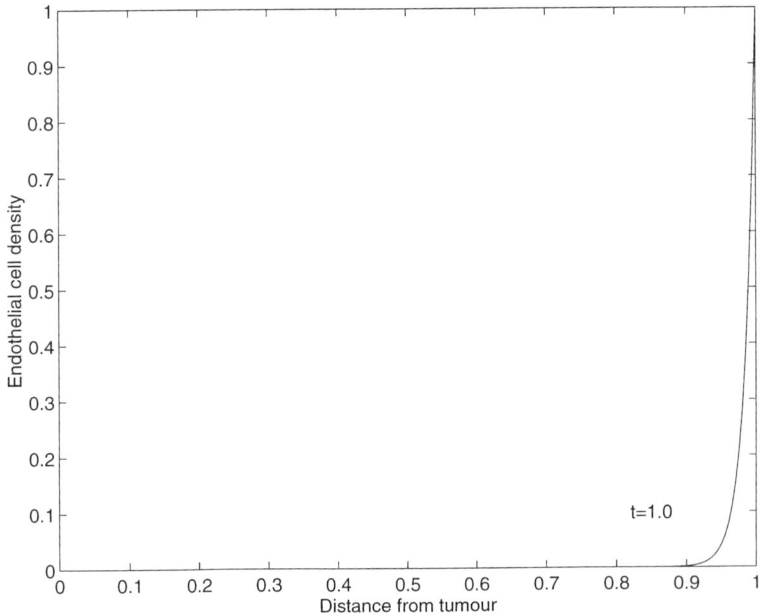

Figure 5.7 — Profile of the endothelial cell density in the external host tissue at $t = 1.0$ when the chemotaxis parameter κ is set to zero. The figure shows very little cell, and hence sprout, growth. This illustrates that cell migration is vital to the complete process of angiogenesis. Parameter values: $\alpha = 10$, $\gamma = 1$, $\delta = 1$, $D = 0.001$, $\kappa = 0.0$, $\mu = 90$, $\beta = 4$, $c^* = 0.2$.

tactic response parameter $\kappa = 0$ and as can clearly be seen, there is very little cell response indicating that chemotaxis, and therefore cell migration, plays a major initiating role in the angiogenic process.

Figure 5.8 shows the endothelial cell density profile when the cell proliferation parameter $\mu = 0$ and once again the effect of this is significant. The figure shows that cell outgrowth, and hence sprout outgrowth, has virtually ceased after $t = 0.4$ which corresponds to a real time of 3.5 days. This is in very good agreement both with experimental evidence [SHO] and with the model of [STOb]. The previous two figures demonstrate that neither cell migration (via chemotaxis) nor cell proliferation alone is sufficient for a completion of angiogenesis which is in agreement with experimental observations. In order for a completion of angiogenesis both events must be included in the model which is what is observed experimentally.

Comparing Figure 5.6 with Figure 5.8 demonstrates a good qualitative agreement with the available experimental evidence. Both simulations give

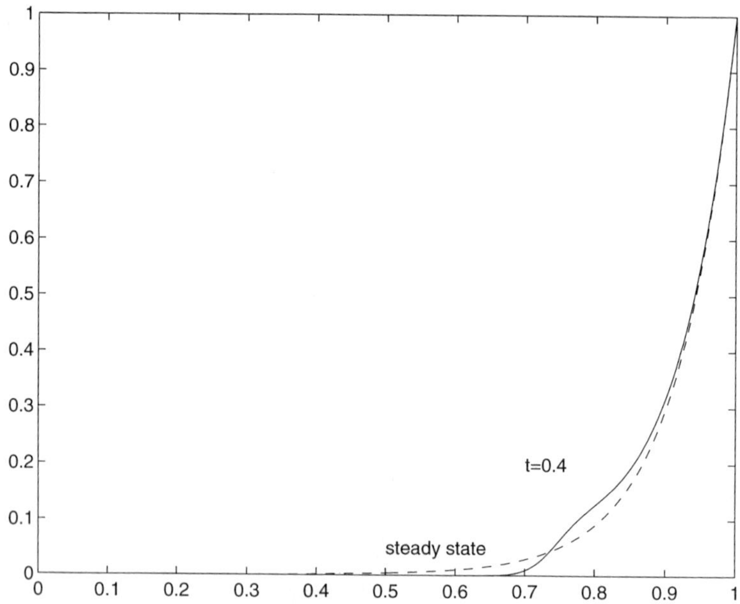

Figure 5.8 — Profile of the endothelial cell density in the external host tissue at $t = 0.4$ (full line) and at steady state (hatched line) when the cell proliferation parameter μ is set to zero. All outgrowth has stopped by steady state. The figure clearly shows that at $t = 0.4$ sprout outgrowth has virtually ceased, which is in agreement with the experimental evidence. This illustrates that cell proliferation is essential for the completion of angiogenesis. Parameter values: $\alpha = 10$, $\gamma = 1$, $\delta = 1$, $D = 0.001$, $\kappa = 0.5$, $\mu = 0.0$, $\beta = 6$, $c^* = 0.2$.

the same profile of cell density for times $0 \leq t \leq 0.4$. This shows that the initial response of the endothelial cells is essentially one of migration with proliferation of the cells occurring at a later time. The form of the function $G(c)$ ensures that there is always a region within the sprouts where there is zero cell proliferation and also that once cells have started to proliferate, the proliferation is mainly confined to a region a short distance behind the sprout tips. Thus the model distinguishes, as far as is possible within its limitations, between proliferating cells near the sprout tip and non-proliferating cells within the rest of the sprout. Also once the cells have started to proliferate the endothelial cell density is greatest (locally) a short distance behind the sprout tips which is what is observed experimentally [PAW], [SHO], [AUS]. Similar results were obtained for different functions

$G(c)$ which were of the same qualitative form as (5.24).

For all numerical simulations carried out we took $c^* = 0.2$. Qualitatively similar results were obtained for various other values of c^* between 0.1 and 0.4. We note that other numerical simulations were carried out with $D = 0$ and $\alpha = 0$. In each case, the profiles of TAF concentration and endothelial cell density remained almost the same as when these parameters were nonzero. In the former case this would seem to confirm the results of the models of [STOb] and [BAL] where diffusion was also seen to have a negligible effect on the results.

5.3.1 Model improvements and extension

Endothelial cell population balance equation

The main events captured in the model of the previous section are the *migration* and the *proliferation* of the EC, with the important processes of *anastomosis* and secondary *budding/sprouting* being accounted for implicitly. We now extend the model by incorporating these two processes explicitly via the function $H(n)$. This function must now incorporate a (spatial) term which models cell loss due secondary sprouting of tips from an existing capillary and at the same time model the effect of anastomosis (tip-tip or tip-branch) on a capillary. It is assumed that the net effect of anastomosis will be to increase the cell density at that particular location of the capillary where fusion takes place. Thus

$$H(n) = -k_p n - s(\mathbf{x})n\,, \tag{5.37}$$

where the function $s(\mathbf{x})$ will be taken to be some appropriate periodic function of the spatial variable $\mathbf{x}$, (e.g. $\cos(a\pi x)$) whose *average* value over a period is zero. Such a function will thus represent the effect of anastomosis for half its period (net increase in cell density due to cell gain) and the effect of secondary budding for the other half period (net reduction in cell density due to cell loss). This means that we assume secondary budding and anastomosis occur in a consecutive, periodic manner and is a reasonable approximation to what are essentially two random processes.

We also assume that the diffusion of the EC is density dependent which also generalises the model of [CHAc]. The flux $\mathbf{J}$ is now written

$$\mathbf{J} = -D_n \left(\frac{n}{n_0}\right)^{\sigma} \nabla n + n\chi_0 \nabla c\,. \tag{5.38}$$

Simple Fickian diffusion is recovered on taking $\sigma = 0$. With the above assumptions we thus have the following population diffusion-chemotaxis equation for the EC

$$\frac{\partial n}{\partial t} = D_n \nabla . \left(\left(\frac{n}{n_0} \right)^{\sigma} \nabla n \right) - \chi_0 \nabla . (n \nabla c) + rn \left(1 - \frac{n}{n_0} \right) G(c) - k_p n - s(\mathbf{x}) n \,. \tag{5.39}$$

Suitable initial and boundary conditions for the EC are prescribed depending upon the precise domain in which the above equations are solved. After a suitable normalization the above equations are solved numerically and the results presented in the following section where the exact form of the boundary and initial conditions will also be given.

Finally, we also note that the numerical simulations of the previous section indicate that the concentration profile for c rapidly reaches a steady state profile. This is not entirely unexpected since the TAF diffuses much faster than the endothelial cells. Thus a reasonable approximation to the TAF concentration profile may be obtained by solving

$$\nabla^2 c - \lambda c = 0 \,, \tag{5.40}$$

subject to $c = 1$ at tumour boundary, $c = 0$ at all other boundaries. This simplification means that now our model is reduced to a single partial differential equation

$$\frac{\partial n}{\partial t} = D_n \nabla . \left(n^{\sigma} \nabla n \right) - \kappa \nabla . (n \nabla c) + \mu n (1 - n) G\big(c(\mathbf{x})\big) - \beta n - s(\mathbf{x}) n \,, \tag{5.41}$$

with appropriate initial and boundary conditions for n. This equation is solved numerically and the results are presented in the following section.

5.3.2 Numerical simulations

We firstly solve our equation in a one dimensional domain, normalized to be $[0, 1]$. We assume the tumour implant is situated at $x = 0$ and the EC at $x = 1$. The solution to (5.40) (in one space dimension) is given by

$$c(x) = \frac{\sinh \left[(1 - x) \sqrt{\lambda} \right]}{\sinh \sqrt{\lambda}} \,. \tag{5.42}$$

It can be shown that a good approximation to the TAF concentration profile with $\lambda = 1$ can be obtained on taking $c = 1 - x$. The equation to be solved is thus

$$\frac{\partial n}{\partial t} = D \frac{\partial}{\partial x} \left(n^{\sigma} \frac{\partial n}{\partial x} \right) + \kappa \frac{\partial n}{\partial x} + \mu (1 - x) n (1 - n) - \beta n - s(x) n \,, \tag{5.43}$$

with initial conditions

$$n(x,0) = \begin{cases} 1, & x = 1, \\ 0, & \text{elsewhere} \end{cases} \tag{5.44}$$

and boundary conditions $n(1,t) = 1$, $n(0,t) = 0$.

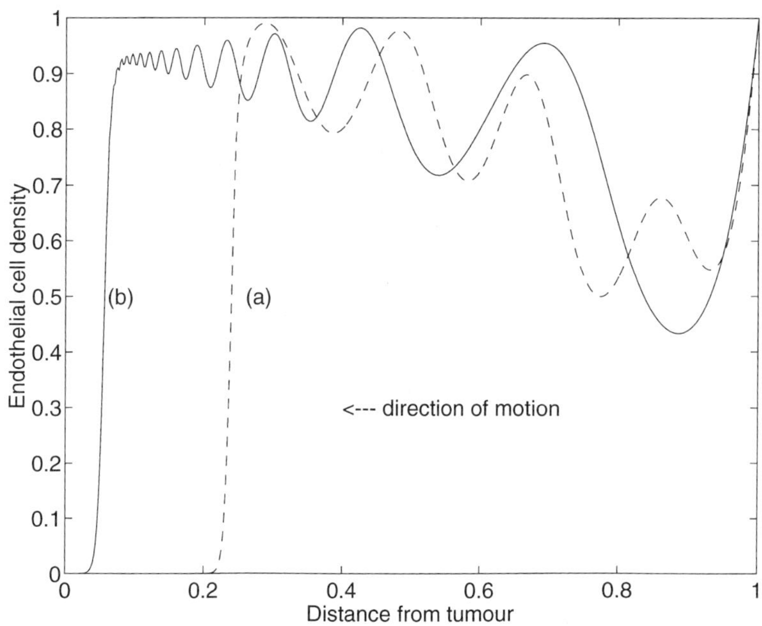

Figure 5.9 — Profile of the endothelial cell density in the host tissue at a time corresponding to 12 days. Profile (a) (hatched line) corresponds to regular anastomosis/side-branching with $s(x) = 5\cos(10\pi x)$, profile (b) (full line) corresponds to more frequent anastomosis/side-branching with $s(x) = 5\cos(2.25\pi x)$. Parameter values: $D = 0.001$, $\sigma = 4$, $\kappa = 0.6$, $\mu = 75$, $\beta = 5$.

Figure 5.9 shows the endothelial cell density profile in the external tissue for two different functions $s(x)$. As can clearly be seen in each case, the results capture qualitatively both the effects of anastomosis (local maxima) and the formation of side branches (local minima) as the capillary sprout migrates towards the tumour. For profile (a) (hatched line) we chose $s(x) = 5\cos(10\pi x)$ representing a regular spatial occurrence of both anastomosis and side-branching. However in profile (b) (solid line)

$s(x) = 5\cos(2.25\pi/x)$ which represents more faithfully the fact that as the capillary network progresses, anastomosis and side-branching occur more frequently. This captures more faithfully the so-called brush-border effect reported by [MUT].

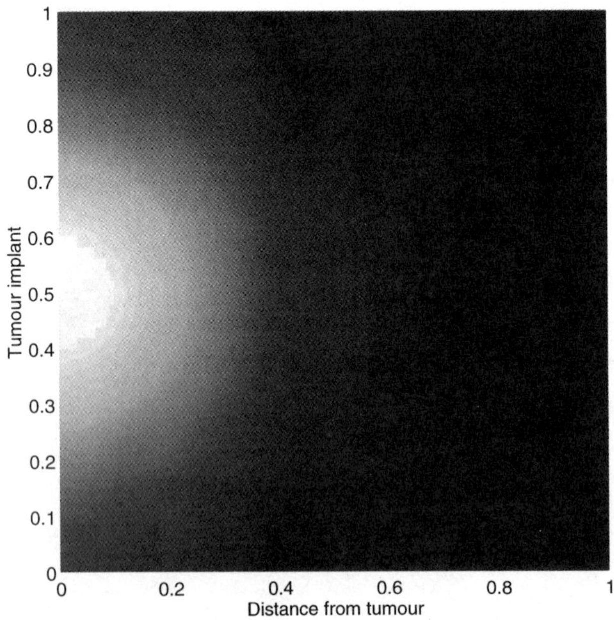

Figure 5.10 — Profile of the steady state TAF concentration profile given by (5.45) used in the 2 dimensional simulations. White = high concentration, black = low.

Experiments are often carried out in very thin regions ($< 50\mu$m) of the cornea or ear chamber of test animals ([GI], [MUT], [STOb]) and so a two dimensional domain is a good approximation of the sprout growth. Using normalized variables, we work on the unit square $[0,1] \times [0,1]$ and assume that the tumour implant occupies the region $(x-0.5)^2 + y^2 \leq 0.1$. We assume that the TAF diffuses in a radially symmetric manner and it can easily be seen that the corresponding solution to (5.40) (in polar coordinates with radial symmetry) is given in terms of Bessel functions but once again we find a very good approximation is given by

$$c(x,y) = c(r) = \begin{cases} 1, & r \leq 1, \\ (1-r)^2/0.81, & r > 1, \end{cases} \tag{5.45}$$

where $r^2 = (x - 0.5)^2 + y^2$. This profile is illustrated in Figure 5.10.

The single equation we now have to solve is given by

$$\frac{\partial n}{\partial t} = D\frac{\partial}{\partial x}\left(n^{\sigma}\frac{\partial n}{\partial x}\right) + D\frac{\partial}{\partial y}\left(n^{\sigma}\frac{\partial n}{\partial y}\right) - \kappa\frac{\partial}{\partial x}\left(n\frac{\partial c}{\partial x}\right) - \kappa\frac{\partial}{\partial y}\left(n\frac{\partial c}{\partial y}\right)$$
$$+ \mu c(x,y)n(1-n) - \beta n - s(x,y)n\,. \tag{5.46}$$

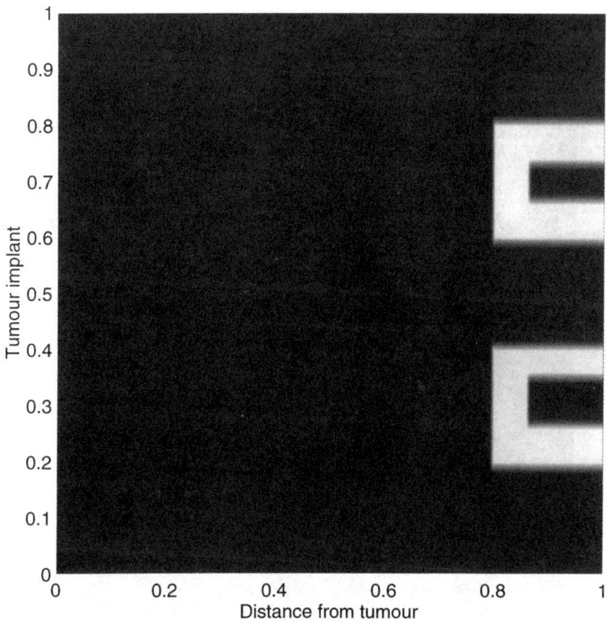

Figure 5.11 — Profile of the initial conditions used for the endothelial cell density simulating the formation of two loops. White = high density, black = low.

We assume that the initial phase of capillary sprout growth has taken place i.e. the cells have secreted enzymes which degrade their basement membrane permitting the formation of small buds [PAW], [PAK]. Indeed, [MUT] do not consider tumour-induced angiogenesis to be initiated until 2 days after implant and only designate a stage I of angiogenesis after 4 days recognising that there may well be some limbal response to the actual preparation of the implant site. [PAW] report two different initial mechanisms from which angiogenesis develops:

- Loops of vessels already present in the parental microcirculation are elongated towards the angiogenic stimulus (TAF) by intercalating EC. They always penetrate the tumour implant as loops. Blood flow is possible within these elongating loops, but is realised only after completion of neovascularization. This kind of growth of new vessels apparently occurs after mild angiogenic stimulation and slow development of vascularization.
- During strong angiogenic induction and rapid growth, mostly sprouts which have to fuse at their tips to develop loops are formed.

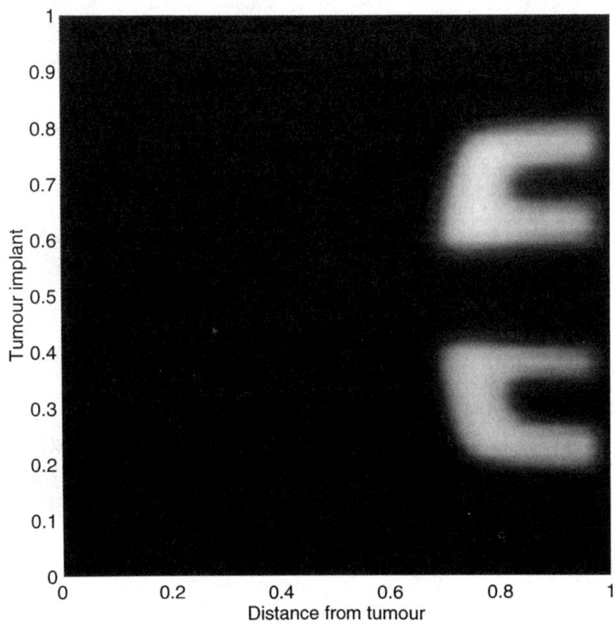

Figure 5.12 — Profile of the endothelial cell density at time $t = 0.3$ showing evolution of the two loops. Parameter values: $D = 0.001$, $\sigma = 1$, $\kappa = 0.6$, $\mu = 75$, $\beta = 0.5$.

We present initial conditions for each of the above scenarios. In the first case, we assume a loop (or loops) have already formed from pre-existing vessels (e.g. in the limbus) and assume that the endothelial cell density within this loop is initially a constant $n_0 = 1$ and zero elsewhere giving initial conditions

$$n(\mathbf{x},0) = \begin{cases} n_0 = 1\,, & \mathbf{x} \quad \text{within loop} \\ 0\,, & \mathbf{x} \quad \text{elsewhere.} \end{cases} \tag{5.47}$$

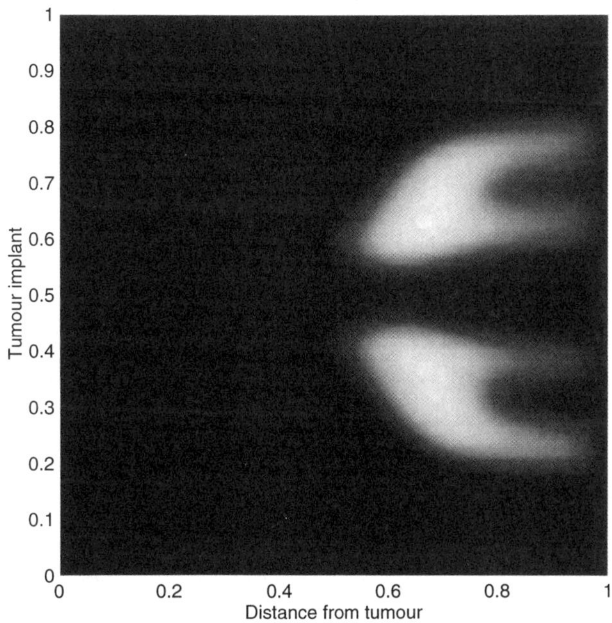

Figure 5.13 — Profile of the endothelial cell density at time $t = 0.5$ showing further evolution of the two loops. Parameter values: $D = 0.001$, $\sigma = 1$, $\kappa = 0.6$, $\mu = 75$, $\beta = 0.5$.

In the second case, we assume that there are several capillary buds which have formed and we focus attention exclusively upon those endothelial cells which are close to the sprout tips since only these cells proliferate. Here the endothelial cell density is initially a constant $n_0 = 1$ and zero elsewhere, giving initial conditions

$$n(\mathbf{x},0) = \begin{cases} n_0 = 1\,, & \mathbf{x} \quad \text{near sprout tip} \\ 0\,, & \mathbf{x} \quad \text{elsewhere.} \end{cases} \tag{5.48}$$

Since we are attempting to focus attention on the EC near to the sprout tips (since these are the cells which proliferate) and also since all the EC

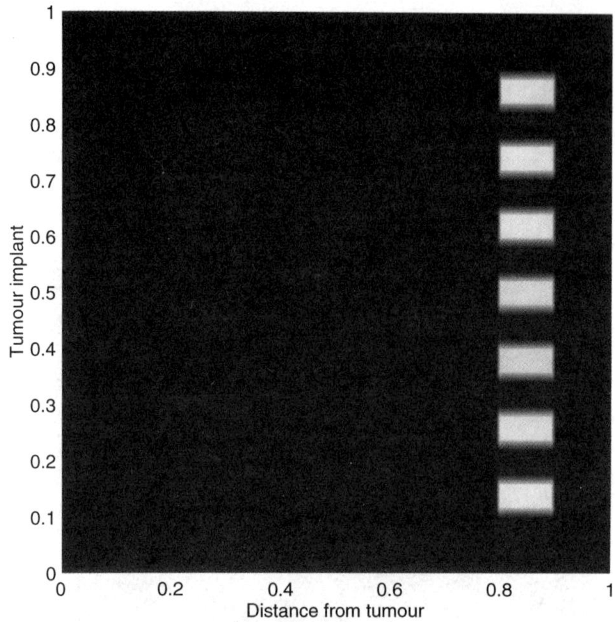

Figure 5.14 — Profile of the initial conditions used for the endothelial cell density simulating the formation of several capillary sprouts. White = high density, black = low.

are confined to within the capillary sprouts, we take the EC density to be zero ($n = 0$) on all boundaries.

Figures 5.11, 5.12 and 5.13 show the evolution of two loops at times $t = 0, 0.3, 0.5$ as they migrate towards the tumour implant with initial conditions as per (5.47). In this case we chose $s(x, y,) = 0$ since anastomosis and side-branching do not appear as frequently in this situation [PAW]. As can be seen from the figures the loops continue to develop and progress as loops. Further figures at later times show that they penetrate the tumour as loops which is what is observed experimentally [PAW].

Figures 5.14, 5.15 and 5.16 show the EC density profile within the capillary sprouts as they migrate towards the tumour with initial conditions as per (5.48). In this case we chose $s(x, y) = 10\cos^6(25\pi x)$, $y < 0.65; s(x, y) = 0$, $y \geq 0.65$, representing explicitly the effect of the brush-border once the initial sprouts/loops have all anastomosed cf. [MUT].

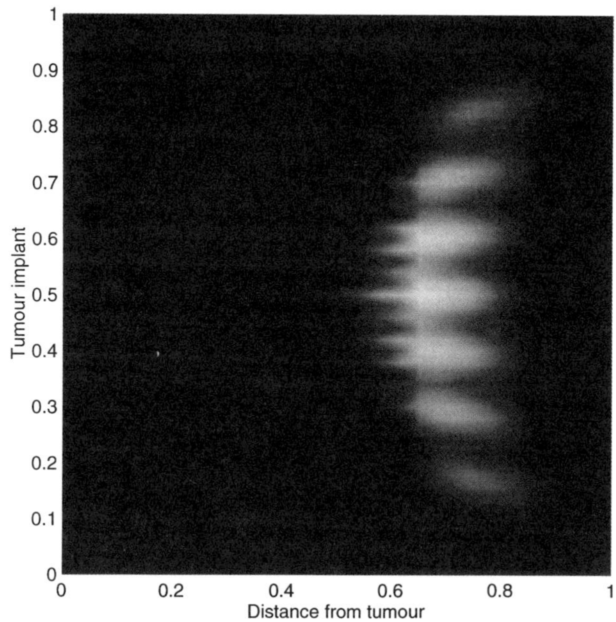

Figure 5.15 — Profile of the endothelial cell density after the capillary network has been established and anastomosis has taken place corresponding to a real time of 5–6 days after initial sprouts have formed as per Figure 5.13. Parameter values: $D = 0.001$, $\sigma = 1$, $\kappa = 0.6$, $\mu = 75$, $\beta = 0.5$.

5.4 Vascular Tumour Growth

While the process of angiogenesis is taking place, the avascular tumour although dormant (or quasi-dormant) with regard to its growth is still in a dynamic state. In this section we consider the possibility of the development of a heterogeneous cellular pre-pattern which takes place prior to successful angiogenesis and which then facilitates the vascular, invasive growth. Experimental results have demonstrated that tumour cells secrete both growth-activating and growth-inhibiting chemicals. The models presented in Section 5.2 have focussed attention on the chemical inhibition of mitosis within multicell spheroids, the main assumption of the modelling being that a growth inhibitory factor (GIF) is produced within the spheroid in some prescribed spatially-dependent manner to reflect the observed cellular heterogeneity within spheroids. As stated in this section,

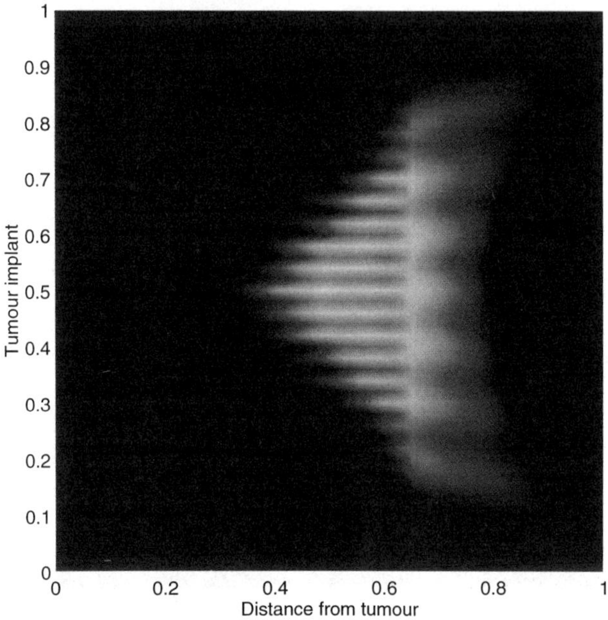

Figure 5.16 — Profile of the endothelial cell density after the capillary network has been established and anastomosis has taken place corresponding to a real time of 7–8 days after initial sprouts have formed as per Figure 5.13. Brush-border effect is clearly visible at the vascular front. Parameter values: $D = 0.001$, $\sigma = 1$, $\kappa = 0.6$, $\mu = 75$, $\beta = 0.5$.

the existence and properties of chemicals which inhibit mitosis are very well documented e.g. [BRU], [HA] and [PAR]. However, there is also much evidence to demonstrate that tumour cells also secrete growth-promoting factors [CHE], [WU].

We consider then the production of growth promoting factors (GPF) and growth inhibitory factors (GIF) by tumour cells during the avascular phase of growth. The theory will be presented for solid spherical tumours, but the analysis goes over equally well to other similar geometries e.g. oblate spheroid, prolate spheroid, ellipsoid etc. It is known, for example, that carcinoma arising in the breast tend to be ellipsoidal in shape. We consider the case whereby the growth factors are produced throughout the interior of the tumour and also the case whereby production of the factors is restricted to the thin layer of live, proliferating cells at the tumour surface. We will discuss the relevance of the resulting spatially inhomogeneous patterns to the experimentally observed cellular heterogeneity within carcinoma and multicell spheroids and also to the well known invasion characteristics of carcinoma.

The system we study is the set of nonlinear partial differential equations which we write in the general form familiar from the theory of reaction-diffusion equations:

$$\frac{\partial \mathbf{c}}{\partial t} = \mathbf{f}(\mathbf{c}) + D\nabla^2 \mathbf{c}\,, \tag{5.49}$$

where $\mathbf{c}$ is the vector of growth factor concentrations, $\mathbf{f}$ represents the reaction kinetics of the chemicals and D is the diagonal matrix of positive constant diffusion coefficients cf. [DIL], [HUNa] and [MUR]. If we denote the permeability of the tumour tissue at the tumour surface by P then appropriate boundary conditions for the above system are of the form

$$D(\mathbf{n}.\nabla)\mathbf{c} = -P\mathbf{c}, \qquad \mathbf{r} \quad \text{on} \quad \partial\Omega\,, \tag{5.50}$$

where $\partial\Omega$ is the closed boundary of the domain i.e. the tumour surface and $\mathbf{n}$ is the outward unit normal. A derivation of these boundary conditions may be found in [CHAg] and [CHAd], and references therein. Appropriate initial conditions will also be prescribed. For our purposes we consider only two chemical species whose concentrations are c_1 and c_2, say, representing some GPF and some GIF respectively. The reaction kinetics governing the system may either be a pure or cross activator-inhibitor mechanism [DIL], [MUR]. The distinction between these two types of kinetics lies in whether the self-activating chemical either activates (pure) or inhibits (cross) the second species. There is experimental evidence which suggests both mechanisms may be applicable in the case of growth factors secreted by tumour cells [MIC]. For our purposes throughout this paper we shall assume that the kinetics are a cross activator-inhibitor mechanism e.g. the prototypical Schnakenberg system, [MUR]. Under appropriate scaling, it can be shown ([DIL], [MUR]) that the above system of equations then reduces to the following:

$$\frac{\partial u}{\partial t} = \gamma f(u,v) + \nabla^2 u\,, \qquad 0 \le r < 1\,, \tag{5.51}$$

$$\frac{\partial v}{\partial t} = \gamma g(u,v) + d\nabla^2 v\,, \qquad 0 \le r < 1\,, \tag{5.52}$$

where, with R an appropriate tumour radius, k an appropriate reaction parameter and D_1, D_2 the diffusion coefficients of the GPF and GIF respectively, $\gamma = R^2k/D_1$ and $d = D_2/D_1$. The boundary conditions for the above system are then given by

$$\frac{\partial u}{\partial r} = -\rho_1 u\,, \qquad \text{on} \quad r = 1 \frac{\partial v}{\partial r} = -\rho_2 v\,, \qquad \text{on} \quad r = 1\,, \tag{5.53}$$

where $\rho_i = RP/D_i$. The homogeneous steady-state (u_0, v_0) of the above equation is the positive solution of

$$f(u,v) = 0\,, \qquad g(u,v) = 0\,. \tag{5.54}$$

Using standard linear stability theory ([DIL], [HUNa]) it can be shown that the stability of the above steady state is governed by the nature of the eigenvalues λ satisfying the following characteristic equation:

$$\lambda^2 + \lambda\Big[\kappa_{nl}^2(1+d) - \gamma(f_u + g_v)\Big] + \Big[d\kappa_{nl}^4 - \gamma(df_u + g_v)\kappa_{nl}^2 + \gamma^2(f_u g_v - f_v g_u)\Big] = 0\,. \tag{5.55}$$

The steady state will be unstable with respect to spatial disturbances if $\mathrm{Re}(\lambda) < 0$. The parameters κ_{nl} are such that they satisfy the eigenvalue problem

$$\nabla^2\psi + \kappa^2\psi = 0\,, \qquad \mathbf{r} \in \Omega \tag{5.56}$$

subject to

$$\frac{\partial\psi}{\partial n} + \rho\psi = 0\,, \qquad \mathbf{r} \;\text{ on }\; \partial\Omega\,. \tag{5.57}$$

Since we are considering the production of the GPF and GIF within a sphere, then the eigenfunctions ψ are given by

$$\psi_{nlm}(r,\theta,\phi) = j_n(\kappa_{nl}r)Y_{nm}(\theta,\phi)\,, \tag{5.58}$$

where $j_n(\kappa_{nl}r)$ are the spherical Bessel functions and $Y_{nm}(\theta,\phi)$ are the (surface) spherical harmonics. From the boundary condition at $r=1$ the wavenumbers κ_{nl} satisfy

$$\kappa_{nl} j_n'(\kappa_{nl}) + \rho j_n(\kappa_{nl}) = 0\,. \tag{5.59}$$

It is well known that for certain conditions on the reaction kinetics and $d > 1$ ([DIL], [MUR]) there exists a range of unstable wavenumbers $\kappa_1^2 < \kappa^2 < \kappa_2^2$ for which $\mathrm{Re}(\lambda) > 0$. Within this unstable range $\mathrm{Re}(\lambda)$ will have a maximum which indicates a fastest growing mode which will eventually dominate over time. This will give rise to a spatially heterogeneous pattern.

5.4.1 Results

From the results of the previous section we assume that all conditions necessary for diffusion driven instability to occur are satisfied and that there exists a dominant, fastest growing mode. As stated previously we also assume that the reaction kinetics are of a cross activator-inhibitor mechanism i.e. regions of high concentration of GPF correspond to regions of low concentration of GIF and vice versa [DIL]. The following figures illustrate what relevance this could have for the growth of solid tumours. We denote the wavenumber of the fastest growing mode by κ^*_{nl} where from (5.59) we have

$$\kappa^*_{nl} j'_n(\kappa^*_{nl}) + \rho j_n(\kappa^*_{nl}) = 0\,. \tag{5.60}$$

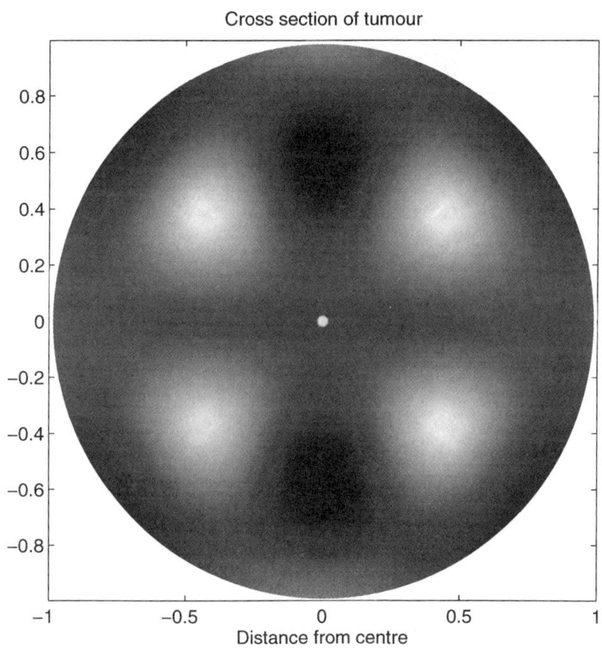

Figure 5.17 — A cross section of a solid tumour showing the prepattern generated when the dominant mode is $j_4(\kappa_{42} r) Y_{42}(\theta, \phi)$, with $\kappa_{42} = 9.84$. The light regions are those where the local concentration of a growth promoting factor is high. It is from these regions that recruitment of the quiescent cells into the proliferating compartment is proposed to take place.

We now give an estimate for the variable $\rho = RP/D$. In [CHAg] and [CHAd] (and references therein) it was demonstrated that reasonable esti-

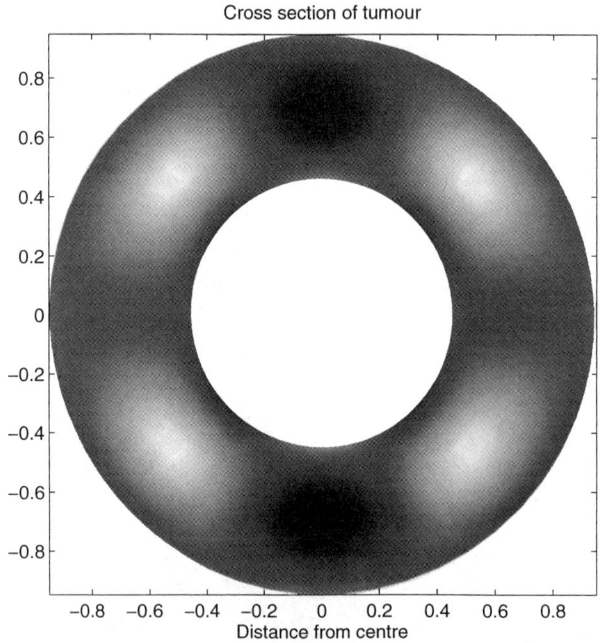

Figure 5.18 — A cross section of a solid tumour showing the prepattern generated when the dominant mode is $j_4(\kappa_{42}r)Y_{42}(\theta,\phi)$, with $\kappa_{42} = 9.84$ under the assumption that chemicals are only produced within the quiescent compartment. The light regions are those where the local concentration of a growth promoting factor is high. It is from these regions that recruitment of the quiescent cells into the proliferating compartment is proposed to take place.

mates for a range of values for the diffusion coefficient D and the permeability P were $10^{-6} - 10^{-8}\text{cm}^2\text{s}^{-1}$ and $10^{-5} - 10^{-6}\text{cms}^{-1}$ respectively. The radius of an avascular multicell spheroid is at most a few millimeters i.e. of the order $10^{-1} - 10^{-2}$cm. Hence within this range of parameters we can choose $\rho = 1$ enabling us to use standard tables to estimate κ^*_{nl}. For illustrative purposes only, Figure 5.17 shows a cross-section of a solid tumour in which the dominant mode prepattern is $j_4(\kappa_{42}r)Y_{42}(\theta,\phi)$, with $\kappa_{42} = 9.84$. This situation is illustrative of growth factors being produced throughout the tumour. As is clearly seen from the figure, there are regions in the interior of the tumour where the concentration of the GPF is high and the GIF low (the light regions). These regions are situated in the area of the interior of the tumour where the quiescent cells are likely to be situated. It is known that these quiescent cells can be recruited to repopulate the proliferating compartment [DUb], [SUc], [WIB]. From Figure 5.17 we suggest that a possible mechanism for this is that the quiescent cells are firstly stimulated into proliferating in those regions of high GPF and are then recruited into the proliferating compartment. A similar situation exists if it is assumed that the chemicals are only produced within the quiescent layer and this is illustrated in Figure 5.18.

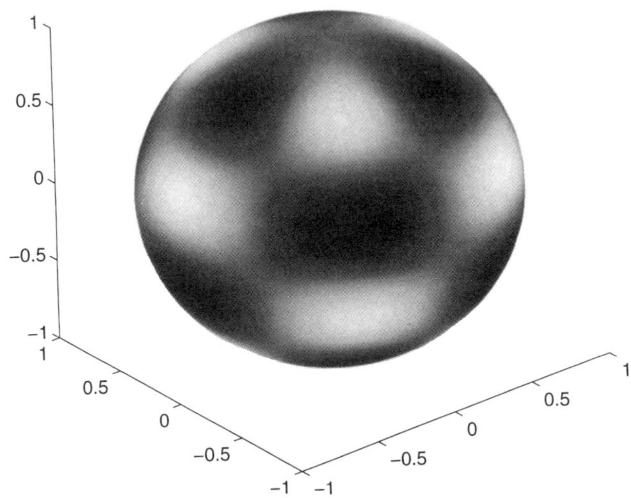

Figure 5.19 — Prepattern observed on the surface of a solid tumour when the dominant mode is $Y_{63}(\theta, \phi)$. Once again the light regions are those in which the concentration of a growth promoting factor is high. It is from these regions that the columns of invading cells are expected to emerge when exophytic growth is taking place. These regions are also expected to influence the local environment through their secretion of growth factor.

If we now consider growth factors being produced only by the live cells at the surface of the tumour, then the problem is essentially a 2-dimensional one in the variables θ and ϕ. The eigenfunctions are simply the surface harmonics $Y_{nm}(\theta, \phi)$ and the wavenumbers in this case are given by $\kappa_n^2 = n(n+1)$. In this case zero flux boundary conditions are assumed. Figure 5.19 illustrates the case when the dominant mode is given by $Y_{63}(\theta, \phi)$. As can clearly be seen once again there are regions on the surface of the tumour where the concentration of the GPF is locally high (dark regions). It is a well-known feature of carcinomas that they invade the surrounding local tissue with columns of cells projecting from the central mass [GI]. We suggest that while in its avascular dormant state a pre-pattern such as is illustrated in Figure 5.19 is set up. Once vascularized the cells which are in regions of high GPF will begin to invade the local tissues. A prepattern of this type is also consistent with the observation that tumours can manipulate the local environment by secretion of growth factors. Thus this prepattern will not only prime the tumour cells but will be affecting the local surrounding tissue as well thus facilitating invasion [KES].

5.5 Discussion and Conclusions

In this paper we have presented a variety of mathematical models describing the various stages of the growth and development of a solid tumour.

In Section 5.2 we focussed attention upon the production of a growth inhibitory factor within a spherical avascular nodule (multicell spheroid) and showed that using a nonlinear, spatially-dependent diffusion coefficient, which reflects the cellular heterogeneity of the interior of multicell spheroids and the heterogeneous intercellular permeability, is alone sufficient to produce a GIF concentration profile within the spheroid which is not incompatible with available experimental evidence. Similar results were also obtained by using a combination of nonlinear diffusion with a nonlinear source term and hence this combination can also account for the experimental observations. These results show that a nonuniform source function is not the only way to produce qualitatively correct GIF concentration profiles within multicell spheroids. Therefore, mathematically it is not possible to distinguish between the effects of nonlinear diffusion and a nonlinear source term. We conclude that more experimental work on the precise mechanisms governing cell cycle kinetics must be done to elucidate the underlying tissue heterogeneity.

In Section 5.3 a mathematical model for tumour angiogenesis was presented which developed and extended the model of [CHAc]. As is apparent from its brief description in the introduction, the complete process of angiogenesis is a complicated one, involving several distinct, and not necessarily related, events. This in turn requires several separate mechanisms which can stimulate each event — e.g. vasodilatation, endothelial cell migration, endothelial cell proliferation and loop formation (anastomosis), to name a few. Despite much research and many advances, many questions still remain unanswered [PAW]. To formulate a single mathematical model which would include all of these processes would be very difficult indeed. In this paper we have chosen to focus attention primarily on the activity of the endothelial cells, since they are always at the heart of the angiogenic process, as well as on the TAF concentration profile. We have modelled in a simple but effective manner two of the three main events concerning the endothelial cells (migration and proliferation) and the results obtained are in good agreement with both experimental evidence and other models ([PAW], [SHO], [STOb]) and represent an improvement upon those obtained by [CHAc]. The model reproduces the experimentally observed facts that the initial response of the endothelial cells is one of migration with proliferation occurring as a secondary response which is nevertheless vital for the successful completion of angiogenesis.

The results also confirm previous assumptions and findings that the endothelial cell migration is almost certainly controlled by some form of taxis rather than diffusion. However, since endothelial cells are known to exhibit different levels of motility on different extracellular molecules ([TER], [UNG], [YOU]) it would certainly be possible to modify the model to account for this variable motility. More specifically we could assume a more general form for the diffusive flux, namely

$$\mathbf{J}_{\text{diffusion}} = -D_n(c)\nabla n\,. \tag{5.61}$$

The diffusion, or motility, coefficient of the cells would now be dependent upon the concentration of the TAF. This means considering a nonlinear diffusion problem.

The extension of the model to 2 spatial dimensions was made in order to take into account explicitly the key features of anastomosis and secondary sprout formation (branching). The numerical simulations show that the basic assumptions of the original model can capture most of the salient features in 2 spatial dimensions with only slight modifications necessary. However, some further points of clarification remain. It was found difficult to simulate two capillary sprout tips moving towards each other (in opposite directions) and fusing together. The features captured by the model are on a rather coarser level. This is perhaps to be expected since certain simplifying assumptions have been made and certain biological details omitted.

Although we have chosen to focus on chemotaxis as the underlying driving mechanism since there is much experimental evidence to support this, there is also experimental evidence that the interaction between the endothelial cells and the extracellular matrix, through which they must move to reach the tumour, may also have a part to play in the angiogenic process. It is known for instance that the EC secrete chemicals which may give rise to haptotaxis (motion up a gradient of increased adhesiveness). From *in vitro* experiments it is known that the mobilization of endothelial cells can be greatly enhanced by adding gangliosides to whatever medium they are cultivated upon. It has been shown that preincubating endothelial cells with trisialogangliosides and then culturing on the same substratum leads to their *binding* to fibronectin being greatly enhanced and their migration is increased five-fold [PAW], [UNG], [ALE]. Including haptotaxis within the model would not be difficult to do from a modelling point of view but would increase the computational time for the simulations drastically since several chemicals would perhaps need to be considered. Also we note that in simulating the brush-border effect, we have not prescribed the precise *mechanism* which gives rise to this event, only assumed that it occurs and incorporated appropriate term in the equation which accounts for this. Investigation of precise mechanisms which give rise to the brush-border and also to the side-branching is a possible line of further research. It may be that a combination of deterministic and stochastic modelling is necessary.

In Section 5.4 we applied standard reaction-diffusion theory (Turing-type models) to a novel situation — that of the growth of solid tumours e.g. carcinoma. We have shown that the spatially heterogeneous patterns which arise in the case of a spherical geometry may play a part and help to explain certain observed phenomenon in carcinoma and multicell spheroids i.e. the characteristic invasive pattern and the recruitment of quiescent cells into the proliferating population. We note that similar results can be obtained for other quasi-spherical geometries which may also be appropriate for solid tumours e.g. oblate spheroid, prolate spheroid, ellipsoid cf. [HUNb,c]. Of course there are many other factors which are involved in tumour growth of this type e.g. nutrient supply, and which are also very important and we certainly do not claim that Turing systems can provide a complete answer in this particular case, but rather may be an important part of the complex overall mechanisms governing solid tumour growth.

We note that there are several features of solid tumour growth which lend themselves naturally to the consideration of a Turing-type model. There are actually present in this system chemicals which both promote and inhibit growth of cells. The time scale for the growth of a solid tumour is very slow in comparison to the time needed for a diffusing substance to reach steady state concentration hence there will be a genuine pre-pattern. There also appears to be a natural critical domain size in this system i.e. the size of carcinoma in its diffusion-limited, avascular state. While in this state no invasion can take place but once vascularized rapid exophytic growth does occur.

We also note that many of the standard problems inherent in Turing models regarding robustness i.e. the same pattern must be repeated faithfully time and time again with the requirement that only a small number of patterns are selected in a robust and controlled manner, are not present for solid tumour growth. The observed "invasion patterns" of *in vivo* carcinoma vary greatly from individual to individual. It is also well known that cellular heterogeneity is not only observed within an individual tumour/multicell spheroid ([DUb], [WIB]) but also varies from tumour to tumour. Also it is worth pointing out that the complex process of invasion is dependent upon many factors such as the actual make up of the surrounding tissue. In view of the latter point regarding the surrounding tissue this may well necessitate a reconsideration of the boundary conditions involved which may lead to even more complex patterning [DIL].

In each of the models presented in this paper, there are strengths and weaknesses. Since each different model focusses on different aspects of solid tumour growth and makes the relevant appropriate simplifying assumptions this is to be expected. However, it is certainly to be hoped that in future, mathematical models of solid tumour growth will develop so as to be of genuine prognostic use to the pathologist.

5.6 References

[ADG] Adam G., Steiner U., Maier H., and Ullrich S., Analysis of cellular interactions in density-dependent inhibition of 3T3 cell proliferation, *Biophys. Struct. Mech.*, **9** (1982), 75–82.

[ADJa] Adam J.A., A simplified mathematical model of tumor growth, *Math. Biosci.*, **81** (1986), 229–244.

[ADJb] Adam J.A., A mathematical model of tumor growth II: Effects of geometry and spatial nonuniformity on stability, *Math. Biosci.*, **86** (1987), 183–211.

[ADJc] Adam J.A., A mathematical model of tumor growth III: Comparison with experiment, *Math. Biosci.*, **86** (1987), 213–227.

[ALE] Alessandri G., Raju K.S., and Gullino P.M., Interaction of gangliosides with fibronectin in the mobilization of capillary endothelium, *Invas. Metast.*, **6** (1986), 145–165.

[AUS] Ausprunk D.H. and Folkman J., Migration and proliferation of endothelial cells in preformed and newly formed blood vessels during tumour angiogenesis, *Microvasc. Res.*, **14** (1977), 53–65.

[BAL] Balding D. and McElwain D.L.S., A mathematical model of tumor-induced capillary growth, *J. Theor. Biol.*, **114** (1985), 53–73.

[BAXa] Baxter L.T. and Jain R.K., Transport of fluid and macromolecules in tumors: I. Role of interstitial pressure and convection, *Microvasc. Res.*, **37** (1989), 77–104.

[BAXb] Baxter L.T. and Jain R.K., Transport of fluid and macromolecules in tumors: II. Role of heterogeneous perfusion and lymphatics, *Microvasc. Res.*, **40** (1990), 246–263.

[BAXc] Baxter L.T. and Jain R.K., Transport of fluid and macromolecules in tumors: IV. A microscopic model of the perivascular distribution, *Microvasc. Res.*, **41** (1991), 252–272.

[BG] Bredel-Geissler A., Karbach U., Walenta S., Vollrath L., and Mueller-Klieser W., Proliferation-associated oxygen consumption and morphology of tumor cells in monolayer and spheroid culture, *J. Cell. Physiol.*, **153** (1992), 44–52.

[BO] Bourrat-Floeck B., Groebe K., and Mueller-Klieser W., Biological response of multicellular EMT6 spheroids to exogenous lactate, *Int. J. Cancer*, **47** (1991), 792–799.

[BRI] Britton N.F. and Chaplain M.A.J., A qualitative analysis of some models of tissue growth, *Math. Biosci.*, **113** (1993), 77–89.

[BRO] Brown J.M. and Gaccia A.J., Tumour hypoxia: the picture has changed in the 1990s, *Int. J. Radiat. Biol.*, **65** (1994), 95–102.

[BRU] Brugal G. and Pelmont J., Existence of two chalone-like substances in intestinal extract from the adult newt inhibiting embryonic intestinal cell proliferation, *Cell Tiss. Kinet.*, **8** (1975), 171–187.

[BRUM] Brümmer F. and Hülser D.F., Intercellular communication in multicell spheroids, *European J. Cell Biol.*, **27** (1982), 108.

[BUL] Bullough W.S. and Deol J.U., The pattern of tumour growth, *Symp. Soc. Exp. Biol.*, **25** (1971), 255–275.

[BUR] Burton A.C., Rate of growth of solid tumours as a problem of diffusion, *Growth*, **3** (1966), 157–176.

[CA] Casciari J.J., Sotirchos S.V., and Sutherland R.M., Mathematical modelling of microenvironment and growth in EMT6/Ro multicellular tumour spheroids, *Cell Prolif.*, **25** (1992), 1–22.

[CHAa] Chaplain M.A.J. and Sleeman B.D., A mathematical model for the production and secretion of tumour angiogenesis factor in tumours, *IMA J. Math. Appl. Med. Biol.*, **7** (1990), 93–108.

[CHAb] Chaplain M.A.J. and Stuart A.M., A mathematical model for the diffusion of tumour angiogenesis factor into the surrounding host tissue, *IMA J. Math. Appl. Med. Biol.*, **8** (1991), 191–220.

[CHAc] Chaplain M.A.J. and Stuart A.M., A model mechanism for the chemotactic response of endothelial cells to tumour angiogenesis factor, *IMA J. Math. Appl. Med. Biol.*, **10** (1993), 149–168.

[CHAd] Chaplain M.A.J. and Britton N.F., On the concentration profile of a growth inhibitory factor in multicell spheroids, *Math. Biosci.*, **115** (1993), 233–245.

[CHAe] Chaplain M.A.J., The development of a spatial pattern in a model for cancer growth, in **Experimental and Theoretical Advances**

in Biological pattern Formation, Othmer H.G., Maini P.K., and Murray J.D. eds., Plenum Press (1993), 45–60.

[CHAf] Chaplain M.A.J. and Sleeman B.D., Modelling the growth of solid tumours and incorporating a method for their classification using nonlinear elasticity theory, *J. Math. Biol.*, **31** (1993), 431–479.

[CHAg] Chaplain M.A.J., Benson D.L., and Maini P.K., Nonlinear diffusion of a growth inhibitory factor in multicell spheroids, *Math. Biosci.*, **121** (1994), 1–13.

[CHE] Chen T.C., Hinton D.R., Apuzzo M.L.J., and Hofman F.M., Differential effects of tumor-necrosis-factor-alpha on proliferation, cell-surface antigen expression and cytokine interactions in malignant gliomas, *Neurosurgery*, **32** (1993), 85–94.

[CLI] Cliff W.J., Observations on healing tissue: A combined light and electron microscopic investigation, *Phil. Trans. R. Soc. Lond. B*, **246** (1963), 305–325.

[DEG] Degner F.L. and Sutherland R.M., Mathematical modelling of oxygen supply and oxygenation in tumor tissues: Prognostic, therapeutic and experimental implications, *Int. J. Radiation Oncology Biol. Phys.*, **15** (1988), 391–397.

[DER] Dertinger H., Hinz G., and Jakobs K.H., Intercellular communication, three-dimensional cell contact and radiosensitivity, *Biophys. Struct. Mech.*, **9** (1982), 89–93.

[DIL] Dillon R., Maini P.K., and Othmer H.G., Pattern formation in generalized Turing systems. I. Steady-state patterns in systems with mixed boundary conditions, *J. Math. Biol.*, **32** (1994), 345–393.

[DUb] Durand R.E., Multicell spheroids as a model for cell kinetic studies, *Cell Tissue Kinet.*, **23** (1990), 141–159.

[DUc] Durand R.E., Cell cycle kinetics in an *in vitro* tumour model, *Cell Tissue Kinet.*, **9** (1976), 403–412.

[FOa] Folkman J. and Hochberg M., Self-regulation of growth in three dimensions, *J. Exp. Med.*, **138** (1973), 745–753.

[FOb] Folkman J., Tumor angiogenesis, *Cancer*, **3** (1975) 355–388.

[FOc] Folkman J., The vascularization of tumors, *Sci. Am.*, **234** (1976), 58–73.

[FOd] Folkman J. and Klagsbrun M., Angiogenic factors, *Science*, **235** (1987), 442–447.

[FRa] Freyer J.P. and Sutherland R.M., Determination of diffusion constants for metabolites in multicell tumor spheroids, *Adv. Exp. Med. Biol.*, **159** (1983), 463–475.

[FRb] Freyer J.P., Role of necrosis in saturation of spheroid growth, *Strahlentherapie*, **160** (1984), 58.

[FRc] Freyer J.P., Tustanoff E., Franko A.J., and Sutherland R.M., In situ oxygen consumption rates of cells in V-79 multicellular spheroids during growth, *J. Cell. Physiol.*, **118** (1984), 53–61.

[FRd] Freyer J.P. and Sutherland R.M., Regulation of growth saturation and development of necrosis in EMT6/Ro multicellular spheroids by the glucose and oxygen supply, *Cancer Res.*, **46** (1986), 3504–3512.

[FRe] Freyer J.P. and Sutherland R.M., Proliferative and clonogenic heterogeneity of cells from EMT6/Ro multicellular spheroids induced by the glucose and oxygen supply, *Cancer Res.*, **46** (1986), 3513–3520.

[FRf] Freyer J.P. and Schor P.L., Regrowth of cells from multicell tumour spheroids, *Cell Tissue Kinet.*, **20** (1987), 249.

[GI] Gimbrone M.A., Cotran R.S., Leapman S.B., and Folkman J., Tumor growth and neovascularization: An experimental model using the rabbit cornea, *J. Natn. Cancer Inst.*, **52** (1974), 413–427.

[GREa] Greenspan H.P., Models for the growth of a solid tumor by diffusion, *Stud. Appl. Math.*, **51** (1972), 317–340.

[GREb] Greenspan H.P., On the self-inhibited growth of cell cultures, *Growth*, **38** (1974), 81–95.

[GREc] Greenspan H.P., On the growth and stability of cell cultures and solid tumours, *J. Theor. Biol.*, **56** (1976), 229–242.

[GRO] Groebe K. and Mueller-Klieser W., Distributions of oxygen, nutrient and metabolic waste concentrations in multicellular spheroids and their dependence on spheroid parameters, *Eur. Biophys. J.*, **19** (1991), 169–181.

[HA] Harel L., Chatelain G., and Golde A., Density-dependent inhibition of growth: inhibitory diffusible factors from 3T3- and Rous sarcoma virus (RSV)-transformed 3T3 cells, *J. Cell Physiology*, **119** (1984), 101–106.

[HO] Hondius-Boldingh W. and Laurence E.B., Extraction, purification and preliminary characterization of the epidermal chalone, *J. Biochem.*, **5** (1968), 191–198.

[HUL] Hülser D.F. and Brümmer F., Closing and opening of gap junction pores between two- and threedimensionally cultured tumor cells, *Biophys. Struct. Mech.*, **9** (1982), 83–88.

[HUNa] Hunding A., Dissipative structures in reaction-diffusion systems: numerical determination of bifurcations in the sphere, *J. Chem. Phys.*, **72** (1980), 5241–5248.

[HUNb] Hunding A., Bifurcations of nonlinear reaction-diffusion systems in prolate spheroids, *J. Math. Biol.*, **17** (1983), 223–239.

[HUNc] Hunding A., Bifurcations of nonlinear reaction-diffusion systems in oblate spheroids, *J. Math. Biol.*, **19** (1984), 249–263.

[IVa] Iversen O.H., Epidermal chalones and squamous cell carcinomas, *Virchows Arch. B Cell Path.*, **27** (1978), 229–235.

[IVb] Iversen O.H., The Chalones, in **Tissue Growth Factors**, Baserga R. ed., Springer-Verlag (1981), 491–550.

[IVc] Iversen O.H., What's new in endogenous growth stimulators and inhibitors (chalones), *Path. Res. Pract.*, **180** (1985), 77–80.

[IVd] Iversen O.H., The hunt for endogenous growth-inhibitory and or tumor suppression factors - their role in physiological and pathological growth-regulation, *Adv. Cancer Res.*, **57** (1991), 413–453.

[JAI] Jain R.K., Barriers to drug delivery in solid tumors, *Sci. Amer.*, **271** (1994), 58–65.

[KAR] Karbach U., Gerharz C-D., Groebe K., Gabbert H.E., and Mueller-Klieser W., Rhabdomyosarcoma spheroids with central proliferation and differentiation, *Cancer Res.*, **52** (1992), 474–477.

[KES] Keski-Oja J., Postlethwaite A.E., and Moses H.L., Transforming growth factors and the regulation of malignant cell growth and invasion, *Cancer Invest.*, **6** (1988), 705–724.

[LA] Landry J., Freyer J.P., and Sutherland R.M., A model for the growth of multicell spheroids, *Cell Tissue Kinet.*, **15** (1982), 585–594.

[LE] Levine A.E., Hamilton D.A., Yeoman L.C., Busch H., and Brattain M.G., Identification of a tumor inhibitory factor in rat ascites fluid, *Biochem. Biophys. Res. Commun.*, **119** (1984), 76–82.

[LIO] Liotta L.A., Saidel G.M., and Kleinerman J., Diffusion model of tumor vascularization and growth, *Bull. Math. Biol.*, **39** (1977), 117–129.

[LO] Loewenstein W.R., Junctional intercellular communication: the cell-to-cell membrane channel, *Physiol. Rev.*, **61** (1981), 829–889.

[MAG] Maggelakis S.A. and Adam J.A., Mathematical model of prevascular growth of a spherical carcinoma, *Math. Comp. Modelling*, **13** (1990), 23–38.

[MAR] Marks F.A., Tissue-specific factor inhibiting DNA synthesis in mouse epidermis, *Natn. Cancer Inst. Monogr.*, **38** (1973), 79–90.

[MCE] McElwain D.L.S. and Ponzo P.J., A model for the growth of a solid tumor with non-uniform oxygen consumption, *Math. Biosci.*, **35** (1977), 267–279.

[MIC] Michelson S. and Leith J., Autocrine and paracrine growth factors in tumour growth: a mathematical model, *Bull. Math. Biol.*, **53** (1991), 639–656.

[MUE] Mueller-Klieser W., Multicellular spheroids: A review on cellular aggregates in cancer research, *J. Cancer Res. Clin. Oncol.*, **113** (1987), 101–122.

[MUR] Murray J.D., Parameter space for Turing instability in reaction diffusion mechanisms: a comparison of models, *J. Theor. Biol.*, **98** (1982), 143–163.

[MUT] Muthukkaruppan V.R., Kubai L., and Auerbach R., Tumor-induced neovascularization in the mouse eye, *J. Natn. Cancer Inst.*, **69** (1982), 699–705.

[PAK] Paku S. and Paweletz N., First steps of tumor-related angiogenesis, *Lab. Invest.*, **65** (1991), 334–346.

[PAR] Parkinson K. and Balmain A., Chalones revisited - a possible role for transforming growth-factor-beta in tumor promotion, *Carcinogenesis*, **11** (1990), 195–198.

[PAW] Paweletz N. and Knierim M., Tumor-related angiogenesis, *Crit. Rev. Oncol. Hematol.*, **9** (1989), 197–242.

[REI] Reidy M.A. and Schwartz S.M., Endothelial regeneration III. Time course of intimal changes after small defined injury to rat aortic endothelium, *Lab. Invest.*, **44** (1981), 301–312.

[SCH] Schoefl G.I., Studies on inflammation III. Growing capillaries: Their structure and permeability, *Virchows Arch. Pathol. Anat.*, **337** (1963), 97–141.

[SHE] Sherratt J.A. and Murray J.D., Models of epidermal wound healing, *Proc. R. Soc. Lond. B*, **241** (1990), 29–36.

[SHO] Sholley M.M., Ferguson G.P., Seibel H.R., Montour J.L., and Wilson J.D., Mechanisms of neovascularization. Vascular sprouting can occur without proliferation of endothelial cells, *Lab. Invest.*, **51** (1984), 624–634.

[SHY] Shymko R.M. and Glass L., Cellular and geometric control of tissue growth and mitotic instability, *J. Theor. Biol.*, **63** (1976), 355–374.

[STOb] Stokes C.L. and Lauffenburger D.A., Analysis of the roles of microvessel endothelial cell random motility and chemotaxis in angiogenesis, *J. Theor. Biol.*, **152** (1991), 377–403.

[STOd] Stokes C.L., Rupnick M.A., Williams S.K., and Lauffenburger D.A., Chemotaxis of human microvessel endothelial cells in response to acidic fibroblast growth factor, *Lab. Invest.*, **63** (1990), 657–668.

[SUa] Sutherland R.M., McCredie J.A., and Inch W.R., Growth of multicell spheroids as a model of nodular carcinomas, *J. Natl. Cancer Inst.*, **46** (1971), 113–120.

[SUb] Sutherland R.M. and Durand R.E., Growth and cellular characteristics of multicell spheroids, *Recent Results in Cancer Research*, **95** (1984), 24–49.

[SUc] Sutherland R.M., Cell and environment interactions in tumor microregions: the multicell spheroid model, *Science*, **240** (1988), 177–184.

[SW] Swan G.W., The diffusion of an inhibitor in a spherical tumor, *Math. Biosci.*, **108** (1992), 75–79.

[TER] Terranova V.P., Diflorio R., Lyall R.M., Hic S., Friesel R., and Maciag T., Human endothelial cells are chemotactic to endothelial cell growth factor and heparin, *J. Cell Biol.*, **101** (1985), 2330–2334.

[UNG] Ungari S., Katari R.S., Alessandri G., and Gullino P.M., Cooperation between fibronectin and heparin in the mobilization of capillary endothelium, *Invas. Metast.*, **5** (1985), 193–205.

[VA] Vaupel P.W., Frinak S., and Bicher H.I., Heterogeneous oxygen partial pressure and pH distribution in C3H mouse mammary adenocarcinoma, *Cancer Res.*, **41** (1981), 2008–2013.

[WAR] Warren B.A., The growth of the blood supply to melanoma transplants in the hamster cheek pouch, *Lab. Invest.*, **15** (1966), 464–473.

[WIB] Wibe E., Lindmo T., and Kaalhus O., Cell kinetic characteristics in different parts of multicellular spheroids of human origin, *Cell Tissue Kinet.*, **14** (1981), 639–651.

[WIL] Williams S.K., Isolation and culture of microvessel and large-vessel endothelial cells: their use and transport in clinical studies, in **Microvascular Perfusion and Transport in Health and Disease**, McDonagh P. ed., Basle:Karger (1987), 204–245.

[WIN] Winter G.D., Epidermal regeneration studied in the domestic pig, in **Epidermal Wound Healing**, Maibach H.I. and Rovee D.T. eds., Chicago Year Book Medical Publishers (1972), 71–112.

[WRI] Wright N.A., Cell proliferation kinetics of the epidermis, in **Biochemistry and Physiology of the Skin**, Goldsmith L.A. ed., Oxford University Press (1987), 203–229.

[WU] Wu S., Boyer C.M., Whitaker R.S., Berchuck A., Wiener J.R., Wienberg J.B., and Bast R.C., Tumor-necrosis-factor-alpha as an autocrine and paracrine growth-factor for ovarian cancer-monokine induction of tumor-cell proliferation and tumor-necrosis-factor-alpha expression, *Cancer Res.*, **53** (1993), 1939–1944.

[YOU] Young W.C. and Herman I.M., Extracellular matrix modulation of endothelial cell shape and motility following injury *in vitro*, *J. Cell. Sci.*, **73** (1985), 19–32.

6

Basic Models of Tumor-Immune System Interactions Identification, Analysis and Predictions

V.A. KUZNETSOV

Center for Biologics Research and Evaluation, FDA
Division of Cellular and Gene Therapies
Laboratory of Molecular Tumor Biology
Bethesda, MD, USA

ABSTRACT. The purpose of this chapter is to consider the basic mathematical models of the interaction of cytotoxic cells and effector molecules of the immune system with tumor cells at the effector stage of an anti-tumor immune response. The logic and design lines of some models relevant for tumor immunology will be reviewed and discussed. Special attention is given to validation problems. Mathematical models of the kinetics of interaction of natural killer cells, lymphokine-activated killer cells, cytotoxic T lymphocytes and tumor will be discussed in detail. Some models of the regulation of cellular cytolytic reactions by nonkiller immune cells and by regulatory immune molecules (antibodies, lectins) will be presented. Predictions of kinetic models by a new theoretical concept describing the recognition of target cells without any specific NK-receptor by NK-like cells will been described. Mathematical models of the propagation and interaction of tumor-specific immune molecules (monoclonal antibodies, cytokines) with tumor cells in multicellular tumors are used for analysis of restriction mechanisms for delivering the toxic factor into a solid tumor.

6.1 Introduction

Research over the past two decades has dramatically increased our understanding of the molecular and cellular basis of cancer growth and of anti-cancer control mechanisms. The surveillance of emerging cancers, metastases, and their dynamic type may depend on their reactive properties, the number of cells called effector cells (ECs) and effector molecules (EMs) of the immune system.

A variety of immune system cells can recognize and kill the autologous tumor cells. It was shown that certain subpopulations of cytolytic T lymphocytes (CTL) such as CD8+, $\gamma\delta$ T cells have capacity to specifically recognize and to destroy cancer cells. A multitude of cell surface molecules, in addition to T cell receptor (TCR) — major histocompatibility (MHC) peptide complexes — involving in the binding and signaling for T lymphocyte mediator lysis of cancer cells have been studied. Two major molecular pathways of CTL mediated destruction of tumor cells are known: the secretion of soluble membrane lytic proteins (perforins and granzymes) from the specialized secretory granules of lymphocytes into the intracellular cleft with target cell (TC) [GRa], and a nonsecretory pathway initiated by receptor-mediated triggering of apoptosis-inducing TC surface Fas-ligand which transduces the killing signal into Fas-bearing TCs [BKb].

In recent years, it has become clear that the negative responses of lymphocyte subsets resulting from antigen contact are at least as important as the positive responses in controlling the quantity and quality of the immune homeostasis and optimal immune response. In particular, apoptosis of CTL may be induced by cross-linking of the T cell surface receptors [BKc]. The human APO-1 and murine Fas are cell surface molecules that transduce a signal for cell inactivation or death. CTL and perhaps other ECs that express APO-1/Fas receptors can be induced to undergo apoptosis by tumor cells during interaction with tumor antigens [FEa].

In addition to CTL, it was shown that cell populations of macrophages, neutrophils and eosinophils, natural killer cells (NK cells), and lymphokine-activated killer cell (LAK cells) nonspecifically can recognize and destroy the cancer cells [BKc], [FRa]. Often these cells provide the first level of immune mediated anti-cancer prevention because they can kill the tumor cells without preactivation by specific antigen, clonal selection and/or proliferation. Some macromolecules produced by immune cells (antibodies, cytokines) are also involved in the recognition and destruction of cancer cells and/or preventing of cancer cells growth. The regulatory mechanisms of the effector immunological cells and molecules are very complex and require intensive study.

The immune system cells are the first host cells to appear within a tumor. Inflammatory cells (macrophages/monocytes and granulocytes) are usually the first to be seen. Later, NK-cells, LAK, T-lymphocytes, B-lymphocytes, nonimmune cells and vascular system components are found in a tumor. Each of the immune cells types is able to produce a large quantity of biologically active substances and to absorb them from a medium. The tumor itself also secrets a large number of biologically active substances, such as angiogenic factor, colony-stimulating factor, chemoattractants, anti-chemoattractants, and the effect of all these factors results in the initiation of leukocyte migration into the tumor. Experimental data indicate that tumor-infiltrating macrophages produce a chemotaxic factor, initiating migration of leukocytes from surrounding tissues into the tumor. Tumor-infiltrating neutrophils are also capable of producing a chemotaxic factor, which attracts T-lymphocytes into the tumor. Thus, the tumor at an early developmental stage already represents a rather complex and heterogeneous tissue. These cellular elements are constantly interacting in a dynamical fashion. From the point of the mathematical population biology it means that an interaction of the cytotoxic effector cells and tumor cells corresponds to "predator-prey" models (see [ADa] and [MCa]).

The dynamics of the anti-tumor immune response *in vivo* are very complicated and are not well understood. Spontaneously arising tumors are known to be of low immunogenicy and usually grow out of control in a organism. However, at the early stages of tumor growth, the cytolytic ECs of the immune system are able to suppress the growth or destroy the host tumor. On the other hand, tumor growth may be stimulated by some molecules and cells of immune system. It was shown that antigen-specific and antigen-nonspecific T lymphocytes, NK-like cells and granulocytes under certain conditions can stimulate tumor growth [COa], [PRa], and [SNa]. Some tumor cells carry on the receptors for growth factors (IL-2, IL-4 etc.) which might stimulate the cell growth. Although mechanisms responsible for "immunostimulation effects" of tumor growth are not clear, the very fact of their existence suggests caution in carrying out of immunotherapy and gene therapy.

Mathematical models may help to increase the informative capacity of certain immunological investigations. Nevertheless, studies in the field of theoretical immunology are still developing in relative isolation from experimental and clinical studies. One of the main reasons is the fact that theoretical immunology remains a border area between experimental immunobiology and clinical immunology on one side, and mathematical biophysics and biochemistry on the other side. Therefore, scientific activity in the field of theoretical immunology requires a high skill in both of the above mentioned areas and close cooperation and collaboration of researchers engaged in mathematical modeling and experimental investigations. Weak cooperation between theoreticians and experimenters does not always produce results stimulating other researchers to expand and verify these predictions. Such situations limit the development of theoretical immunology to being a subdiscipline of immunology [LMa], [KZf].

The other important reason for this current situation is that the majority of mathematical models in immunology are not compared directly with the available experimental data. In order to compare mathematical models with the experimental data and to select non-contradictory models, it is necessary to plan experimental research in such a way that a correct comparison is made. The purpose of this survey is to discuss the experimental validation of basic mathematical models describing the interaction of the different immune effector cells and molecules with tumor cells.

The methodological uniqueness of this survey is the consideration of the nonlinear processes at different levels of complexity of systems: single cells, heterogenic cell populations and spatio-temporally distributed cells in tumor tissue. We will describe and analyze the mathematical models of the effector stage of immune response. Methods of quantitative comparison with experimental data are an important feature of this survey.

The development of mathematical models of complicated dynamic processes and verification of their relevance to observations is a natural and essential stage in their formulation. This will entail the necessity of solving problems of structural and parametric identification. Structural identification means selection of the class and order of the model, a mathematical description of structure within the parameters. Parameter identification means determination of parameters of the model selected by experimental data.

At present, many methods of parameter identification of dynamical systems have been developed and subsequently used in mathematical immunology and tumor biology [KUa], [PAa], and [HGa]. The results in structural identification are much more modest, evidenced by the nontriviality of the problem [KZi]. However, some effective computer methods of structural identification of algebraic, dynamical and parabolic nonlinear systems were proposed and successfully used for the estimation of parameters of the tumor-immune system models by kinetics experimental data [KZh], [KZi]. Results on the identification of the mathematical models and their biological interpretation will facilitate some of the problems of the tumor immunology.

The content of this review is organized in seven sections. The second section deals with the description of some basic kinetic models of effector stage of CTL, and with the discussion on the activity of NK cells and LAK cells. The third section describes a model of cell-mediated regulation of cytolytic reactions. The fourth section deals with a description of the models of the lectin/antibody dependence cellular-mediated cytolyticity (LDCC/ADCC) and a kinetic switch model of the mechanism of the differential cytolytic activity regulated by soluble bispecific macromolecules. The fifth section deals with the theoretical analysis of the biophysical mechanism of recognition of the target cells by NK-like cells without specific NK-receptors. The sixth section refers to the analysis of spatio-temporal dynamics of the propagation and interaction of monoclonal antibodies in the multicellular tumor spheroids (MTS). Some conclusions will be reported in the last section.

6.2 Kinetics Models of Cellular Cytotoxic Reactions at the Effector Stage of Immune Response

Tumor-infiltrating T lymphocytes (TIL), NK cells, LAK and macrophages are the main ECs involved in the effector stage of cellular mediated immune reactions against malignant cells. These ECs are able to infiltrate a growing tumor causing its destruction. Moreover, new cells and gene therapy methods based on the use of NK, LAK or TIL cells hold great promise for therapy in various tumors. Therefore, it is very important to elucidate and compare the mechanisms involved in the binding, killing and detachment of various killer cells. Determination of the kinetic parameters of these processes and elucidation of their mechanics may be extremely effective in developing theoretical models, which must subsequently be subjected to experimental verification.

Mathematical modeling is an obligatory component of kinetic studies in biological sciences. Kinetic studies of the effector stage of cell mediated immune reactions against TCs is one of the areas of experimental immunology in which fruitful cooperation has appeared between mathematicians and experimenters.

In the past 20 years, mathematical modeling have been applied to studies of immune processes, in particular, to cytotoxic reactions of various types of killer cell *in vitro*, e.g. [BLa], [CAa,b], [CUa], [IVa], [KZe], [KZf], [LEa], [MAa], [MIa], [MLa,b], [PEa,b], [PLa], [PSa], [TRb,c], and [VOa].

Irrespective of the molecular basis of the mechanisms for EC–TC interactions, four stages of the effector phase can be distinguished in the lytic process:

i) binding of EC and TC leads to the formation of the ET-TC conjugate(s),
ii) activation of EC cytolytic mechanism(s),
iii) the lethal hit of the target cell; TC disintegration,
iv) detachment of the EC from the TC.

Kinetic studies have shown that these processes mediated by CTL, NK, and LDCC/ADCC effectors *in vitro* can be described in a manner analogous to enzyme-catalyzed reactions.

Initial studies of the kinetics of cellular cytotoxicity reactions have generally applied models for enzyme kinetics originally developed in [CAa], [CUa], [MIa], [TRb], and [ZEa]. Based on this analogy, it has been proposed that lysis obeys the Michaelian-like rate law

$$v = \frac{d}{dt}T^* = \frac{V_{\max}^{\text{app}}T}{K_m^{\text{app}} + T}, \tag{6.1}$$

where the velocity, $v(t)$, represents the number of targets killed per unit time, T the initial number of TCs, $V_{\max}^{\text{app}}$ and K_m^{app} are the cellular analogs of the apparent maximal enzymatic reaction rate and of the apparent Michaelis constant.

Formula (6.1) was usually used to compare mathematical models of cytotoxic reactions with experimental data. However, for this equation to be correct certain restrictions must be observed. Some of those are the quasi-stationary of the process, which is realized at large time intervals from initiation of the process, beginning with definite conditions which are required for process constants and initial concentrations of the ECs and the TCs [KZf], [SEa]. If these special conditions are not experimentally controlled, using Eq. (6.1) for fitting of experimental data may lead to results for the reaction mechanisms which are not correct.

Analysis of experimental data has shown that these conditions are not always implemented. The apparent problem concerning the accuracy of the constants determined by comparison of approximate formulae remains unclear. As usual, this is due to the fact that under real experimental conditions differences exist between the approximate solution of the model and the exact solution. Additionally, it is well known from enzyme kinetic theory that kinetic curves reflect the limiting stages only for a quasi-stationary process and these curves does not provide information about rapid early and rapid intermediate stages of the process. This means that, in some cases, an asymptotic, quasi-stationary equation may correspond to several kinetic mechanisms of the reactions. More accurate and objective information on the mechanism reaction is provided by high-resolution nonstationary kinetics analysis.

Deterministic nonstationary models of the cytotoxic reaction meditated by CTL NK-like cells can be applied to study of kinetic experiments over broad intervals of time and cell concentrations. In this case, fitting mathematical models to experimental data will provide a more correct estimation of the parameters of the models. On the other hand, stochastic models of cytolytic reactions will not be discussed here. Some stochastic models of cytotoxic cellular mediated immune reactions have been presented in the literature (see for references [CUa], [MAa], and [PEb]).

More in detail, Garay and Lefever [GAa] have suggested that binding of EC and TCs is a disequilibrium process and that cytotoxic reaction of

CTL and NK cells may be described by the kinetic scheme

$$x + y \overset{k_1}{\to} [xy] \overset{k_2}{\to} x + y^* , \tag{6.2}$$

where the terms x, y, $[xy]$, and y^* represent effector, target, effector-target conjugate, and a target cell that has been programmed for lysis respectively. k_1 and k_2 are the rate constants for the step binding and lytic programming. It was proposed in [KZb] that EC can dissociate from TC without killing of TC. This assumption allows an accurate fitting of the model with experimental data.

TC are homogeneous populations, and initial concentrations are large for each population in a fixed volume (the case of *in vitro*). Suppose that a loss of EC activity is small during the characteristic testing period. If a detachment of EC from TC without cell damage occurs, then a cytolytic process is described, see [KZa] and [KZd], by equations

$$\begin{cases} \dfrac{dz}{dt} = k_1(x^0 - z)(y^0 - z - y^*) - (k_{-1} + k_2)z \, , \\ \dfrac{dy^*}{dt} = k_2 z \, , \\ \dfrac{dm}{dt} = k_2 \theta(t - \tau_0) \displaystyle\int_{\tau_0}^{t} F(t-s) z(s) \, ds \, , \end{cases} \tag{6.3}$$

with initial conditions *in vitro*

$$x(0) = x^0 \, , \quad y(0) = y^0 \, , \quad z(0) = z^0 \, , \quad y^*(0) = m(0) = 0 \, , \tag{6.4}$$

and where the conservation equations

$$x^0 = x(t) + z(t) \, , \qquad y^0 = y(t) + z(t) + y^*(t) \, ,$$

have been used towards the derivation of the model. Here, $x(t)$, $y(t)$, $z(t)$, and $y^*(t)$ are the concentration of free ECs, free TCs, EC–TC pairs, and dying TCs; $m = m(t)$ is the radiation label (or other constituent TC parts, for example, ATP, nicotinamide, nucleic acids) which is released in medium from destroyed TC; t is the time. k_1, k_{-1}, and k_2 are the means of rate coefficients of adsorption EC to TC, detachment EC from living TC and of TC EC recycling in the lytic cycle. According to observations of [BKb], the ECs do not adhere to dying TCs. System (6.3) is similar to the Briggs–Holdein model of the simple enzyme-substrate kinetics [CRa], [MUa]. The third equation in (6.3) determines a relationship between a TC death rate and a change of radioactive label (or other constituent TC parts) in the medium. τ_0 is the value of lag-period that is recorded experimentally, and $\theta(t)$ is Heaviside's function. The cytotoxic reaction model (6.3) will be named the "minimal" one, see [KZd].

In many experimental systems, direct measurements of outcome variables, such as the number of dying TC, $y^*(t)$, are not available. The chromium-release kinetic assay is one of the typical example of such cytotoxicity assays [BLb], [MTa].

6.2.1 Solutions of the model at quasi-stationary approximation

System (6.3) has been known for 70 years in enzyme kinetics, being the model for a one-product enzyme reaction. Despite its simplicity, model (6.3) does not have exact solutions because of its nonlinearity. Nevertheless a few approximate solutions, which correspond to the different initial conditions, have been obtained in [KZc], [MLa,b], [SEa] by methods of singular perturbation theory [VAa].

It was shown that the rate of TC death, at the quasi-stationary condition

$$\mu = \frac{x^0}{K_M} \ll 1\,, \qquad t \gg \tau_1 = \frac{1}{k_1(y_0 + K_M)}\,, \qquad K_M = \frac{k_{-1} + k_2}{k_1}\,,$$

is given by the differential equation

$$\frac{dy^*}{dt} = k_2 {x^0} y \, \frac{1 + \mu\,\xi(y) + O_3(\mu^2)}{K_M + y}\,, \tag{6.5}$$

where

$$y = y(t) = y^0 - K_M \ln\left(\frac{y}{y^0}\right) - k_2 {x^0} t\,, \tag{6.6}$$

and where $\mu\,\xi(y)$ is the first-order small correction given by $\mu\xi = \hat{z}_1/\hat{z}_{0|t\gg\tau_1}$. Approximate evaluation of the maximum value of $\mu\xi(y)$ yields

$$\mu\,\xi_{\max}(y) = \frac{x^0}{K_M\left(1 + \dfrac{y}{K_M}\right)^2}\,. \tag{6.7}$$

In studies of the cytolitic activity of ECs in blood or immune tissues the fraction of the killer cells ($\nu = x^0/X^0$) is usually small. In this case, the strong inequality $x^0/K_M \ll 1$ applies, so that the cytolitic kinetics quickly approach the quasi-stationary solution (6.1). For $x^0 \ll y^0$ or $x^0 \ll K_M$, an approximate solution of Model (6.3–6.4) (expressed in terms of experimental values) can be obtained using Eq. (6.5)

$$-\frac{t}{\ln\left(1-\dfrac{y^*}{y^0}\right)} \equiv -\frac{t}{\ln(P)} \approx \frac{K_M+\nu X^0}{k_2\nu X^0} - \frac{y^*}{k_2\nu X^0 \ln\left(1-\dfrac{y^*}{y^0}\right)}. \tag{6.8}$$

Numerical experiments have shown that Eq. (6.8) provides a good approximation to the exact solutions of (6.3) under typical experimental conditions and for typical parameters of the cell mediated cytolytic processes.

In some experiments, the kinetics of cytotoxic reactions are studied at the transitional stage of the process. Such experiments can be analyzed by means of the following approximate solution:

$$y^*(t) \approx \frac{k_2\,\nu X^0 y^0}{K_M+y^0}\left(t+\frac{\exp\left[-k_1(K_M+y^0)t\right]-1}{k_1(K_M+y^0)}\right). \tag{6.9}$$

This equation may be used when $x^0 \ll K_M$ or $x^0 \ll y^0$.

Consider now the case when ECs are bound TCs but TC cytolysis does not take place. Such a situation occurs frequently in experiments. Mathematically this is expressed with coefficient $k_2 = 0$ in Eq. (6.3). The exact solution describing the binding kinetics of EC with TC is then

$$z(t) = l_1 l_2 \frac{e^{k_1(l_1-l_2)t}-1}{l_1 e^{k_1(l_1-l_2)}-l_2}, \tag{6.10}$$

where

$$l_{1,2} = \frac{1}{2}\left(x^0+y^0+\frac{k_{-1}}{k_1}\right) \pm \frac{1}{2}\sqrt{\left(x_0+y^0+\frac{k_{-1}}{k_1}\right)^2 - 4x^0y^0}\,.$$

In space variables x, y, z as $t \to \infty$ only one singular point occurs; this point is the knot having coordinates (x^0-l_2, y^0-l_2, l_2). It means that not all of the EC are bound to TC as $t \to \infty$ if the EC and TC binding stage is reversible. Such a result was observed in [CAc] and [PZa].

6.2.2 Comparison of the minimal model with experimental data

Migration of immune cells and formation of the cellular conjugate are required in the initial stages of lytic reaction of cytotoxic lymphocytes [CAc]. Flow cytometry is used to investigate the strength of lymphocyte-TC interaction, as well as the kinetics of conjugate formation and dissociation. Only a small fraction of conjugate-forming lymphocytes in human peripheral blood exhibit NK lytic activity. Therefore using cloned NK cells or

LAK provides a more accurate fit of the model with the experimental data. In particular, Callewaert et al. [CAc] have shown that fresh human peripheral blood lymphocytes, as well as cloned human NK cells and human LAK cells, form conjugates with cultured cell lines that are not susceptibility to lysis. For example, cloned NK3.3 cells, which cannot lyse Daudi or RPMI-766 cells, readily form conjugates with these cell lines. Comparable values were also obtained for the conjugation of human LAK cells with LAK-resistent RPMI-766 cells as LAK-susceptible K-562 or Daudi cells.

Figure 6.1 shows the kinetics of conjugate formation by human LAK cells. Model (6.10) was used for analysis of the kinetics binding-dissociation of these effector cells [CAc]. Table 6.1 shows the parameters which were estimated from the fitted model. The dissociation rate constants were calculated from kinetics curves presented in [CAc].

Effector-Target Cell	Parameters		
	k_1, min^{-1}	ν, %	k_1, min^{-1}
LAK-K562	0.67	49.2	.0085
LAK-Daudi	0.91	53.1	.0200
LAK-RPMI 766	0.85	39.2	.0081

Table 6.1 — Parameters for LAK interactions with tumor cell lines: binding rate, frequency of cytolytic effector cells, and dissociation rate.

The rates of binding of human LAK cells are 3–4 times higher than in human NK cells and frequency of the killer cells in LAK cells is twice as high as in NK cells. However, the frequency and kinetic binding-dissociation of the LAK cells were independent of the relative susceptibility of the target cells to lysis (Table 6.1). Thus, conjugate formation alone cannot be used as a measure of the specific recognition interaction between NK or LAK cells and tumor cells. In the Section 6.5 the possible mechanisms of susceptibility of tumor cells to NK- and LAK-mediated lysis will be discussed.

In order to compare mathematical models of lymphocyte cytotoxic reaction with experiments, an investigation on the interaction of human peripheral blood NK cells with NK-sensitive leukemic human cell lines K-562 and Molt-4 in cytotoxicity assays was carried out in [KZd], [KZf].

Figure 6.2 shows a typical result of cytotoxic reaction of NK cells from the blood of the healthy volunteer. An estimation of the coefficients of the model was obtained using the algorithm of interval estimation of unknown kinetic parameters [PAa]. Numerical estimations yield: $\nu = [0.027 - 0.034]$,

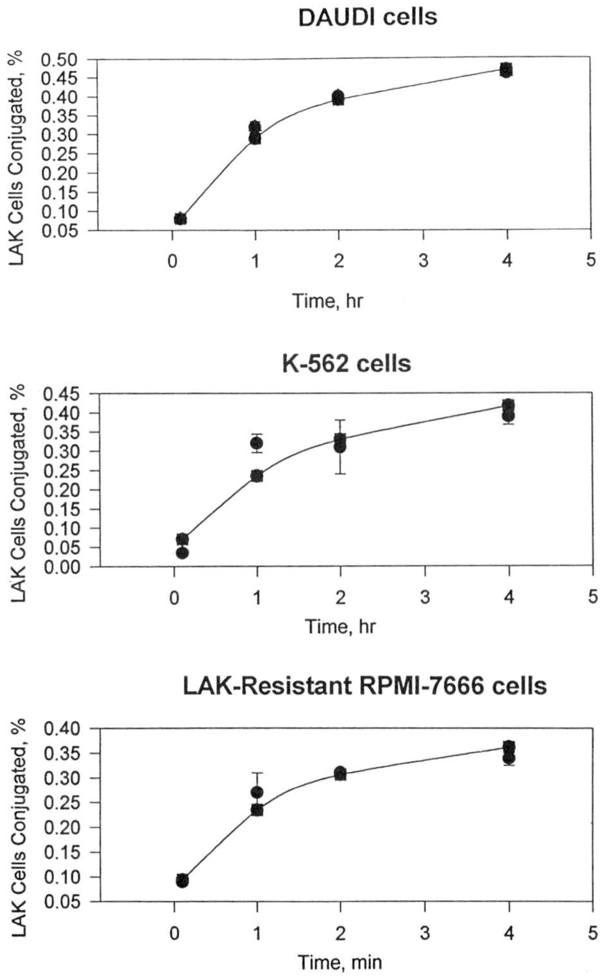

Figure 6.1 — Kinetics of conjugate formation by human LAK cells. Experimental points (black circles) represent the means of three measurements [CAc]; theoretical prediction (squares) corresponds to the model (6.10). LAK cells were generated by culture of blood lymphocytes for 3 days in 600 IU/ml recombinant IL-2. Labeled LAK cells and hydroethidine labeled target cells (Daudi, K-562, RPMI-766) TCs were pre-chilled to 0^0C, mixed in several chilled microtubes, and centrifuged in the cold. Pairs of tubes were transferred to 37^0C and incubated for the indicated time intervals, after which the pelleted cells were resuspended by gentle pipetting. Aliquots were immediately removed and the percentage of LAK cells determinated by flow cytometry. Error bars represent standard deviations.

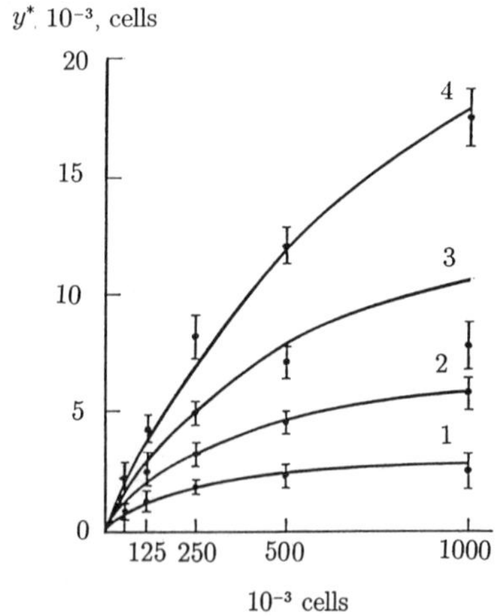

Figure 6.2 — "Dose-effect" curves were determined by ^{51}Cr release from leukemia K-562 cell line (i.e. TC) for 3.5 hr cytolytic reaction by NK cells. The initial numbers of TC per well (0.2 ml) which equaled 0.5 10^4 (1), 10^4 (2), 2 10^4 (3), 4 10^4 (4) were used, respectively. Four sets of experimental points (with $\pm SD$) for NK-activity of peripheral blood lymphocytes of healthy volunteer (V.K.) are presented. Data are represented as mean ± 1 SD of triplicate determination (black circles); bars, SD shown when large than symbols. The initial number of the lymphocytes (X^0) are along X axis, the TC number which are "programmed for death" (y^*) is along Y axis. Curves are theoretical solutions after fitting the model.

$k_2 = [0.37 - 0.42]$ 1/hr, $K_M = [49.5 - 99.5]\,10^3$ cells/ml. This figure shows that the nonstationary solutions of the system (6.3) fit closely the experimental data.

Table 6.2 shows the parameters of the minimal models for cytotoxic reaction of the NK cells of healthy volunteers against NK-sensitive leukemia TC K-562 and against thymoma Molt-4 cell lines [IVa], [KZf]. About 3–10% of lymphocyte population obtained from blood of healthy persons exerted NK-activity as against K-562 as against Molt-4. The estimations of kinetic constants are also similar. These numerical results are consistent with those which were determined in other investigations [PSa], [TIa], and [ULa]. For instance, the portion of NK cells in the blood lymphocytes of healthy human is about 2–7%, see [ULa].

The ability of killer cells to move actively and to enter repeatedly the lytic reaction may prove to be an effective method for monitoring foreign

Parameter	Cell line		U-criterion
	K-562	Molt-4	
$K_M * 10^{-3}$ cell/well	10.7 ± 2.1	21.0 ± 13.2	< 0.1
$\nu, \%$	4.9 ± 0.9	4.6 ± 0.2	none
t_{rec}, hr	2.5 ± 0.5	1.1 ± 0.4	< 0.07
CI, %	34 ± 3.6	56.1 ± 9.8	< 0.05

Table 6.2 —Kinetic parameters of cytolytic reaction of the NK cells from mononuclear blood cells.

cells in the body. The recycling time may be estimated as $t_{\text{rec}} = 1/k_2$. Table 6.2 shows that each NK cell is able to kill three Molt-4 cells; however, the question of the recycling of NK cells in the reaction against K-562 cells remains open. Most published data indicated that the one and the same cytotoxic T lymphocyte can be involved many times in the lytic cycle [BKb], [ZUa]. However, experimental results suggest that NK cells and some cloned CTL do not readily recycle and lyse additional TCs [ABa,b], [CAb], and [KZe].

In order to determine whether NK cells may be repeatedly involved in the lytic cycle against K-562, after onset of the reaction (using estimated parameters ν, k_2, K_M) we measured dose-effect relationships for mononuclear cells of seven healthy subjects during two time intervals (3–4 hrs and 16–18 hrs). The results summarized in Table 6.4 show that the rate of NK cell recycling (k_2^{app}) becomes drastically slower. This means that the cytolytic process is practically completed after one or two lytic cycles.

Notice, that parameter K_M^{app} has a similar value in both cases. On the other hand $K_M = k_2/k_1 + k_{-1}/k_1$. This indicates that the NK cell avidity $A = k_1/k{-}1$ is also diminished during the cytotoxic reaction.

In summary, in contrast to the most CTL, NK cells, at least *in vitro*, have a restricted capability to be recycled in the course of the cytolytic reaction. Our results correlate well with studies by other authors, e.g. [ABa] and [MHa]. The data of Mahle et al. [MHa] suggest that cloned NK3.3 cells cannot readily recycle and kill multiple TCs. Thus, the recycling ability may be determinant from the type of NK-sensitive tumor cells (K-562, but not Molt-4 cells) and from properties of NK cell themselves.

The mechanisms of these changes can be attributed to the inhibitory effect of local toxic actions of live tumor cells on the EC membrane during binding of the TC and NK cells. The deleterious effect of biologically active compounds released by NK cells themselves, as a result of their interaction

Parameter	Length of test, (hr)	
	3	18
$K_M * 10^{-3}$ cell/well	8.2 ± 1.60	9.8 ± 1.1
ν, %	4.9 ± 0.30	4.2 ± 0.4
k_2^{app}, hr^{-1}	0.5 ± 0.14	0.1 ± 0.6

Table 6.3 — Kinetic parameters of the 3-th hr and 18-th hr cytolytic reaction of NK cells against K-562 cell.

with TC or the loss of some necessary components of "effector recognition mechanism"(binding receptors, perphorin vesicles etc.), or inhibition of the biosynthesis of some components of recognition mechanism of NK cell can contribute to this phenomenon.

As can be seen from these results, the minimal mathematical model quite adequately describes the experimental data for short times (about 3 hr), since it provides a good description for the dose versus effect curves. In the case of longer experiments, the minimal model may have to be slightly modified according to the following scheme:

$$x + y \underset{k_{-11}}{\overset{k_{11}}{\rightleftharpoons}} [xy] \xrightarrow{k_{21}} x + y_1^*, \tag{6.11}$$

$$x + y \underset{k_{-12}}{\overset{k_{12}}{\rightleftharpoons}} [xy] \xrightarrow{k_{22}} x_2 + y_2^*, \tag{6.12}$$

where x_1 and x_2 are the NK cells after the first and the second binding with TCs respectively. In this model $k_{21} > k_{22}$, $A_1 >> A_2$, where $A_i = k_{1i}/k_{-1i}$, $i = 1, 2$.

When the tumor grows, enlarges and disseminates beyond a local focus, the probability of NK encounters with TC increases as well as the frequency of NK–TC binding events. If our findings obtained *in vitro* prove to be true for *in vivo*, then it can be predicted that tumor growth will be accompanied by a decline in NK cell activity. At the effector stage of the process, this decline is necessarily associated with inhibition of the processes that occur after the NK–TC binding event. This hypothesis was verified by studying NK activity of mononuclear cells from blood of patients with corpus uteri carcinoma of stages I–IV [KZf]. Figure 6.3 shows the cytotoxic index measured with respect to ^{51}Cr yield from TC K-562 cells, in which the mononuclear cells and TCs were incubated in the ratio 50: 1 during a 18 hr. It can be seen that as the cancer disease progressed, the activity of NK

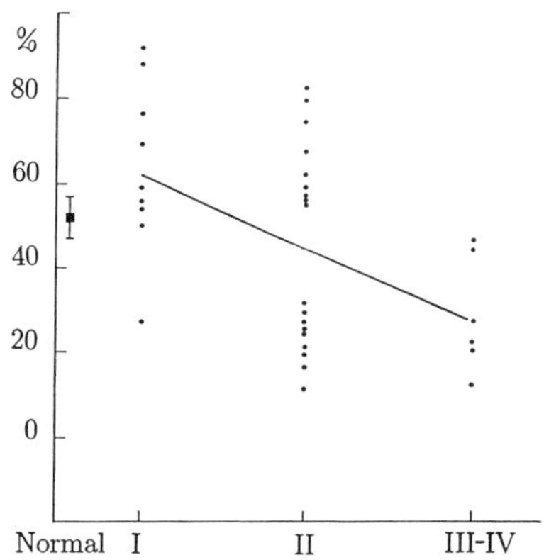

Figure 6.3 — NK-activity of mononuclear cells from the blood of healthy volunteers and of the patients with uteri carcinoma cells at different stages (I–III–IV) of this disease. The cytolytic activity was determined as a percentage of dead K-562 cells.

cells declined.

What is (are) the mechanism(s) of this decline? In order to find an answer to this question, the data of the dose-effect curves for the above patients were averaged and the parameters ν, k_2^{app} and K_M^{app} were identified. The computation results are summarized in Table 6.4, which shows that at the advanced stage of disease, i.e. stages III–IV, NK-cell activity was lowered due to the decrease of k_2^{app}, characterizing the rate of events taking place after NK–TC binding. Similar disorders in NK cell activity were found in the investigations of many solid tumors and chronic lymphocytic leukemia of human.

Thus, the minimal model (6.3) describes well the kinetics of NK-cell mediated cytotoxic reactions *in vitro* during the first three hours. The modified model (6.11–6.12) allows to describe cytolytic reaction by NK cells accurately for larger observation times. Based on the numerical fitting of the model to experimental data, it can be concluded that the stages following after primary NK cell / TC binding are most vulnerable and can be easily affected at the dissemination of tumor.

Moreover, Figure 6.4 shows experiments by Martz [MTa] and the theoretical curves after fitting of the model (6.3). Only a portion of the immune lymphocytes from the peritoneal cavity can kill the TC. According

Parameter	Group			
	Norm	Stage of cancer		
		I	II	III–IV
$K_M^{\text{app}} * 10^{-3}$ cells/well	9.8 ± 1.7	21.9 ± 6.7	9.8 ± 2.4	13.8 ± 3.5
$\nu, \%$	4.2 ± 0.3	5.1 ± 0.5	9.4 ± 2.0	8.2 ± 2.2
k_2^{app}, hr^{-1}	0.09 ± 0.03	0.08 ± 0.2	0.04 ± 0.01	0.03 ± 0.01
$V_{\max}$, hr^{-1}	0.37 ± 0.12	0.41 ± 0.14	0.37 ± 0.11	0.23 ± 0.10
$\frac{k_2^{\text{app}}}{K_M^{\text{app}}} 10^3$ $((\text{cells/well})\ \text{hr})^{-1}$	10.0 ± 2.3	3.7 ± 0.9	4.1 ± 0.8	2.5 ± 0.8

Table 6.4 — Kinetic parameters of the 18th hr cytolytic reaction of NK cells of patients with corpus uteri carcinoma against K-562 cells. See Figure 6.3 for details.

to [MTa], this portion of killer cells (ν) in the population of peritoneal lymphocytes was estimated as 0.3. Kinetics parameters were calculated for specific binding of the CTL with allogenic TCs and of lytic reaction in same experimental system. According to our estimations the constants of the model are $k_1 = 0.075$ $(10^3 \text{ cells min})^{-1}$, $k_{-1} = 0.082$ 1/min, $k_2 = 0.31$ 1/min.

Notice that in the cases $y^0 \ll x^0$ or $x^0 \ll y^0$, more complex kinetic models of cytotoxic reaction may be needed for agreement of theory with experimental data [GAa], [PEb]. However, within the framework of standard experimental conditions such models often do not provide any higher accuracy than the minimal model. The fitting of some mathematical models to the measurements of the CTL and TC binding kinetics illustrates this point, see Figure 6.5, [KZf]. In the investigation by Perez et al. [PZa] the detailed data on temperature kinetics of the binding CTL and TCs was presented using the dual parameter flow cytometry. The variable $x_p(t)$, $y_p(t)$, and $z_p(t)$ i.e. percent of free EC, TC and correspondence pair conjugates of EC–TCs were determined.

The relationship between observed and model variables of Eq. (6.3) were determined, see [KZf], by

$$x_p = \frac{x}{x^0 + y^0 - (y^* + z)}, \qquad y_p = x_p \frac{y}{x}, \qquad z_p = y_p \frac{z}{y}.$$

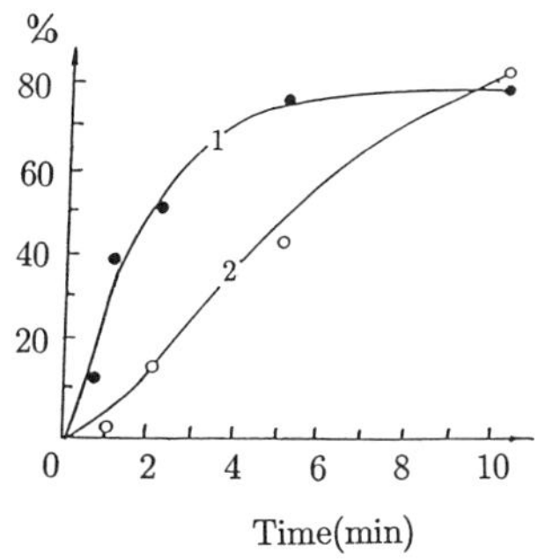

Figure 6.4 — Kinetics of the specific cell binding (1) and cytolytic reaction (2) against allogenic P815 tumor cell line ($H - 2^d$) by peritoneal immune CTL of mice C57Bl/6 ($H - 2^b$). $y^0 = 10 - 10^3$ cells, $x^0 = \nu X^0 = 60 - 10^3$ cells per well (0.2 ml). Points are experimental data, curves are numerical solutions of the minimal model.

Figure 6.5 shows that the experimental points and theoretical curves are practically coincident. The mean relative deviation of theoretical values from experimental values did not exceed 4%. It is interesting that experimental values corresponding to 30 min and 60 min time intervals in experiments carried out at 37^0C were not used in calculations. Nevertheless, the values at these time points are prognostically correct from the model. Table 6.5 shows the parameter estimations calculated by computer after fitting the model to experimental data. The dimension of the parameter k_1 was $(\text{min})^{-1}$ because the cell concentrations were determined in dimensionless units. The dimensionless parameter $\hat{A} = k_1/k_{-1}$ characterizes the avidity of EC to TC.

Perez et al. [PZa] noted that the population of cloned CTL is as heterogeneous as is the lymphocytes capacity for TC lysis. About 20–25% of lymphocytes bound with TC at 37^0C did not induce injury during the experimental time interval. The data from other investigations [THa] and [TRa,b] indicate the existence of such cells in the populations of ECs. Taking into account these data, the modified model of cytotoxic reaction can be used if one proposes that the cell subpopulation capable of cytolytic reaction is presence in the CTL population. Then, the kinetic scheme of the reaction can be written as

$$x_1 + y \underset{k_{-1}}{\overset{k_1}{\rightleftharpoons}} z_1 \overset{k_2}{\rightarrow} x_1 + y^* , \qquad x_2 + y \underset{k_{-1}}{\overset{k_1}{\rightleftharpoons}} z_2 , \tag{6.14}$$

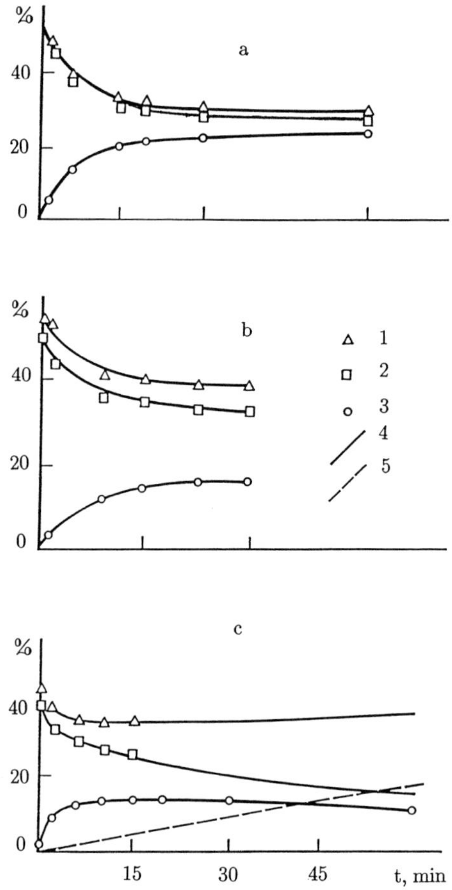

Figure 6.5 — The temperature-dependent time-kinetic of conjugate formation between cloned mice CTL (BM10-5.6 (anti-K^b)) recognizing the I class $H2 - K^b$ MHC antigens and mouse splenic TCs from the B6-CH-2^{bm10}) were studied. CTL (10^7 cells) and TC (10^7 cells) were labeled by different fluorochromes and were mixed in 1 ml of medium in equal parts. Then the cells from 50 ml of the medium were sedimented shortly by centrifugation (for 1 sec) and were incubated for different times at 24^0C (a), 30^0C (b) and 37^0C (c). After certain time intervals, the relative contents of free CTL ($1, \triangle$), free TC ($2, \square$), and pairs of cell conjugates between EC and TC ($3, \circ$), were determined by means of cell sorting. The measurement of the dead TC number was not carried out. The lines represent the numerical solutions of Model (6.3). Dotted lines on the lower panel indicate the numerical prediction of dead cell number.

Parameter	Temperature, ^{0}C		
	24	30	37
k_1 1/min	0.1040	0.135	0.229
k_{-1} 1/min	0.3400	0.083	0.114
k_2 1/min	0.0024	0.014	0.027
$\hat{A}$	3.0600	1.630	1.700

Table 6.5 — Temperature kinetics parameters of cytolytic reaction of cloned CTL.

where x_1, x_2, z_1, and z_2 are the number of capable and non-capable lymphocytes for cytolytic activity and coupling conjugates of these EC with TC. In this *in vitro* process the conservation laws are maintained as

$$x^0 = x_1 + x_2 + z_1 + z_2\,, \qquad y^0 = y + y^* + z_1 + z_2\,.$$

It was found that the model (6.14) describes the experimental data with the same accuracy as the model (6.3). At the initial conditions $y(0) = y^0 = 0.44$, $z_1^0 = 0.04$, $z_2^0 = 0.01$, $x_1^0 = 0.41$, $x_2^0 = 0.08$, and $y^* = 0.0$, the calculated values of kinetic parameters have following values: $k_1 = 0.173$, $k_{-1} = 0.114$, $k_2 = 0.031$. These parameters do not differ considerably from the parameters reported in Table 6.5.

Thus, using this scheme of experiments, it appears impossible to distinguish between models (6.3) and (6.14) (even by increasing the number of experimental points and the precision of measurements) within the framework of the kinetic approach. This is a known restriction in biological kinetics [BRa], which can be overcome by additional investigations that have to be planned in other ways. For example, by CTL subpopulations separated by strength of binding with TC or by killing activity, etc.

Mathematical modeling permits one to obtain quantitative and qualitative information about temperature-dependence of the separate stages of the cytolytic process. Lifetime of the CTL–TC cell conjugate ($\tau_{KT} = 1/k_{-1}$) decreases, approximately by a factor two, for each increase of medium temperature by 7^0C (see Table 6.5). Independent of temperature, the rates of the CTL binding and detachment are considerably faster than the rate of TC programming for lysis. The effect of the cell conjugate number decreasing, when the temperature increases, depends not only on the increase of TC lysis rate, but directly depends on the binding-dissociation ratio. The normal temperature is optimal for the cytolytic stage of the

CTL mediated immune reaction. Undoubtedly, the analogous mathematical analysis would be interesting in the cases of NK and LAK cells.

Referring to the problems of parameter estimations, the use of the singular-perturbation methods permits one to estimate the difference between exact and quasi-stationary solutions. The maximum error which occurs if the exact solution of Model (6.3) is substituted in the quasi-stationary solution was estimated in [KZf]. For cellular-mediated cytolysis rate this estimation is

$$\mu\,\xi_{\max} = \frac{x^0}{K_M(y+K_M)^2}\,, \qquad t > \tau\,, \qquad \tau = \frac{1}{k_1(y^0+K_M)}\,.$$

If one defines the function P in Eq. (6.9) as a probability of finding an uninjured TC at time t, then the approximate Eq. (6.9) coincides with the formula offered by Chu [CUa] and obtained by a stochastic consideration of cytolysis process. The comparison allows one to connect the fundamental kinetic and probability features of the killer cell mediated immune reaction

$$k_2 = \frac{q}{\tau_{KT}}\,, \qquad K_M = \frac{1}{a\,\tau_{KT}}\,,$$

where a is the constant proportional to the probability that the EC and TC contact brings to its binding; q is the probability of TC death after attachment to EC; t_{KT} is the mean time during which EC and TC are in the bound state after its attachment. Note that the formula offered by Chu is correct when $x^0 a\tau_{KT} \ll 1$, i.e. $x^0 \ll K_M$. However, the last inequality is the condition for a quasi-stationary process.

It is interesting to compare the kinetic parameters of interaction of NK-like cells and CTL. The results presented here for interaction of fresh NK cells, as well as cloned NK and LAK cells (Table 6.2) and cloned allogenic CTL (Table 6.5) with their TCs indicate that the rates of conjugate formation (k_1) for fresh NK cells and cloned CTL are similar, and that both rates are at least 3–4 times slower than the rate formation of LAK-TC conjugates. These differences in the rate of conjugate formation are apparently not related to TC specificity, since LAK cells form conjugates with susceptible and resistant cell lines at comparable rates (Table 6.2).

The lifetimes of conjugates between effector cells and TC at the 37^0C for NK and LAK cells are 6–12 times longer than for CTL. These differences suggest that different molecular mechanisms are involved in dissociation of NK-like cells and CTL from their TCs. The rate of TC lysis for CTL varies from 2–3 min to 1–2 hrs, see Tables 6.2–6.5 and Figure 6.4.

6.3 Regulatory Cells at the Effector Stage of the Cellular Immune Response

This section deals with the kinetic analysis of the role of nonkiller immune cells in processes of regulating the interaction of killer cells with their target cells (tumors, transplants, virus-infected cells).

It has been indicated above that a killer cell subpopulation (x) shares a fraction of cells ν of the entire EC population X^0. Any influence of cells from the rest of the population $(1-\nu)X^0$ has been neglected. However, in a number of cases, in order to fit a theoretical value to an experimental one, it was necessary to expand the model (6.3) including "the 3rd type" cell which in various studies were identified as normal splenocytes [TRb] and monocytes or erytrocytes [IVa], [KZe], [SUa], [THa], [VOa], and [ZEa].

Merrill [MLa] derived a modified model (6.3) for the analysis of the kinetics of cellular mediated cytotoxicity reaction by considering that cytotoxic and not cytotoxic immune cells in the assay mixture may bind to TCs. This model gives rise to the following expression for the maximum cytotoxic reaction rate

$$V_{\max} = k_2 \alpha f X^0 ,$$

where f is the fraction of the lymphocytes that bind to the TCs (i.e. form conjugates), and α is the fraction of conjugate-forming cells that are cytolytically active. However, the expression for the analogue of apparent K_M^{app} that results from considering nonlytic conjugate-forming cells in this model was very complex.

Consideration of the competition mechanisms of other immune cells, and the kinetics of the intercellular interactions in cellular mediated cytolytic reactions, have permitted us to suggest that the whole complex of experimental data may be described by the kinetics scheme [KZd]:

$$x + y \underset{k_{-11}}{\overset{k_{11}}{\rightleftharpoons}} [xy] \xrightarrow{k_{21}} x + y^* , \tag{6.15}$$

$$x + m \underset{k_{-3}}{\overset{k_3}{\rightleftharpoons}} [xm] , \tag{6.16}$$

$$[xm] + y \underset{k_{-12}}{\overset{k_{12}}{\rightleftharpoons}} [xym] \xrightarrow{k_{22}} [xm] + y_1^* , \tag{6.17}$$

$$[ym] + x \underset{k_{-15}}{\overset{k_{15}}{\rightleftharpoons}} [xym] , \tag{6.18}$$

$$[xy] + m \underset{k_{-4}}{\overset{k_4}{\rightleftharpoons}} [xym] , \tag{6.19}$$

$$y + m \underset{k_{-5}}{\overset{k_5}{\rightleftharpoons}} [ym], \tag{6.20}$$

$$[xym] \xrightarrow{k_{23}} [xm] + y_2^*, \tag{6.21}$$

where x, y, and m are the concentrations of free ECs, TCs and modulator cells m (or "3rd type cells" population); $[xm]$, $[xy]$, $[ym]$, and $[xym]$ are concentrations of pair or triple complexes; k_{11}, k_{-11}, k_{12}, k_{-12}, k_{13}, k_{-13}, k_{22}, k_3, k_{-3}, k_4, k_{-4}, k_5, and k_{-5} are kinetic constants.

Some reduced variants of this scheme were used in studies of the regulation of enzymes catalysis, muscular contraction, protein-receptor interactions [CRa], [KOa]. Scheme (6.15–6.21) was applied in [KZd] to the study of mechanisms of cellular regulation at an effector stage of cytolytic immune reaction. The exact solution of the model corresponding to Scheme (6.15–6.21) cannot be obtained analytically. However, some relevant special cases can be analyzed in what follows.

If the reaction (6.20) is absent (meaning that the modifier cells did not bind directly with TC) we have the following analysis. According to the kinetic scheme (6.15–6.21), the process is described by a system of three conservation laws for cell number:

$$x^0 = x + [xy] + [xym] + [xm], \tag{6.22}$$

$$y^0 = y + [xy] + [xym] + y^*, \tag{6.23}$$

$$m^0 = m + [xm] + [xym], \tag{6.24}$$

and by four differential equations:

$$\frac{d[xy]}{dt} = k_{11}xy - (k_{-11} + k_{21})[xy] + k_{-4}[xym] - k_4 m[xy], \tag{6.25}$$

$$\frac{d[xm]}{dt} = -k_3[xm] + k_{-3}mx - k_{12}y[xm] + (k_{-12} + k_{22})[xym], \tag{6.26}$$

$$\frac{d[xym]}{dt} = k_{12}y[xm] - (k_{-12} + k_{22})[xym] + k_4 m[xy] - k_{-4}[xym], \tag{6.27}$$

$$\frac{dy^*}{dt} = k_{21}[xy] + k_{22}[xym], \tag{6.28}$$

where x^0, y^0, and m^0 are initial concentrations of ECs, TCs, and MCs.

When the process reaches a quasi-stationary state (i.e. when $x^0 \ll y^0$, $x^0 \ll m^0$), the rate process is written as follows

$$\frac{dy^*}{di} = \frac{k_{21}x^0 y}{\Delta}\left[(a_1 + a_2 m + a_3 y) + \frac{k_{22}}{k_{21}} m\,(a_4 + a_5 m + a_6 y)\right], \tag{6.29}$$

where

$$\Delta = (a_7 + a_8 m + a_9 y) + y(a_1 + a_2 m + a_3 y) \\ + my(a_4 + a_5 m + a_6 y) + m(a_{10} + a_{11} m + a_{12} y)\,, \qquad (6.30)$$

with a_i , $i = 1, \ldots, 12$ suitable constants.

If the processes described by Scheme (6.19) are absent ($k_4 = k_{-4} = 0$), then Eq. (6.29) reduces to the simple form

$$v(t) = \frac{dy^*}{dt} = \frac{Vy}{K + y}\,, \qquad (6.31)$$

where

$$V = x^0 k_{21} \frac{sr + pm}{sr + m}\,, \qquad K = sK_{M1} \frac{r + m}{sr + m}\,,$$
$$s = \frac{K_{M2}}{K_{M1}}\,, \qquad p = \frac{k_{22}}{k_{21}}\,, \qquad K_{Mi} = \frac{k_{-1i} + k_{2i}}{k_{1i}}\,. \qquad (6.32)$$

It is possible to show by Eq. (6.31) that the cytolysis is accelerated when the RC concentration increases, if $dy^*/dm > 0$ and cytolysis is hindered if $dy^*/dm < 0$. Such a situation takes place when the following conditions occur during experiment:

$$y > \tilde{y} = \frac{K_{M1} sr(s - p)}{p - 1}\,, \qquad 1 < p < s\,. \qquad (6.33)$$

In this case, if the RC concentration exceeds a certain threshold value

$$\tilde{m} = \frac{(1 - p)y}{K_{M1}(p - s)} - sr\,, \qquad (6.34)$$

then, when $m < \tilde{m}$, the TC lysis process is accelerated and when $m > \tilde{m}$ it is hindered. In a similar manner, it is possible to show the conditions under which small MC concentrations can inhibit (and large concentrations can accelerate) TC cytolysis by ECs.

A number of model sequences can now be compared to experimental data. In the study by [BLa] the presence of "cooperative" interactions between NK receptors of the human blood and the cells of erythroleukemia K-562 cell has been noted. These cooperative interactions manifest themselves in the presence of a bend on a "dose-effect" curve (S-wise form of the curve $y^* = y^*(x^0)$) when low TC concentrations are used. If the S-wise form of the curve is not conditioned by differences in EC mobility, then it is possible to explain this cooperative effect by a certain character of cellular interactions in a three-cellular system, and not by cooperative interactions of NK receptors themselves. Indeed, when

$$x^0 = \nu\bar{x}^0\,, \quad m^0 = (1-\nu)\bar{x}^0\,, \quad x^0 \ll y^0\,, \quad k_{-4} = k_4 = k_{-5} = k_5 = 0\,,$$

an initial section of the lytic curve may be either convex or concave, depending on a ratio of the model constants on the "dose-effect" curve, which is interpreted by the authors as a manifestation of cooperative interactions in the TC reception by NK. In other words, cooperative interactions occur at the level of cell-cell interactions.

The mechanisms of how monocytes effect TC P815-X2 lysis using human peripheral blood cells have been studied in [VOa] and [ZEa], where the authors concluded that monocytes show a suppressor activity and inhibit steps occurring after NK binding to TC. According to our analysis of these data using Eqs. (6.22–6.28), the following inequalities occur:

$$\frac{\Delta V}{\Delta m} < 0\,, \qquad \frac{\Delta K}{\Delta m} < 0\,, \qquad \frac{1}{\Delta m}\Delta\left(\frac{V}{K}\right) < 0\,,$$

thus, the inhibiting effect of monocytes is more complicated, i.e., it is necessary to suppose that monocytes hinder both EC binding to TC and the following TC cytolysis stages. Within the framework of our model these conditions take place if concentration of the ECs is relatively low ($x^0 \ll m^0$, $m^0 \ll y^0 + K_{M2}$) and under conditions:

$$k_4 = k_{-4}\,, \qquad k_{22} < k_{21}\,, \qquad K_{M2} < K_{M1}\,, \qquad \frac{k_{22}}{K_{M2}} < \frac{k_{21}}{K_{M1}}\,.$$

These results can be verified experimentally.

The model also permits one to describe more complicated situations. An effect determined by initial concentrations of cells and kinetic constants occurs when the same population of MC may act both as a helper and a suppressor. For instance, if $y(t) > \tilde{y} = \text{const} > 0$, then a reversal of the sign in one of the above conditions (i.e. $k_{22} > k_{21}$) allows us to show the stimulating and suppressing effect of MCs on the rate of cytolitic reaction. At the relatively low concentration of ECs, the introduction of a small number of the MCs ($m < \tilde{m}$) accelerates the cytolytic process and the introduction of high doses of the MCs ($m > \tilde{m}$) inhibits of the rate of cytolytic reaction. These predictions follow from Eqs. (6.32–6.34). Such nonlinear dependencies coincide with those described in the experimental study of the effect of monocytes/macrophages on the proportion of EC–TC conjugates, and rate of cytolytic reaction mediated by NK cells [BLb],

[DVa]. Regulation of the effects of monocytes/macrophages on the NK-activity depends strongly on the ratio of monocytes EC and requires close cellular proximity at the single cell level [BLb]. [DVa] have shown that autologous monocytes accelerate K-562 TC lysis by human peripheral blood NK when the monocyte concentration is small; while with larger doses monocytes inhibit the NK-activity.

Condition $k_{22} < k_{21}$ means that monocytes accelerate the cytolytic stage. However, the inequality

$$\frac{k_{22}}{K_{M2}} < \frac{k_{21}}{K_{M1}}$$

means that the cytolytic reaction on the whole is less effective by EC–MC conjugates as by the ECs alone. The last inequality is possible, for instance, if the time needed for the EC+MC+TC conjugate formation is larger than that for the EC–TC conjugate formation. These predictions may be tested experimentally.

Note that the model ensures a reversible EC activity regulation; a MC does not induce or totally abolish EC activity. It is interesting that not only monocytes/macrophages, but also some other cell types are capable of dramatically modifying the cytotoxic reactions. Granulocytes, erythrocytes, epithelial cells posses such a modulating activity. For instance, it was shown that peripheral blood erythrocytes in low doses amplify the NK-cell mediated cytolytic activity; however, in large doses they inhibit such activity [SUa].

6.4 Modeling of the Recognition Mechanisms of Tumor Cells by NK-like Cells

NK lymphocytes are the main subpopulation of the natural immune effector cell population, termed NK-like lymphocytes. Natural killer cells form a distinct heterogenic population of lymphocytes that do not express the CD3 molecular complex (which are associated with T cell receptors) or TCR for antigen ($CD3^-$ TCR^-). These cells exert killer activity "spontaneously" against tumor cells, virus-infected cells, some microorganisms, aged cells and some normal cells [BZa], [HEa].

Additionally, populations of NK cells have been shown to respond to interleukin-2 (IL-2) by acquiring the ability to lyse many target cells (TCs), such as freshly isolated autologous tumors that are resistant to inactivated NK cells. This activity has been termed lymphokine activated killer (LAK) cell function. The phenotype of LAK may be the same as of NK or T lymphocytes. In addition to their cytotoxic function, several other regulatory functions of NK-like cells have been reported. These cells have multiple activities in the development and regulation of the immune system network such as the production of cytokines and a direct cytostatic effect on some cells.

The NK cells are ubiquitously distributed among various species ranging from phylogenetically low invertebrates to man. This phylogenetic conservation of NK cells supports the view that they play an important role in the basic defense and preservation of the organism. It seems NK cells are evolutionary forerunners of T lymphocytes and represent a primitive immune system [CPa]. The NK-like lymphocytes represent a quite heterogeneous group both morphologically and phenotypically. It includes NK cells, killer cells, natural cytotoxic cells, major histocompatibility complex (MHC)-unrestricted T cells, and LAK [HEa], [MOa], [VIa]. All these cells display characteristics that fit well the requirements for a tumor surveillance function. This function includes a rapid oncolytic activity without sensitization with antigen and the ability to recognize a broad spectrum of target cells including the poorly immunogenic tumors. This cytolytic activity is not restricted by MHC class I antigens. Several days or weeks are required after antigen priming *in vitro* and *in vivo* for the generation of mature MHC-restricted cytotoxic T-lymphocytes (CTL) from their precursors. At variance with the MHC-restricted CTL response via TCR, the NK-like cells can recognize and kill their target cells (TCs) within 1–30 min without preliminary stimulation by antigens or mitogens. This is one of the most notable features of the NK-like cells.

How does an NK-like cell, without classical immune activation by antigen, clonal selection and expansion, know which cells to attack? The answer to this question remains unknown [GUa]. The nature of the receptor which NK cells use to recognize their target molecules and the nature of ligands for these receptor are unknown. The cell surface structures allowing for LAK activity also have not been clearly defined.

Three types of the NK-recognition models are discussed in the literature: immunologically "specific" non-self-recognition, self-recognition, and nonspecific recognition. The first model is a classical one for immunology. It is conditioned by the presence of certain specific receptors on an NK cell and by the appropriate ligands on the surface of the TC [MOa], [ORa], [YOa]. The second model assumes loss or lack of some "protection antigens" on the TC surface, for instance, loss of MHC class I antigen which protects certain TCs from NK lysis [GUa], [KAa], [MOa]. The third model presumes that certain stable NK-receptor and their counter-structures do not exist on the surfaces of a NK cell and a TC [KIa], [KZg].

Recently, a new theoretical model describing the recognition of target cells by NK cells (or NK-like cells) without any specific NK-receptor has

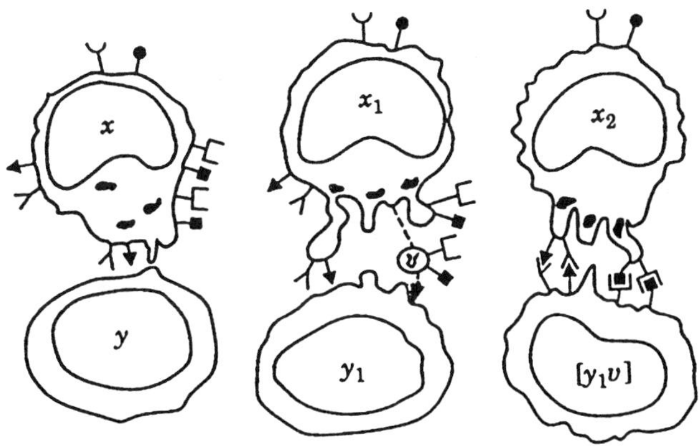

Figure 6.6 — The sequence of events in the NK/LAK cell recognition of target cells (TC). x and y are the free intact effector cell (EC) and TC, respectively; $x - y$ (or $[xy]$) is the initial conjugate between intact EC with TC; x_1 is the EC quickly activated to the exocytosis of receptor and anti-receptor molecules exocytosis from the NK cell surface; y_1 is the TC activated quickly after contact with a EC; v is the vesicle and/or the membranophilic substance shed from the NK cell surface; $v - y$ (or $[vy]$) is the TC that have received receptors and anti-receptors; $x - v - y$ (or $[x[vy]]$) is a EC–TC strong conjugate: after that the transfer of vesicles and/or membranophilic substances from the surface of an activated EC to the TC surface is complete and TC is programmed for lysis.

been described [KZf], [KZg], [KZn]. In Figure 6.6 some details of the model are drawn. There it is proposed that the exchange of small lipid vesicles (or membrane fragments) between the NK and TC surfaces after an initial contact of NK-like cells with TC is very important. These vesicles or membrane fragments can carry different types of receptors and counter-receptor molecules (for instance, different types of adhesion receptors and ligands, lymphokine receptors and lymphokines etc.). After the fusion process of vesicles (or membrane fragments) on the membrane of a TC, the local lipid composition of the TC membrane can be changed and, in addition, the TC can receive receptors and counter-receptors, so that the TC can be bound and lysed by the NK-like cell. This cell-cell interaction model is named the "harpoon recognition model"(HR model). Our suggestion for nonspecific NK recognition is associated with selective "harpooning" of the TC by lipid vesicles of the cells which express multiple disorders in structure and organization of the extra-membrane macromolecular framework, lipid-membrane submembrane cytoskeleton assembly. These aberrations are expressed by many primary tumor cells, metastatic cells, virus-infected cells, some immature normal cells and old cells.

Many non-NK killer cells (clones of T cells, for example) can bind to the NK-sensitive TCs. However, most of these cells do not kill the TCs. As follows from many experimental data, the close binding of NK-like cell with TC is only a necessary condition for NK-mediated TC lysis. The connection is determined by the interaction of specific macromolecules of receptors and ligands localized on the surfaces of EC and TC. However, the formation of a stable linking between EC and TC is a dynamic process, more complicated than a simple physical-chemical interaction between two or more types of molecules with a high affinity to each other localized on cell surfaces [HIa].

According to the foregoing theory, the kinetics of the cytotoxic reaction is described in the following scheme:

$$x + y \underset{k_{-1}}{\overset{k_1}{\rightleftharpoons}} [xy] \overset{k_2}{\rightarrow} x_1 + y_1 \,, \tag{6.35}$$

$$x_1 \overset{k_8}{\rightarrow} x_2 + v \,, \tag{6.36}$$

$$y_1 + v \underset{k_{-3}}{\overset{k_3}{\rightleftharpoons}} [y_1 v] \overset{k_3'}{\rightarrow} y_1 \,, \tag{6.37}$$

$$[y_1 v] + x_2 \underset{k_{-4}}{\overset{k_4}{\rightleftharpoons}} \Big[[y_1 v] x_2\Big] \overset{k_5}{\rightarrow} x_3 + y^* \,, \tag{6.38}$$

$$[y_1 v] + x_1 \underset{k_{-4'}}{\overset{k_4'}{\rightleftharpoons}} \Big[[y_1 v] x_1\Big] \overset{k_5}{\rightarrow} x_3 + y^* \,, \tag{6.39}$$

$$x_2 \overset{k_6'}{\rightarrow} x \,, \tag{6.40}$$

$$x_3 \overset{k_6}{\rightarrow} x \,, \tag{6.41}$$

$$y_1 \overset{k_7}{\rightarrow} y \,, \tag{6.42}$$

$$v \overset{k_9}{\rightarrow} v^* \,, \tag{6.43}$$

where

- x and y refer free resting NK cells and TCs respectively;
- x_1 is the activated NK cells after their primary contact with TCs;
- y_1 is the TCs after their primary contact with NK cells. The surface of these cells do not carry the receptor and counter receptor molecules

transferred from NK cells;

- x_2 is the NK cells after shedding some of the small vesicles and/or membranophilic substance (carrying the sets of receptor and counter receptor molecules) from the NK cell plasma membrane;
- x_3 is the NK cells after "programming" of TCs for lysis and NK cell detachment from the disintegrating TC;
- y^* is the disintegrating TCs;
- v is the small vesicles and/or membranophilic substance shed by NK cells and localized in the intercellular cleft area and/or in the environment medium;
- v^* is the inactivated vesicles;
- $[xy]$, $[y_1v]$, $[[y_1v]x_1]$, and $[[y_1v]x_2]$ are the conjugates of the component of reaction;
- k_1, k_2, $\ldots k_9$, k_{-1}, k_{-3}, k_{-4}, k'_{-3}, k'_{-4}, and k'_6 are kinetic constants.

This scheme takes into account a binary type of cell-cell interaction. Such types of conjugates usually dominate in *in vitro* experiments. The scheme also takes into account that NK cells and LAK can be detached easily without damage to the TC, see [BKb] and [MHa]. It may be suggested that after primary contact with an intact TC and following detachment of a NK from this cell, the NK-like cells have a higher probability to interact with the cell type y_1, but not with TC y (possibly, because the distance to cell y is short or/and some attractors between NK and TC type y may have appeared). The NK cell in state x_1 sheds its vesicles and/or membranophilic substances (v) quickly, which either perish (or become inactivated) spontaneously at rate k_9, or are taken up by the closest activated TC at rate k'_3 [KZn].

The kinetics of lysis of both a highly and weakly sensitive TC mediated by NK-like cells which have a rapid or slow restoration rate in their cytolytic potential. Numerical values of kinetic parameters and concentrations of cells were estimated on the basis of information about kinetic parameters of cytolytic reactions, and proceeded from several preliminary calculations of the typical times for stages in NK/LAK cytotoxic reactions *in vitro* [BKb], [KZe], [KZf], [KZg], and [MHa].

The case of a LAK (or NK cell) which can recycle in the lytic cycle at least a few times will be analyzed in the sequel. The following values of the constants were used:

$$\begin{aligned}
&k_1 = 0.5\,, \quad k_{-1} = 0.14\,, \quad k_2 = 0.35\,, \quad k_3 = 10.0\,, \quad k_{-3} = 0\,, \\
&k_4 = 0.7\,, \quad k_{-4} = 0.1\,, \quad k'_3 = k'_4 = k'_{-4} = k'_6 = 0\,, \\
&k_5 = 0.2\,, \quad k_6 = 0.5\,, \quad k_7 = 0.2\,, \quad k_8 = 0.5\,, \quad k_9 = 0.2\,. \qquad (6.44)
\end{aligned}$$

Cell numbers are normalized by the initial number of EC+TC, so they have dimension $(\text{min})^{-1}$. Initially, the ratio between NK-like cells and their TC is one.

We will focus on the simplified case $k_6' = k_4' = k_{-4}' = k_5' = 0$, i.e. when reactions (6.39) and (6.40) are relatively slow, and exocytosis/pinocytosis of NK-derived vesicles by TCs is absent.

Figure 6.7 shows the result of a numerical solution of the initial value problem for ordinary differential equations corresponding to the kinetic scheme (6.35–6.44) in the case of highly sensitive TCs. The typical initial conditions *in vitro* correspond to the nonzero positive values only for free nonactivated LAK and TC. It follows from Figure 6.7 that the model describes well both the qualitative and quantitative peculiarities of the cytolytic reaction kinetics, including the S-shape curve for the number of TCs "programmed" to lyse (y^*), the presence of the relatively short lag-period on this curve followed by rapid accumulation of EC–TC complexes, and the rapid decline in the rate of TCs lysed after 1–2 hrs. Note that at the selected parameter values (6.44) the cytolytic reaction is completed by the destruction of all TC (i.e. $y^* \approx y^0$ at $t = 16$ hr). This estimation corresponds well to the typical times for the completion of the cytolytic process by LAK or by NK cells from the peripheral blood.

It follows from comparisons of the solutions in Figure 6.7 with quasi-stationary solutions at $t > 15$ min that these solutions become close to each other in value. For example, the exact value $v(t)$ at $t > 15$ min differs only slightly from the quasi-stationary solution determined by the equation

$$v(t) \approx \frac{k_7}{k_9}\, y_1(t)\,. \tag{6.45}$$

In its turn, (6.45) requires that variables y_1 and x_2 should also be relatively fast. This statement can be easily proved if the right hand sides of Eqs. (6.38), (6.41), and (6.45) are set to 0 and then variables $[xy]$ and $[y_1 v]$ are excluded from the system of ordinary differential equations. It can be assumed based on equation (6.45) that a linear relation is established between a number of activated TCs and a number of free vesicles shed from ECs. This prediction can be confirmed experimentally. Moreover, suitable calculations show that the kinetics of the cytotoxic reaction change remarkably when the parameters k_3 and k_7 vary.

Some implications of the HR model can be experimentally verified. Several of its consequences and predictions will be considered below [KZf], [KZg], and [KZk]. Let us identify some of them.

• It follows from the model that the resistance of cells to NK cell cytotoxicity may be modified by means of natural or artificial damage of the structure and organization of the "extracellular matrix-membrane-submembrane cytoskeleton" framework [KNa]. If such changes are preserved for a sufficient time, NK-resistant cells may become NK-sensitive. Damage to the

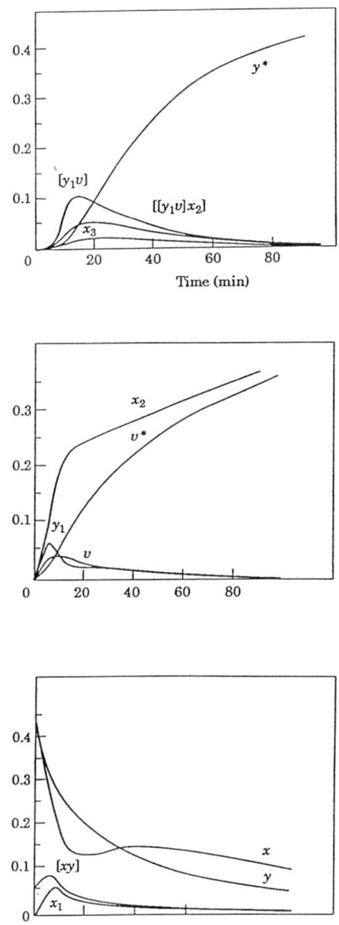

Figure 6.7 — Kinetics of the cytotoxicity reaction in the case of a "highly sensitive" TC ($k_7 = 0.2$ 1/min). The terms x, y, $[xy]$, x_1, y_1, v, v^*, $[y_1v]$, x_2, x_3, and y^* represent ECs, TCs, initial effector-target conjugates, the ECs which are quickly activated after initial collision with TCs, TCs after their initial contact with NK cells, free vesicles and/or membranophilic substance, inactivated vesicles, ECs that have received vesicles, ECs that have shed vesicles from the NK/LAK cell plasma membranes; ECs that have lost vesicles; ECs after EC killing that restore their surface receptor and counter-receptor molecules and their lytic potential, EC–TC strong conjugate that have transferred vesicles from the surface of activated EC to the TC surface, TCs that have been programmed for lysis, respectively. All variables are normalized on the total initial cell number. Initial EC:TC ratio equals 1.

structural organization of this framework can be achieved by using various preparations which perturb the components of the plasma membrane, or by means of a mechanical influence on the cell. Indeed, it has been found that desialylation of the cell surface of low-sensitive or NK-resistant cells makes them highly sensitive to lysis by NK-cells [KIa]. It seems that some mechanical processing of target cells, e.g. by ultrasound, could increase the sensitivity of TC to recognition by NK cells. if membrane integrity is preserved.

• A series of studies on the effects of viscous-elastic properties of the membrane of NK cells and of their TC have been presented by several research groups [KNa], [PVa], [RZa–c]. The results of these studies find their natural interpretation within the point of view of the HR model, which predicts that a decrease in the membrane viscosity of NK-sensitive TC, which have expressed disorder in the structure and organization of the "extracellular matrix-membrane-submembrane cytoskeleton" framework will not influence the frequency of NK–TC conjugate formation significantly, since near-membrane areas on the TC surface are already accessible to NK microfilaments. On the contrary, a decrease of the membrane viscosity of NK-resistant TC (e.g. by implanting membrane fragments of NK-sensitive TC) should heighten the frequency of attachment of TC with NK cells and accelerate the cytotoxic reaction in NK–TC conjugates. The observed data ([REa], [RZb]) correspond to these ideas. On the other hand, a relatively small increase in the membrane viscosity of NK-sensitive TC, according to the theory, should not lead to major changes in the formation of NK–TC pairs, but its influence on intercellular attraction pathways could consequently after the cytotoxic activity of a NK cell. It is probable that a significant increase in the TC membrane viscosity will become an obstacle for the processes that follow the initial NK–TC linking. Namely this would be the implantation of vesicles and fragments of the NK-cell surface into the TC membrane, and the formation and shedding of similar TC structures. Therefore the adhesive force in the NK–TC pairs will be lowered by a significant increase of the TC membrane viscosity, and consequently it will also lower the probability of TC lysis in such complexes. It was shown that an increase of the TC membrane viscosity of the K-562 line by lydocaine and colhicine enhances the NK-sensitivity of these cells [KNa]. When the membrane viscosity for the K-562 TCs is too high, the frequency of NK–TC conjugates was not changed significantly, but the TC lysability was reduced.

• The reversible diminution of the avidity of NK cells to TCs and of cytolytic activity after direct interaction between a NK cell and a TC *in vitro* and *in vivo* are well-known peculiarities of NK cells, but not CTLs [ABa,b], [KZe], [MHa]. The mechanisms of this phenomenon are unclear. According to the HR model the post-binding inactivation effect may result from at least two mechanisms: a loss of some receptor and counter-receptor molecules from the surface of the NK cell and/or the change of "optimal" lipid composition in the NK membrane after transfer of lipid vesicles from NK cell to TC. In this respect, it would be important to detect the fate of the receptor and counter-receptor pairs on the NK surface and the vesicle transport proteins during the binding and killing stages at NK–TC interaction. On the other hand, it would be interesting to determine the dynamics of the cholesterol level in the membrane of a NK cell; the kinetics of low- and high-density lipoprotein exocytosis; and the rate of lipoprotein production in a NK-cell before its binding with a TC, in the single NK–TC conjugate and in the NK cell after cytolytic reaction. As a consequence of both mechanisms, the recognition potential of a NK cell will be reduced.

Recently, some experimental data supporting the HR model were presented. It has been found that both anti-CD11a/CD18 MAb directed at LFA-1 and anti-CD54 MAb directed at ICAM-1 can inhibit the formation of the conjugate of NK-like cells and TCs and cytolysis at the effector cell level [ROa], [TIa]. These data indirectly suggest the importance of both receptors and counter-receptors in the process of recognition by NK cell. In addition, human cord blood lymphocytes lack of NK-function correlates with low level of LFA-1 and ICAM-1, CD2 and LFA-3. However, NK cells can express these antigens quickly after *in vitro* activation of the NK cells. Prompt and short-lived changes in the avidity of LFA-1 together with the activation-dependent expression of ICAM-1 [FIa] are also thought to provide the dynamics of autoregulation of these cell adhesion molecules in the process of cell-cell attachment and detachment, allowing recirculation of the ECs. Thus, lymphocytes require a certain level of activation (expression of these membrane molecules) to exert the lysis of TCs. Additionally, increases in the number of molecules (LFA-1, ICAM-1, CD2 and LFA-3) on the surface of NK cells were associated with enhanced formation of EC–TC conjugates, enhanced killing of NK-sensitive targets, and with the induction of LAK-susceptibility of previously resistant targets (LAK activity) [ROa]. Iho and Shaw [IHa] have investigated the role of ICAM-1 (CD54), LFA-1 (CD11a-c), β2-integrins (CD18), LFA-3 (CD58), CD2, CD56 antigens in the binding and cytotoxic activity of IL-6-treated LAK cells. None of the MAbs to CD11c, CD2, CD56 or CD58 used in this study caused significant changes in binding or cytotoxicity of untreated or IL-6-treated LAK cells. Only LFA-1 (CD11a/CD18) and ICAM-1 (CD54) molecules on surface of EC cells are involved in the standard LAK activity of IL-6 unregulated thymocytes against the NK-resistant melanoma UCLA-50-M14-cell line. M14 TCs did not express CD11a/CD18 and was CD54$^+$. However, pretreatment of M14 with anti-CD54 MAb did not inhibit LAK function (adhesion and killing of the TC). Pretreatment of LAK cells with anti-CD54 MAb decreased their cytotoxicity and binding capacity. Furthermore, these authors have observed that the combination of anti-CD11a and anti-CD54

MAbs inhibited stronger target conjugation and cytotoxicity of LAK cells than MAb alone. Therefore, CD54 molecules on the LAK effector cells, but not on the M14 TCs, were involved in binding and cytolysis.

These observations did not explain the reasons for recognition by LAK cells of their TC based on classic self-recognition or nonself recognition models. The EC (LAK) expresses the cytolysis-involved adhesion receptor (LFA-1) on the cell surface and the counter-receptor (ICAM-1), but TCs (melanoma cell line M14) did not express LFA-1, and ICAM-1, which were not involved in the adhesion of LAK with M14 TCs. According to the self or nonself recognition theory, ECs cannot recognize the TC because a specific ligand was not expressed on the TC surface. However, the counter-receptor and receptor molecules were present on the EC before the cell-cell interaction only. Taking into account the possibility of exchange of membrane LFA-1 macromolecules between conjugated CTL and TC [FOa], the experimental results of Iho and Shaw [IHa] can be explained naturally according to the HR model but cannot be explained by classical models of nonself and self recognition [BUa].

In conclusion, the harpoon model permits the interpretation of a wide variety of experimental observations. A "specific" NK-receptor analogous to a T or B cell receptor, which has proved elusive despite many attempts to find it, is not required in this model. The HR model permits a novel experimental way to study questions regarding mechanisms of NK-like cell recognition and its regulation by physical and biological factors and modifiers as well as those about the nature of a wide variety of cell types attacked by NK-like cells. In addition, the harpoon recognition mechanism may offer a basis for interaction of the antigen-presenting cells among others with their TCs.

6.5 Switch of Cytolytic Mechanisms: Effector Cells, Target Cells and Bispecific Regulating Molecules

Various types of cytotoxic/cytostatic cells (CCs) of the immune system (NK cells, CTLs, cytotoxic macrophages) bind to target cells (TCs) through soluble bispecific "regulating molecules" (BRMs) (for example, monoclonal antibodies (MAbs), lectins, artificial bispecific MAbs), which carry connection sites both for these effector cell and target cells. These molecules can be used for redirecting CCs to TCs. We suggest a model for the interaction kinetics of CCs and TCs through direct cell-cell contact or with BRMs, which are able to bind the surface of both CC and TC. It has been shown that a certain difference in the avidity of BRM to receptors on the TC and CC is needed for a maximum efficiency of antibody-dependent cell cytolysis (ADCC), bispecific MAbs (bi-ADCC), or lectin-dependent cell cytolysis (LDCC). Cytotoxic/cytostatic activity in all these reactions is described by a bell-like curve with an increase in the concentration of BRM in the media. The optimum ratios have been defined between kinetic parameters and reaction component concentrations, at which the same CC (a subpopulation of NK cells with ADCC activity, for example) may utilize either a direct cell-cell recognition mechanism or an indirect recognition mechanism resulting from the BRM binding.

6.5.1 Kinetics of multiple cytotoxic reactions

It was established that among immune cytotoxic/cytostatic ECs at least some ECs carry several types of receptor molecules of diverse specificity on their surface, through which the same cell can utilize several cytolytic mechanisms. Thus, CTL-recognizing MHC antigens may realize their cytolytic potential as the result of their linking to TC by the T cell receptor, the receptor to sheep erythrocytes (CD2-antibodies), the NK-like receptor, the CD45 antigen and other cell surface receptors [LOa], [TEa]. Moreover, on the surface of many cytotoxic ECs (CTLs, NK cells, LAKs, activated macrophages) there are receptors to Fc-portions of antibodies. Therefore, the EC cytolytic reaction may be initiated as a result of linking Fc-receptors of killer cells with Fc-portions of antibodies specifically linked to any antigenic determinants of TC surface molecules. The second type of cytotoxic reaction is called antibody-dependent cell cytolysis (ADCC). ADCC consists of several stages. However, similar to other effector mechanisms, a necessary phase of the reaction is firm linking of EC with TC. TC lysis is implemented during subsequent stages of the reaction. Cross-linking of Fc-receptors by MAbs on the surface of the EC has been shown to lead to the rapid stimulation of protein trosine kinase (PTK) activity and to activate of the signal trasduction pathways. Activated oxygen metabolites, e.g. H_2O_2, NO are involved in TC lysis, mediated by ADCC mechanism.

EC sensibilising antibodies used in the process of ADCC are usually IgG. The Fc receptors (FcRs) represent one of the most important receptor elements of the immune system, as they create a bridge of communication between the humoral and cellular immune compartments. FcRs are a diverse group represented by multiple members, many of which are in the multigene families. Three classes of Fc receptors for IgG have been established on the cell surface — FcRI, FcRII and FcRIII — which differ in their molecular mass, avidity, their number at the surface of various types of EC. ADCC can be implemented by killer cells, most CTL, NK cells, LAK, macrophages, polymorpho-nuclear leukocytes [LOa]. Usually, the Fc receptors are transmembrane proteins which bind a polymeric or monomeric Ig with low affinity. Cell surface Fc receptors are capable of receptor-mediated endocytosis of immunoglobulins [GOa]; exocytosis of Fc receptors by a cell may also take place [GEa].

Besides IgG molecules, the third necessary component in the linking of cytolytic EC of diverse origin with TC may be represented by monosaccharides, glycolipides, lectin-like molecules, soluble forms of ligand-receptor complexes and other molecules of the medium [BKa], [LOa].

The TC lysis mechanism is well characterized when it is implemented by the activation of EC cells (CTL, NK, K cells, macrophages), by lectins and glycoproteins linking hydrophylic carbohydrate groups. LDCC may play an essential role in tumor surveillance [LOa], [SHa]. Antigen is determinant on TC for lectins or lectin-like molecules may be components of tumor-associated glycolipids which are targets for NK-like receptors. For instance, GD2 and GD3 gangliosides are present on surface of solid tumor cells and these molecules are targets for binding of NK-like cells [HRa].

The presence of lectin in a medium does not heighten the frequency of pair EC:TC conjugates or the frequency of EC conjugates with two or more TC. The mechanism of lectin effect on EC is conditioned by an increase in the avidity of linking cells and/or the following induction of the potential lytic mechanism, which has no visible effect in the EC linking with TC in the absence of lectin [BOb], [JEa].

A novel way of cytolytic induction activation of "resting" CTL has been found in the recent years. Non-MHC-restricted CTL cytotoxicity with respect to TC may be induced if BRM are represented by monoclonal antibodies specific to CD3 molecules of the T cell receptor complex, or by heteroconjugates consisting of two monoclonal antibodies, one of which is specific to the CD3 antigen, and the other to some definite antigen on the TC surface [JUa], [LWa], [LUa], [TUa]. In the first case, EC link with TC if the latter express Fc receptors, in the second case the linking is implemented with TC, on the surface of which the heteroconjugate of two antibodies finds specific determinants. Note that the CTL cytolytic reaction is initiated as the result of physical linking and micro-clustering of CD3 molecules on the CTL membrane in the area of contact with the TC surface antigen [BKb,c].

Thus, the three-component interaction between EC, TC and BRM is a rather common phenomenon in immune processes *in vivo*.

The presence of several independent pathways linking cytotoxic EC with TC and the following cytolytic processes offers great difficulties for experimental study of a "pure" form of a single mechanism of recognition by EC, and for understanding of regulation processes governing of these mechanisms on the cellular level.

What particular features in the course of EC–TC reaction may result if at least two different types receptors are expressed on the same surface of EC: If one of them recognizes corresponding counter-receptors on the surface of TC directly, and the other can recognize the TC through the soluble bispecific molecule? What is the relationship of the cytolytic reaction intensity with the ratio of the components involved? What are the control mechanisms leading to the dominance of a certain mechanism of TC recognition by cytotoxic EC? Why would some subpopulations of FC-positive ECs be activated and other inactivated by the Ig in certain experimental models of ADCC?

To answer these questions, a mathematical model for the reaction of EC capable of the realization of their cytolytic potential either through direct linking with TC by a specific receptor, or indirectly through soluble bispecific molecules is described in what follows.

6.5.2 General model

Mechanisms for triggering various cytolytic processes by a killer cell and the possibilities of their sequential or parallel realization on the level of single EC:TC conjugates are unknown. However, within the framework of the biological kinetics approach, the main stages and kinetic features of the cytotoxic reaction following the initial linking of EC with TC in the cases ADCC, LDCC, anti-CD3-induced cytotoxic reaction are similar to those in the case of direct specific interactions mediated by ligand-receptor linking of CTL, NK cells with corresponding TCs [BKa], [HKa], [ZEa].

Therefore, we propose that the kinetics of the interaction of cytotoxic cells with TC may be described by simplified kinetic schemes which were presented in the previous section. In the mathematical consideration of the problem, let us restrict ourselves to the case in which we may neglect EC inactivation and the appearance of "refractory" TC in the process of BRM and EC interaction, i.e. TC which have partly or entirely lost their surface antigens recognized by EC. We will analyze the kinetic scheme:

$$x + y \underset{k_{-11}}{\overset{k_{11}}{\rightleftharpoons}} [xy] \xrightarrow{k_{21}} x + y_1^* , \qquad (6.46)$$

$$x + z \underset{k_{-12}}{\overset{k_{12}}{\rightleftharpoons}} [xz] , \qquad (6.47)$$

$$[xz] + y \underset{k_{-13}}{\overset{k_{13}}{\rightleftharpoons}} [xyz] , \qquad (6.48)$$

$$y + z \underset{k_{-14}}{\overset{k_{14}}{\rightleftharpoons}} [yz] , \qquad (6.49)$$

$$[yz] + x \underset{k_{-15}}{\overset{k_{15}}{\rightleftharpoons}} [xyz] , \qquad (6.50)$$

$$[xyz] \xrightarrow{k_{22}} x + y_2^* + z^* , \qquad (6.51)$$

$$[xy] + z \underset{k_{-16}}{\overset{k_{16}}{\rightleftharpoons}} [xyz] , \qquad (6.52)$$

where variable x is the free (unbound) ECs, y is the free TCs, and z is the soluble bispecific number of regulating molecule which is involved in EC and TC binding. Variables $[xy]$, $[xz]$, $[yz]$, and $[xyz]$ are the cell-cell, cell-molecule and cell-molecule-cell conjugates; y_1^* and y_2^* are the TCs programmed for dying; z^* is the degrading BM; k_{1i}, k_{-1i}, k_{21}, and k_{22} are the kinetic constants of binding, detachment of reaction components, while k_{21} and k_{22} are the rates of the cytolytic reactions.

The system of ordinary differential equations corresponding to the above scheme, is

$$\frac{dx}{dt} = -k_{11}xy + (k_{-11} + k_{21})[xy] - k_{12}xz + k_{-12}[xz] + k_{22}[xyz] \\ - k_{15}x[yz] + k_{-15}[xyz]\,, \tag{6.53}$$

$$\frac{dy}{dt} = -k_{14}yz + k_{-14}[yz] - k_{13}y[xz] + k_{-13}[xyz] \\ - k_{11}xy + k_{-11}[xy]\,, \tag{6.54}$$

$$\frac{dz}{dt} = -k_{12}xz + k_{-12}[xz] - k_{14}yz + k_{-14}[yz] \\ - k_{16}z[xy] + k_{-16}[xyz]\,, \tag{6.55}$$

$$\frac{d[xy]}{dt} = k_{11}xy - k_{-11}[xy] - k_{21}[xy] + k_{-16}[xyz] - k_{-16}z[xy]\,, \tag{6.56}$$

$$\frac{d[xz]}{dt} = k_{12}xz - k_{-12}[xz] + k_{-13}[xyz] - k_{13}y[xz]\,, \tag{6.57}$$

$$\frac{d[yz]}{dt} = k_{14}yz - k_{-14}[yz] + k_{-15}[xyz] - k_{15}x[yz]\,, \tag{6.58}$$

$$\frac{d[xyz]}{dt} = k_{13}y[xz] - (k_{-13} + k_{-15} + k_{-16} + k_{22})[xyz] \\ + k_{15}x[yz] + k_{16}z[xy]\,, \tag{6.59}$$

$$\frac{dy_1^*}{dt} = k_{21}[xy]\,, \tag{6.60}$$

$$\frac{dy_2^*}{dt} = k_{22}[xyz]\,, \tag{6.61}$$

$$\frac{dz^*}{dt} = k_{22}[xyz]\,, \tag{6.62}$$

where variables and parameters are the same as the previous kinetic scheme.

Under *in vitro* conditions, the conservation laws are valid for these kinetics:

$$x^0 = x + [xy] + [xz] + [xyz]\,, \tag{6.63}$$

$$y^0 = y + [yx] + [yz] + [xyz] + y_1^* + y_2^* \,, \tag{6.64}$$

$$z^0 = z + [xz] + [yz] + [xyz] + z^* \,. \tag{6.65}$$

6.5.3 Kinetics of ADCC/LDCC reactions

The model is nonlinear and consists of many components. In order to make the qualitative features of behavior of the model solutions easier to comprehend, some special cases can be dealt with.

Let us select for analysis the reactions corresponding to the ADCC or LDCC process *in vivo*, when a binding of MAb with free EC is also permitted:

$$x + z \underset{k_{-12}}{\overset{k_{12}}{\rightleftharpoons}} [xz] \,, \tag{6.66}$$

$$[xz] + y \underset{k_{-13}}{\overset{k_{13}}{\rightleftharpoons}} [xyz] \,, \tag{6.67}$$

$$y + z \underset{k_{-14}}{\overset{k_{14}}{\rightleftharpoons}} [yz] \,, \tag{6.68}$$

$$[yz] + x \underset{k_{-15}}{\overset{k_{15}}{\rightleftharpoons}} [xyz] \,, \tag{6.69}$$

$$[xyz] \xrightarrow{k_{22}} x + y^* + z^* \,. \tag{6.70}$$

It might be expected that the relationship of the kinetic parameters of binding/detachment of BRM, EC and TC produces a rather important effect on the intensity of the cytotoxic reaction. This expectation was confirmed by numerical experiments [KZf]. Conversely, if the BRM avidity to EC decreases, the reaction effectivity essentially increases. Such a nonlinear phenomenon was explained as the result of a fast increase in the concentration of $[xz]$ and $[yz]$ complexes which rapidly diminishes the unbound EC (x) and TC (y). In this case, BRMs rapidly bind the available binding sites as on surface of EC and of TC. Then, the further formation of three-component complexes TC–BRM–EC and, consequently, realization by the EC of the cytotoxic reaction became impossible. Thus, the high avidity of BRM as to antigen on TC and to antigen on EC is not optimal for the realization of the cytotoxic response in ADCC/LDCC. If the difference between A_2 and A_4 is increased, the cytotoxic reaction efficiency increases.

Note that Fc receptors (FcR-III) type III, which are expressed on NK-like cells and mediated ADCC, have a much lower affinity for Fc-fragments of antibodies than the typical specific binding site affinity on Ig [GEa]. These differences are well explained by the model.

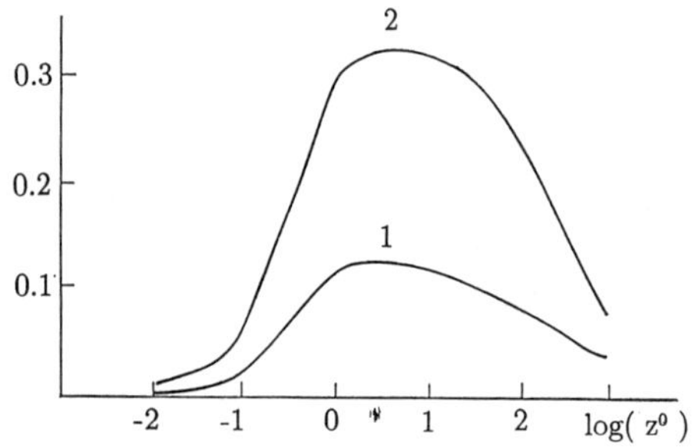

Figure 6.8 — Dose relationship of three-component $[xyz]$ complexes formation (1), ADCC y^* (2) at various initial levels of antibodies in a medium ($\log(z^0)$) and fixed value of $t(t = 4\text{hr})$. Initial values: $x(0) = 0.5$, $y(0) = 0.5$, $[xy] = [xz] = [yz] = [xyz] = 0$. Kinetic parameters: $A_2 \ll A_4$; $k_{12} = 0.01$, $k_{-12} = 0.1$, $k_{14} = 5.0$, $k_{-14} = 0.1$; $k_{22} = 0.5$, $k_{13} = 0.5$, $k_{-13} = 0.14$, $k_{15} = 3.0$, $k_{-15} = 0.14$. The dimension of all kinetic parameters equals t^{-1} (hr^{-1}).

Now, we analyze the "dose versus effect" dependence which corresponds to $A_2 \ll A_4$ in the model. The results of a numerical analysis of the dose relationship of a cytotoxic reaction with the initial number of BRM are presented in Figure 6.8, which shows that the "low" and "high" BRM concentrations are less effective than "average" ones. This phenomenon is explained by the fact that with a lack of BRM in a medium most of these molecules are bound on the part of TCs which then are destroyed by ECs, and the other part of TC which did not bind enough BRM will not be recognized by ECs and a lytic reaction will stopped before it can be completed; with excess BRM in the medium, free EC and TC rapidly disappear leading to inhibition of the cytolytic reaction.

This important theoretical result has received experimental confirmation. For example, the presence of a soluble form of a specific antigen in a medium during ADCC of T lymphocytes causes the inhibition of the reaction [MEa]. Liu et al. [LUa] have established a bi-phasic dose relationship of the CD3-dependent T cell cytotoxic reaction when various concentrations of a heteroconjugate of two antibodies are used. The specificity of one the two conjugated antibodies was directed against the CD3 molecule of the T cell receptor complex; the other antibody was directed against a certain antigen of TC cell surface. The threshold concentration of the antibody conjugate is $4 \cdot 10^{-11}M$, the optimum concentration is $10^{-10}M$, and the blocking concentration is $10^{-8}M$.

6.5.4 One effector cell and two molecular mechanisms recognition

Consider the kinetics of the effector reaction in the case of simultaneous existence of two EC mechanisms for TC recognition. Let the first mechanism be realized due to the direct interaction of receptors and their ligands on surfaces of opposite cells; the second mechanism can be realized through the BRM-mediated linking of EC with TC.

It is evident that at low BRM concentration the first mechanism will dominate in the reaction. This result comes from computer-aided calculations of the Eqs. (6.46–6.52). When the BRM concentration is low ($z^0 \ll x^0$, $z^0 \ll y^0$), both TC binding pathways provide a comparable cytotoxic effects, see Figure 6.9. As the BRM initial concentration grows, at a small BRM in excess of $z^0 \geq 2.0$, the direct EC reaction is intensely inhibited and it does not influence the results of the cytotoxic process. Note that these conditions are optimum for the manifestation of the ADCC reaction (Figure 6.8). It should be mentioned that if the reaction of the $xz + yz \rightleftharpoons [xyyz] \rightarrow [yz]^* + \ldots$ type is permissible in Eqs. (6.46–6.52), then the dose-effect curves may not have a bell-like shape and the mechanism of switching on two types of cytotoxic reactions may not be kinetically "eroded".

Thus, if in the system EC–BRM–TC, cooperating under simple chemical kinetics laws takes place, then it is possible to flexibly regulate TC lysis at varying BRM concentrations. For example, by varying the initial BRM concentration it is possible to make dominant either the direct TC recognition mechanism, through specific receptors and their ligands on opposite cells, or through ADCC type mechanisms in the TC lysis. Moreover, sufficiently high BRM concentrations inhibit ADCC as well.

Notice that the Eqs. (6.53–6.65) model is the summarized mathematical formulation of autoregulation processes in three-component biochemical and metabolytic systems [KOa], [KWa]. Several results of the mathematical aspects corresponding to the above particular cases may be found in [BAa,b], [KOa], [KZf], and [SOa].

In the kinetic analysis we have not considered effector immune processes in the case of formation of complexes of a single EC with two or more TC, a single TC with two or more EC etc. However, under *in vitro* conditions ([BDa], [BOa], [PZa]) and possibly often *in vivo* as well [LKa], cytolytic reactions occur primarily in the process of the formation of pair EC:TC cellular conjugates. Nevertheless, if the initial ratio between EC and TC is much more or less than one, then a minor fraction of the three-cellular and larger multi-cellular clusters of the TCs and the ECs are formed. The mechanisms of multicellular conjugate formation and the switch of lytic

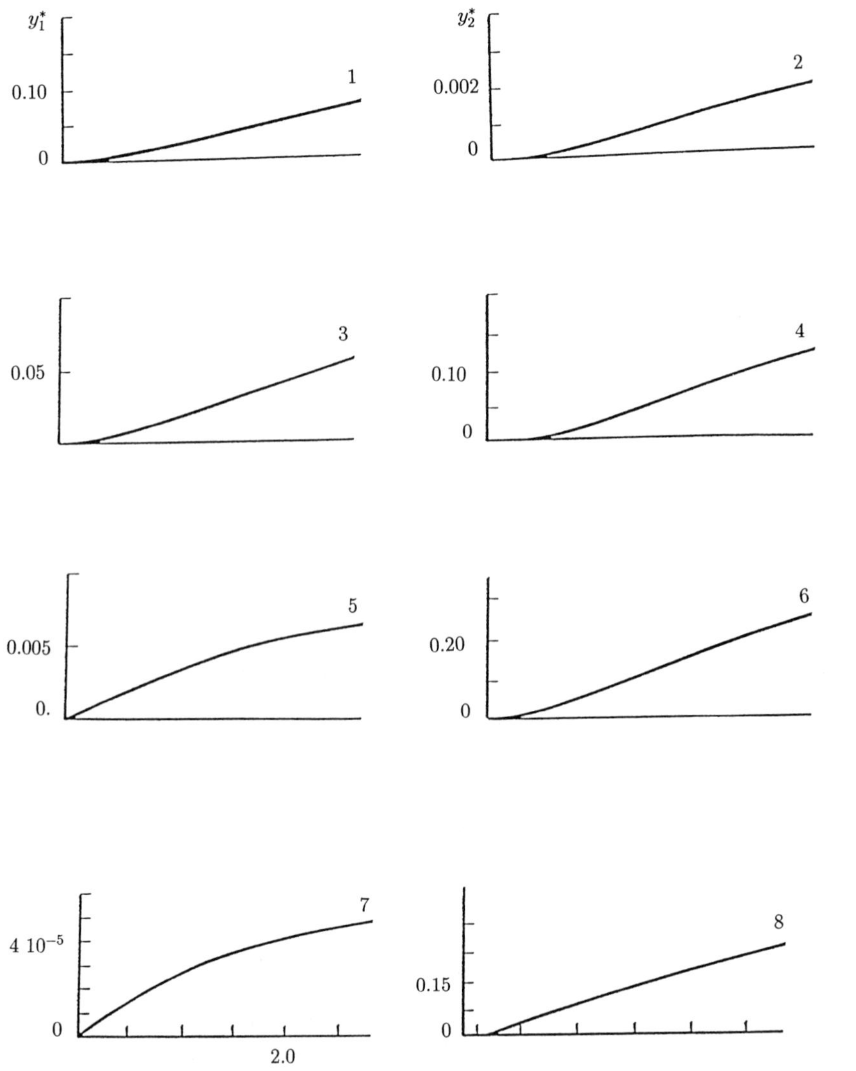

Figure 6.9 — Kinetics of a EC cytotoxic reaction with two TC recognition mechanisms present and at various levels of the BRMs in the medium $z_1(0) = 0.05$ (curves 1, 2), $z_2(0) = 0.2$ (curves 3, 4), $z_3(0) - 2.0$ (curves 5, 6), $z_4 = 250$ (curves 7, 8). $x(0) = y(0) = 0.5$, $k_{11} = 0.5$; $k_{-11} = 0.14$; $k_{21} = k_{22} = 0.5$. Other parameters are the same as in Figure 6.8.

reaction in these conjugates are of a great theoretical and practical interest. Experimental and theoretical aspects of EC interaction with TC are described in [BDa], [MKa], and [PEb].

6.5.5 Conclusion

Various types of cytotoxic/cytostatic EC can bind to TC with the help of soluble "helper molecules" present in a medium, which carry sites for binding with both EC and their TCs. The process of TC cytolysis by EC involving bispecific molecules (in ADCC, LDCC or cytotoxic reactions mediated by bispecific antibodies) and (depending on the ratio between EC, TC, and BRM concentrations) may have a complicated nonmonotonous character and a nonlinear relationship with kinetic parameters and reaction component concentrations. This hypothesis has been verified using the mathematical model presented. Within the framework of the model, an explanation has been provided for nonlinear effects observed in cytotoxic cellular reactions involving BRM. Optimum ratios were determined between reaction component concentrations, at which the same EC may lyse TC either primarily as the result of a direct cell-cell binding, or involving bispecific medium molecules mediating the formation of cell-molecule-cell complexes.

Equations (6.53–6.65) may serve as basic models for a quantitative analysis of the effects of the biological response modifiers, drugs on the pathways and stages of cytotoxic reactions of ECs with TCs *in vitro*, and also it may by used for construction of more complex mathematical models of immune response *in vivo*.

6.6 Propagation and Interaction of Tumor-Specific Macromolecules in Multicellular Tumors

Although cytotoxic lymphocytes that have the capability for recognition and killing tumor cells can be detected in the peripheral blood of cancer patients, and in some tumors, these cells often are not sufficiently active to control the growth of tumors. Experimental data suggest that the state of nonreactivity or tolerance of the cytotoxic lymphocytes has been attributed to the existence of defects on the level of expression of tumor-associated antigens (TAAs), in the presentation of TAA by tumor cells, or in kinetic and space restrictions for interaction of the cytolytic cells with the cells in the tumor. The spatio-temporal restrictions for lymphocytes may be very important in the case of the solid tumors. Solid tumors are known to progress through two distinct phases of growth — the avascular phase and the vascular phase. This topic is dealt with in [ADa] and [CHa].

Typically, avascular tumor nodes or tumor foci in tissue grow to a few millimeters in diameter. The density of the solid tumor and the intra-tissue pressure in these tumors are strong restrictions for free migration of immune cells into tumor tissue. Therefore, infiltration of avascular solid tumors by immune cytotoxic cells may be an extremely slow process. Obviously, the spatio-temporal restrictions may be somewhat reduced in the case of diffusion of the immune macromolecule. Monoclonal antibodies (MAbs) directed to TAAs, and some cytokines are often discussed in the literature as potential tools for delivering cytotoxic factors into solid tumors [JNa].

In this section mathematical models describing propagation of specific macromolecules (MAbs, cytokines, anti-growth factors etc.) in multicellular tumors, and the interaction of these macromolecules with tumor associated antigens will be discussed.

Targeted damage of tumor cells by specific antibodies (Abs) against TAAs is a promising method in the therapy for small tumors and metastases in the body. In order to increase the damage, Abs or cytokines are bound to radioactive labels or toxins [BXa], [JNa], [JWa], [KKb], [ONa], [WEa]. Such complexes are often called "magic bullets". Processes of interaction of high-affinity MAbs with cells in a fluid medium are well studied *in vitro*. The kinetics of these interactions is determined by various processes: Ab molecule diffusion in the medium, reversible linking with specific sites on cell surface antigens (Ags), clusterization of the complexes formed, their internalization by a cell and/or shedding into a medium. Diffusion limits ("diffusion obstacles") mostly have no essential effect on the kinetics of the process in homogenous systems, since the rate of macromolecules collisions with linking sites on cells under experimental conditions exceeds the rate of their specific interaction. Compact distribution of Ag takes place in the case of tumor. Then as "magic bullets" are introduced in the body, reacting components are separated in the space and "diffusion obstacles" may prove crucial and cause substantial deceleration in the accumulation of "magic bullets" in a tumor. Such restrictions lead to nonuniform distribution of macromolecules in a tumor and consequently to nonuniformity of damage of the TCs in the tumor.

The kinetic study of the propagation and interaction of MAb in solid tumors is extremely important for quantitative comparison of the mathematical models with the real process, and in the search for critical parameters which can determine the outcome of the interaction of cytotoxic molecules. Mathematical analysis of the role of diffusion restrictions of MAb and MAb affinity in the process of the MAb accumulation in solid tissues was presented in [JWa], [MFa], [NUa], [ONa], [SAa], and [WEa]. To optimize the therapeutic effect, the process of distribution of specific macromolecules and their interactions with TC in biological tissues is studied in phenomenological models. Usually, models of these processes are written in the form of a nonlinear diffusion model, and describe the propagation of macromolecules into the tumor, and their binding to tumor-associated antigens expressed on the surface of tumor cells. In this section we will use kinetic and spatio-temporal experimental data for construction of minimal physico-mathematical models of the uptakes of specific MAb in small multicellular tumor spheroid (MTS).

The MTS growth *in vitro* are widely used as experimental models to study the interaction of macromolecules and drugs with solid tumors. Such tumors can be regarded as an *ex vitro* model of avascularized micrometastases or primary tumor.

One study [KKa] presents the results of detailed kinetic measurements of uptake of specific MAbs by human melanoma MTS. MTSs of the CaCl 73–36 melanoma cell line of the $300\mu m$ or $500\mu m$ diameter were put into the nutrition medium with a high concentration of AB96.5 MAb (IgG2a) isotype previously labeled with ^{125}I . Experimental tubes were placed on a slowly rotating plate at 37^0C. The Ab concentration in the medium was usually 0.2 μg/ml. No significant effect on the growth of the spheroids was observed resulting from these tracer dose concentrations. This experimental model is considered by the present author to be a special case of reversible specific binding of macromolecules in the absence of convection and metabolism of macromolecules.

Aliquots of MTSs were sampled at t_c = 1, 4, 8, 11, 14 and 24 hrs at 37^0C. At the end of each of the designated incubation times, some of the spheroids were sampled and washed with phosphate buffered saline (PBS) without MAb for a brief period (about 5 seconds). This rinsing removed any residual Ab adhering to the surface of the spheroid. After the brief wash of the tumor spheroids, the following occurred:

a) an aliquot was placed into a gamma-radiometer to measure radioactivity accumulated in spheroids in time t_c;

b) micro-radiography of spheroids was carried out, thus fixing the spatial distribution of radioactive Abs in MTS at a fixed time t_c;

c) an aliquot of ATSs was placed into pure medium for $\tau_1 = 1$ hour or $\tau_2 = 24$ hours; after τ_1 and τ_2 the amount of Ab effluxes during the reincubation process and the amount of MAb retained in the spheroids were measured by gamma counting.

The number of spheroids in each sample contributing to the radioactive measurement was counted on a microscope. Ab uptake was measured in 50 MTSs and normalized per spheroid. The effluxed radioactivity was examined by trichlorocetic acid precipitation. Spatial distribution of radiolabeled MAb in some MTSs at fixed time points was determined radiometrically.

Thus, the experiments of MAb interaction with MTS consist of two phases:

1) Initial incubation: When MAbs penetrate the MTS from the medium. At a high concentration of MAb in the medium the concentration of

these molecule at the MTS surface is practically constant in time;

2) Reincubation: During this phase of experiment the MAbs (which have already accumulated in the MTS at the first phase of experiment) flowed out from the MTS into a large amount of MAb-free medium.

The Ab used in the experiments had a valence of binding n equal to 2. However, if the concentration of the Ab is much higher than the concentration of the binding sites, then the most of the Ab could use only one of the binding sites and in reality $n = 1$. This may happen in the region near surface of the spheroid during incubation. On the contrary, if the concentration of Ab is equal to or smaller than the concentration of binding sites, than n would appear to 2. This is may well happen near the center of the MTS. In [KKa] the concentration of MAb in the medium was much higher than the concentration of free binding sites; for fitting the model the case $n = 1$ will be used.

According to the above considerations, we suggested a kinetic scheme for the interaction and distribution of specific MAb in the MTS:

$$u(r,t) + w\left(\overset{D_w\downarrow}{r}, t\right) \underset{k_{-1}}{\overset{k_1}{\rightleftharpoons}} [u,w](r,t)\,, \tag{6.71}$$

where u, w, and $[uw]$ denote distribution densities of free specific binding sites on the cells (receptors), free MAbs and complexes of the binding sites and MAbs; k_1 is the rate of specific MAb binding with the binding sites, k_{-1} is the dissociation rate of such complexes, D_w is the diffusion coefficient of MAb in the spheroid; t is time, r is a space variable.

It may be assumed that a conservation law for components of the reaction applies, i.e. a sum of the ligand-receptor complexes and unbound receptors is equal to the initial amount of receptors in the tumor $(u^0(r))$. In this case

$$\Big[u(r,t)w(r,t)\Big] = u^0(r) - u(r,t)\,. \tag{6.72}$$

We may describe the processes of incubation and reincubation of MAbs with the MTSs by the same system of equations. However, the initial and boundary conditions will be different. The two separate phases of the experiment documented by [KKa] are the following:

The 1st phase of kinetic experiments: MAb accumulation assay

This process can be described by the following simple mathematical model:

$$\begin{cases} \dfrac{\partial u}{\partial t} = k_{-1}u^0(r) - u\Big(k_1 w + k_{-1}\Big)\,, \\[2ex] \dfrac{\partial w}{\partial t} = \dfrac{D_w}{r^2}\dfrac{\partial}{\partial r}\left(r^2\dfrac{\partial w}{\partial r}\right) + k_{-1}u^0(r) - u(k_1 w + k_{-1})\,, \end{cases} \tag{6.73}$$

where $u = u(r,t)$, $w = w(r,t)$, $t \in [0, t_c]$, and $r \in [0, R]$.
Initial conditions are written as:

$$u(r,0) = u^0(r)\,, \qquad w(r,0) = W^0 \exp\left(\gamma(r^2 - R^2)\right)\,, \tag{6.74}$$

where W^0 is the MAb concentration at $r = R$, and $\gamma \gg 1$ is a constant.
Boundary conditions for the diffusion equation in the incubation experiment are:

i) at $r = 0$ the boundary condition is symmetrical in the center of the spheroid

$$\frac{\partial w}{\partial r}(0,t) = 0\,, \tag{6.75}$$

ii) at the outward surface of the tumor spheroid (at $r \geq R$) the MAb concentration is generally related to time. The MAb concentration out of the spheroid is maintained constant in the *in vitro* experiments

$$w(R,t) = W^0\,. \tag{6.76}$$

The 2nd phase of kinetic experiments: MAb efflux assay

The partial differential equations are written as

$$\begin{cases} \dfrac{\partial u'}{\partial t} = k_{-1}u^0(r) - u'\left(k_1 w' + k_{-1}\right)\,, \\ \dfrac{\partial w'}{\partial t} = \dfrac{D_w}{r^2}\dfrac{\partial}{\partial r}r^2\left(\dfrac{\partial w'}{\partial r}\right) + k_{-1}u^0(r) \\ \qquad - u'\left(k_1 w' + k_{-1}\right)\,, \end{cases} \tag{6.77}$$

where $u' = u'(r,t)$, $w' = w'(r,t)$, $t \in [t_c, t_{c+\tau j}]$, and $r \in [0, R]$.
The initial conditions are

$$u'(r,t_c) = u(r,t_c)\,, \qquad w'(r,t_c) = w(r,t_c)\,. \tag{6.78}$$

Boundary conditions for the diffusion-kinetic system are the following:

i) the condition of symmetry in the center of the sphere;

ii) zero concentration of free MAb is maintained at the outward surface of the MTS at $r = R$

$$w'(R,t) = 0\,, \tag{6.79}$$

where t is time, r is the spatial variable in spherical coordinates; $u(r,t)$ and $u'(r,t)$ are volume densities of free receptors at cell surfaces of tumor cells in the spheroid, for the processes of incubation and reincubation, respectively; $w(r,t)$ and $w'(r,t)$ are volume densities of free MAb molecules in the spheroid measured in molecular units (m.u.) or receptors in ml; dimension of k_1 is $\text{ml} \cdot \text{hr}^{-1} \cdot \text{m.u.}^{-1}$, the dimension of k_{-1} is hr^{-1} (both are kinetic constants); D_w is the diffusion coefficient of MAb molecules, measured in cm^2/hr.

As already mentioned, this model has shown good agreement with experimental data.

6.7 Conclusion

Interaction between the immune system and a tumor is an extremely complicated phenomenon involving several interrelated processes. In this survey some basic and relatively simple mathematical models of the interactions of effector cells and macromolecules of the immune system with tumor cells have been reviewed. The discussed mathematical models include minimal numbers of components and realistic physical and biochemical propositions on the mechanisms of their interactions. Nevertheless, these "minimal" models were well fitted to a set of experimental data and these models allow for some nontrivial predictions. It seems that such models could provide the basis for future experimental studies and for mathematical modeling of more complex situations in the interactions of tumor and immune system. These models may be used in the experimental studies of the interaction of immune effector cells and molecules against other types of antigens (virus-infected cells, parasites etc.). Further, one can develop studies related to bifurcation analysis [KZj] and diagnostics [KZl]. The development of suitable comparisons, and validation, between mathematical models and experimental results can be regarded as the guideline of this survey.

Recently, several new methods have been reported in the literature for isolation and propagation of cloned CTL, NK and LAK cells. New quantitative kinetics methods for monitoring cellular and molecular transport, conjugation, intracellular biochemical and biophysical processes on the level of the isolated effector cell, target cell and their conjugates have also appeared. Further examination of kinetics binding/dissociation and killing by cloned cytotoxic cells and immune macromolecules is necessary in order to confirm the validity of the models and conclusions presented above. Quantitative kinetic studies together with cellular and molecular biology methods will provide valuable information regarding the basic mechanisms involved in anti-cancer cytolytic processes. The existing literature can be recovered by the chapters of this book.

6.8 Acknowledgment

I deeply acknowledge Dr. G. Marti for his valuable comments about a preliminary draft of the manuscript and for essential notes making the survey more readable.

6.9 References

[ABa] Abrahms S.I. and Brahmi Z., The functional loss of human natural killer cell activity induced by K-562 is reversible via interleukin-2-dependent mechanisms, *Cellular Immunology*, **101** (1986), 558–570.

[ABb] Abrahms S.I. and Brahmi Z., Mechanism of K562-induced human natural killer cell inactivation using highly enriched effector cells isolated via a new single-step sheep erythrocyte rosette assay, *Ann. Inst. Pasteur Immunology*, **139** (1988), 361–381.

[ADa] Adam J.A., General aspects of modeling tumor growth and immune response, in **A Survey of Models for Tumor-Immune System Dynamics**, Adam J.A. and Bellomo N. eds., Birkhäuser (1996).

[BAa] Bardsley W.G., The quantitative analysis of ligand binding and initial rate data for allosteric and other complex enzyme mechanisms, *Biochem. J.*, **153** (1975), 101–117.

[BAb] Bardsley W.G., Simple enzyme kinetic mechanisms that can give all possible velocity profiles with chemically reasonable rate constant values, *J. Theor. Biol.*, **104** (1983), 485–491.

[BDa] Bradley T.P. and Bonavida B., Mechanism of cell-mediated cytotoxicity at the single cell level, *J. Immunology*, **129** (1982), 2260–2265.

[BKa] Berke G., The cytolytic T lymphocyte and its mode of action, *Immunology Letters*, **20** (1989), 169–178.

[BKb] Berke G., The binding and lysis of target cells by cytotoxic lymphocytes: Molecular and cellular aspects, *Ann. Rev. Immunology*, **12** (1994), 735–773.

[BKc] Berke G., Unlocking the secrets of CTL and NK cells, *Immunology Today*, **16** (1995), 343–347.

[BLa] Bloom E.I. and Korn E.L., Quantification of natural cytotoxicity by human lymphocyte subpopulations isolated by density: Heterogeneity the effector cells, *J. Immun. Meth.*, **58** (1983), 303–335.

[BLb] Bloom E.I. and Babbitt J.T., Monocyte-mediated augmentation of human natural cell-mediated cytotoxicity, *Cellular Immunology*, **91** (1995), 21–32.

[BOa] Bonavida B., Bradley T.P., and Grimm E.A., The single-cell assay in cell-mediated cytotoxicity, *Immunology Today*, **4** (1983), 196–200.

[BOb] Bonavida B., Lebow L.T., and Bradley T.P., Mechanism of cell-mediated cytotoxicity at all single cell level. Direct assessment of the cytotoxic potential of human peripheral blood non-lytic effector-target cell conjugates, *J. Immunology*, **132** (1984), 594–598.

[BRa] Berezin I.V. and Varfolomeev S.R., **Biokinetics**, Nauka (1979) (in Russian).

[BUa] Burnet F.M., **Cellular Immunology**, Melbourne University Press (1969).

[BXa] Baxter L.T. and Jain R.K., Transport of fluid and macromolecules in tumors. Role of interstitial and convection, *Microvasc. Res.*, **37** (1989), 77–104.

[BZa] Bezouska K., Yuen C.-T., O'Brien J., Childs R.A., Chai W., Lawson A.M., Drbal K., Riserova A., Pospisil M., and Feizi T., Oligosaccharide ligands for NKR-P1 protein activate NK cells and cytotoxicity, *Nature*, **372** (1994), 150–157.

[CAa] Callewaert D.M., Johnson D.F., and Kearney J., Spontaneous cytotoxicity of cultured human cell lines mediated by normal peripheral blood lymphocytes. I. Kinetic parameters, *J. Immunology*, **121** (1978), 710–717.

[CAb] Callewaert D.M., Meyers P., Hiernaux J., and Radcliff G., Kinetics of cellular cytotoxicity mediated by cloned cytotoxic T lymphocytes, *Immunobiology*, **178** (1988), 203–214.

[CAc] Callewaert D.M., Radcliff G., Waite R., LeFevre J., and Poulik M.D., Characterization of effector-target conjugates for cloned human natural killer and human lymphokine activated killer cells by flow cytometry, *Cytometry*, **12** (1991), 666–676.

[CLa] Chaplain M., From mutation to metastasis: The mathematical modelling of the stages of tumour development, in **A Survey of Models for Tumor-Immune System Dynamics**, Adam J.A. and Bellomo N. eds., Birkhäuser (1996).

[COa] Colmeraver M.E., Loziol I.A., and Pilch V.H., Enhancement of metastasis development by BCG immunotherapy, *J. Surg. Oncology*, **15** (1980), 235–241.

[CPa] Cooper E.L., Phylogenesis of cytotoxicity, *Endeavors*, **4** (1980), 160–165.

[CRa] Cornish–Bowden A., **Principles of Enzyme Kinetics**, Butterworths (1976).

[CUa] Chu G., The kinetics of target cell lysis by cytotoxic T lymphocytes: A description by Poisson statistics, *J. Immunology*, **120** (1978), 1261–1267.

[DVa] De Vries J.E., Mendelson J., and Bont A., The role of target cell monocytes and Fc receptor bearing lymphocytes in human spontaneous cell-mediated, *J. Immunology*, **125** (1980), 396–405.

[FEa] Ferrarini M., Heltai S., Toninelly E., Sabbadini M.G., Pellicciari C., and Manfredi A.M., Daudi lymphoma killing triggers the programmed death of cytotoxic $V\gamma9/V\delta2$ T lymphocytes, *J. Immunology*, **154** (1995), 3704–3712.

[FIa] Figdor C.B., van Kooyk Y., and Keizer G.D., On the mode of action of LFA, *Immunology Today*, **11** (1990), 277–280.

[FOa] Foa C., Bongrand P., Galindo J.R., and Golstein P.J., Unexpected cell surface labeling in conjugates between cytotoxic T lymphocytes and target cells, *Histochem. and Cytochem.*, **33** (1985), 647–657.

[FRa] Forni G., Parmiani G., Guarini A., and Foa R., Gene transfer in tumor therapy, *Annals of Oncology*, **5** (1994), 789–794.

[GAa] Garay R.P. and Lefever R., A kinetic approach to the immunology cancer stationary state properties of effector-target reaction, *J. Theor. Biol.*, **73** (1978), 417–438.

[GEa] Gergely J. and Sarmay G., IgG-Fc-receptors: Ligand binding and lysis induction, *Immunology Letters*, **20** (1989), 1–4.

[GOa] Goud B. and Antoine J.C., Emergence of a surface immunoglobulin recycling process during B lymphocyte differentiation *J. Cell. Biol.*, **48** (1984), 1238–1246.

[GRa] Griffiths G.M., The cell biology of CTL killing, *Current Opinion in Immunology*, **7** (1995), 343–348.

[GUa] Gumpertz J.E. and Parhan P., The enigma of natural killer cell, *Nature*, **378** (1995), 245–248.

[HEa] Herberman R.B., Vujanovic N., Rabinowich H., and Whitside T.L., Natural killer cells and interleukin-2-activated killer cells, in **Lymphohaemotopoietic Growth Factors in Cancer Therapy, II**, Mertelsmann R. ed., Springer (1993), 11–27.

[HGa] Hoang T., Tsodikov A., Yakovlev A., and Asselain B., Modeling breast cancer recurrence, in **Mathematical Population Dynamics: Analysis of Heterogeneity**, Vol. II, Arino O., Axelrod D., and Kimmel M. eds., Wuerz Publishing Ltd. (1995), 283–296.

[HIa] Hiserodt J.C., Britvan L.J., and Targan S.R., Characterization of the cytolytic reaction mechanism of the human natural killer (NK) lymphocyte: Resolution into binding, programming and killer cell-independent steps, *J. Immunology*, **131** (1983), 2710–2713.

[HKa] Herrick M.V. and Pollack S.B., Kinetic analysis of antibody dependent cellular cytotoxicity: Evidence for noncompetitive inhibition by autologous lymphoid cells, *J. Immunology*, **121** (1978), 1348–1352.

[HRa] Herlyn M. and Koprowski H., Melanoma antigens: Immunological and biological characterization and clinical significance, *Ann. Rev. Immunology*, **6** (1988), 299–308.

[IHa] Iho S. and Shau H., Role of enhanced cellular adhesion in IL-6-augmented lymphokine-activated killer-cell function, *Scand. J. Immunol.*, **39** (1993), 233–240.

[IVa] Ivshina A.V., Kuznetsov V.A., and Kadagidze Z.G., Interaction of the human natural killer cells with target cells. The quantity estimations, in **Dynamics of Biological Populations**, Goryachenko D.D. ed., Gor'ki State Univ. Press (1985), 72–83 (in Russian).

[JEa] Jenski L.J., Kinetic assay of cytotoxic T lymphocyte clones II: Comparison of primary and secondary responses and lectin-dependent cytotoxicity. *J. Immunol. Meth.*, **117** (1989), 191–198.

[JNa] Jain R.K., Barriers to drug delivery in solid tumors, *Sci. Amer.*, **271** (1994), 58–65.

[JUa] Jung G. and Eberhard H.J.M., An *in vitro* model for tumour immunotherapy with antibody heteroconjugates, *Immunology Today*, **9** (1988), 257–260.

[JWa] Juweid M., Neumann R., and Paik Ch., Micropharmacology of monoclonal antibodies in solid tumors: Direct experimental evidence for a binding site barrier, *Cancer Res.*, **52** (1992), 5144–5153.

[KAa] Karre K., Hanson M., and Kiesling R., Multiple interactions at the natural killer workshop, *Immunology Today*, **12** (1991), 343–345.

[KIa] Kimber I. and Moore M., Mechanism and regulation of natural cytotoxicity, *Exp. Cell. Biol.*, **53** (1985), 69–84.

[KKa] Kwok C.S., Cole S.E., and Liao S.K., Uptake kinetics of monoclonal antibodies by human malignant melanoma multicell spheroids, *Cancer Res.*, **48** (1988), 1856–1863.

[KKb] Kwok C.S., Crivici A., MacGregor W.D., and Unger M.W., Optimization of radioimmunotherapy using human malignant melanoma multicellspheroids as a model, *Cancer Res.*, **49** (1989), 3276–3281.

[KNa] Konev C.B., **Structural Liability of Biological Membranes and Regulatory Processes**, Nauka & Technika (1987) (in Russian).

[KOa] Kometiany Z.P. and Vekua M.G., **Kinetics of Membrane Enzymes**, Vysshaya Shkola (1988) (in Russian).

[KUa] Kunisch K. and Schelch H., Parameter estimation in a spatial reaction diffusion system modelling man-environment diseases, *J. Math. Biology*, **27** (1989), 633–665.

[KWa] Kawade Y., Neutralization of activity of effector protein by monoclonal antibody: Formulation of antibody dose-dependence, of neutralization for an equilibrium system of antibody, effector and its cellular receptor, *Immunology*, **56** (1985), 497–504.

[KZa] Kuznetsov V.A., The dynamics of cellular immunological antitumor reactions. I. Synthesis of a multi-level model, in **Mathematical Methods of Systems Theory**, Fedorov V.D. ed., Kyrghiz State Univ. Press, **1** (1979), 57–71 (in Russian).

[KZb] Kuznetsov V.A. and Volkenshtein M.V., Dynamics of immunological cellular antitumor reactions. II. Qualitative analysis of the model, in **Mathematical Methods of Systems Theory**, Fedorov V.D. ed., Kyrghiz State Univ. Press, **1** (1979), 72–100 (in Russian).

[KZc] Kuznetsov V.A., Asymptotics of solutions of the singular perturbation problems in study of the enzyme-like kinetics equation system, in **Studying of Integral Differential Equations**, Imanaliev M. ed., Ilym, **15** (1982), 262–270 (in Russian).

[KZd] Kuznetsov V.A., Analysis of population dynamics of cells exhibiting natural resistance to tumors, *Soviet Immunology*, **3** (1984), 58–68.

[KZe] Kuznetsov V.A., Ivshina A.V., and Kadaghidze Z.G., Computerized determination of the number of active natural killer cells, their avidity and rate of recycling during lytic cycle, *Soviet Immunology*, **5** (1988), 33–38.

[KZf] Kuznetsov V.A., **Dynamics of Immune Processes During Tumor Growth**, Nauka (1992) (in Russian).

[KZg] Kuznetsov V.A., The NK cell recognition of target-cells without specific NK-receptor: A biophysical model, *Immunologiya*, **3** (1992), 8–13 (in Russian).

[KZh] Kuznetsov V.A. and Stepanova L.A., Space-time waves and dissipative structures in a model of growth of tumors infiltrated by immune lymphocytes, in **Lecture Notes of the ICB Seminars Biosystems**, Marchuk G. and Werynski A. eds., Intern. Center of Biocybernetics (1992), 68–111.

[KZi] Kuznetsov V.A., Zhivoglyadov V.P., and Stepanova L.A., Kinetic approach and estimation of parameters of cellular interaction between immune system and a tumor, *Archivium Immunologiae et Therapie Experimentalis*, **41** (1993), 21–32.

[KZj] Kuznetsov V.A., Makalkin I., Taylor M.A., and Perelson A.S., Nonlinear dynamics of immunogenic tumors: Parameter estimation and global bifurcations analysis, *Bull. Mathem. Biology*, **56** (1994), 295–321.

[KZk] Kuznetsov V.A. and Borisova L.P., Kinetics model of the interleukin-4 (IL-4) binding to high affinity IL-4 receptor and their internalization, in **Differential Equations and Applications to Biology and to Industry**, Martelli M., Cooke K., Cumberbatch E., Tang B., and Thieme H. eds., World Scientific (1995), 271–280.

[KZl] Kuznetsov V.A., Ivshina A.V., Sen'ko O.V., and Kuznetsova A.Z., Syndrome approach for computer recognition of fuzzy systems and its application to immunological diagnostics and prognosis of human cancer, *Math. Comput. Modeling*, **23** (1996), 92–112.

[KZn] Kuznetsov V.A., "Harpoon" model for cell-cell adhesion and recognition of target cells by the natural killer cells, *J. Theor. Biol.* (1996) to appear.

[LEb] Lefever R., Hiernaux J., Urbain J., and Meyers P., On the kinetics and optimal specificity of cytotoxic reactions mediated by T lymphocyte clones, *Bull. Math. Biol.*, **54** (1992), 839–873.

[LKa] Look A.T., Schriber T.J., Nawrocki J.F., and Murphy W.H., Computer simulation of the cellular immune response to malignant lymphoid cells logic of approach model design and laboratory verification, *Immunology*, **43** (1981), 677–690.

[LMa] Lumb J.R., The value of theoretical models in immunological research, *Immunology Today*, **4** (1983), 209–210.

[LOa] Lomakin M.S., **Immunobiological Surveillance**, Medicine (1990) (in Russian).

[LUa] Liu M.A., Kranz D.M., Kurnick J.T., Boyle L.A., Levy R., and Eisen H.N., Maintenance and cure of the L5178 murine tumour dormant state by Interleukin-2: *In vivo* and *in vitro* effects, *Proc. Natl. Acad. Sci. USA*, **82** (1985), 3648–8652.

[LWa] Leeuwenberg J.F., Spitz H., Tax W.J., and Capel P.J.A., Induction of nonspecific cytotoxicity by monoclonal anti-T3 antibodies, *J. Immunology*, **134** (1985), 3770–3775.

[MAa] Macken C.A. and Perelson A.S., Aggregation of cell surface receptors by multivalent ligands, *J. Immunology*, **132** (1984), 1614–1624.

[MCa] Michelson S. and Leith J.T., Tumor heterogeneity and growth control, in **A Survey of Models for Tumor-Immune System Dynamics**, Adam J.A. and Bellomo N. eds., Birkhäuser (1996).

[MEa] Meuer S.C., Hussey R.E., Hodgon J.C., Hercend T., Schlossman S.E., and Reinherz E.L., Lymphocyte mediated lysis, *Science*, **218** (1982), 471–473.

[MFa] McFadden R. and Kwok C.S., Mathematical model of simultaneous diffusion and binding of antitumor antibodies in multicellular human tumor spheroids, *Cancer Res.*, **48** (1988), 4032–4037.

[MHa] Mahle N.H., Radclif G., Sevella C.L., Kornbluth J., and Callewaert D.M., Kinetics of cellular cytotoxicity mediated by a cloned human natural killer cell line, *Immunobiol.*, **179** (1989), 230–243.

[MIa] Miller R.G. and Dunkley M., Quantitative analysis of the Cr release cytotoxicity assay for cytotoxic lymphocytes, *Cellular Immunology*, **14** (1974), 284–292.

[MKa] McKinnon D. and Hodgkin P.D., A model of a T cell-target interaction leading to lymphokine release, *Immunol. Cell. Biol.*, **65** (1987), 443–451.

[MLa] Merrill S.J., Foundation of the use of enzyme kinetic analogy in cell-mediated cytotoxicity, *Math. Biosciences*, **62** (1982), 219–236.

[MLb] Merrill S.J. and Sathananthan S., Approximation Michaelis–Menten kinetics displayed in a stochastic model of cell-mediated cytotoxicity, *Math. Biosci.*, **80** (1986), 223–238.

[MMa] Mellman J. and Plutner P., Internalization and rapid recycling by macrophage Fc-receptors with monovalent antireceptor antibodies a possible role of relysomal compartment, *J. Cell. Biol.*, **98** (1984), 1163–1169.

[MOa] Moretta A., Vitale M., Sivori S., Bottino C., Morelli L., Angagliaro R., Bararesi M., Pele O., Ciccone E., Lopez-Bolet M., and Moretta L., Human natural killer cell receptors for HLA-class I molecules. Evidence that the Kp 43(CD 94) molecule functions as receptors for HLA-B alleles, *J. Exp. Med.*, **180** (1994), 454–555.

[MTa] Martz E., Mechanism of specific tumor cell lysis by alloimmune T lymphocytes: Resolution and characterization of descreate stages in cellular interaction, *Contemporary Topics in Immunology*, **7** (1977), 301–361.

[MUa] Murray J.D., **Lectures on Nonlinear Equation Models in Biology**, Clarendon Press (1977).

[NUa] Nugent L.J. and Jain R.K., Extravascular diffusion in normal and neoplastic tissues, *Cancer Res.*, **44** (1984), 238–244.

[ONa] Ong G.L. and Mattes M.J., Penetration and binding of antibodies in experimental human solid tumors grown in mice, *Cancer Res.*, **49** (1989), 4264–4273.

[ORa] Ortaldo J.R., Glenn G.M., Yong H.A., and Frey J.L., Natural killer (NK) cell dysfunction and putative NK cell receptor expression abnormality in members of a family with chromosome 3p-linked von Hippel-Lindau disease, *J. Natl. Cancer Inst.*, **84** (1992), 1897–1902.

[PAa] Pankov P.S., Kuznetsov V.A., and Kenenbaeva G.M., Algorithm of the global search and the program package for approximation of kinetic experimental data at known measure errors, Preprint Inst. of Chem. Phys. of USSR Acad. of Sciences, Moscow (1990), 42 (in Russian).

[PEa] Perelson A.S. and Bell G.I., Delivery of lethal hits by cytotoxic T lymphocytes in multicellular conjugates occurs sequentially but at random times, *J. Immunology*, **129** (1982), 2796–2801.

[PEb] Perelson A.S., Macken C.A., Grimm E.A., Roos L.S., and Bonavida B., Mechanism of cell-mediated cytotoxicity at the single cell level. V. Kinetics of lysis of target cells bound by more than one cytotoxic T lymphocyte, *J. Immunology*, **132** (1984), 2190–2198.

[PLa] Pollack S.B. and Emmons S.L., Kinetic analysis of human spontaneous cell-mediated cytotoxicity, *J. Immunology*, **123** (1979), 160–165.

[PRa] Prehn R., Stimulatory effects of immune reactions upon the growth of untransplantated tumors, *Cancer Res.*, **54** (1994), 908–914.

[PSa] Pross H.F., Callewaert D., and Rubin P., Assays for NK cell cytotoxicity: Their values and pitfalls, in **Immunobiology of Natural Killer Cells**, Lotzova E. ed., CRC Press (1986), 1–20.

[PVa] Provinciali M., Fabris N., and Pieri C., Improvement of natural killer cell activity by in vitro active lipids (AL 721) administration in old mice, *Mechanisms of Aging and Development*, **52** (1990), 245–254.

[PZa] Perez P., Bluestone J.A., Stephany D.A., and Segal D.M., Quantitative measurements of the specificity and kinetics of conjugate formation between cloned cytotoxic T lymphocytes and splenic target cells by dual parameter flow cytometry, *J. Immunology*, **134** (1985), 478–485.

[REa] Reiter Z., Reiter Y., Fishelson Z., Shinitzky M., Kessier A., Loyter A., Nussbaum O., and Rubinstein M., Resistance to NK cell mediated cytotoxicity (in K-562 Cells) does not correlate with Class I MHC antigen levels, *Immunology*, **183** (1991), 23–39.

[ROa] Robertson M.J., Caliguiri M.A., Manley T.J., Levine H., and Ritz J., Biphasic responses, signals and cellular behaviour, *J. Immunology*, **145** (1990), 3194–3201.

[RZa] Roozemond R.C. and Bonavida B., Effect of altered membrane fluidity on NK cell-mediated cytotoxicity. I. Selective inhibition of the recognition or post recognition events in the cytolytic pathway of NK cells, *J. Immunology*, **134** (1985), 2209–2214.

[RZb] Roozemond R.C. and Bonavida B., Effect of altered membrane structure on NK-mediated cytotoxicity: Conversion of NK-resistant tumour cells into NK-sensitive targets upon fusion with liposomes containing NK-sensitive membranes, *J. Immunology*, **136** (1986), 3921–3928.

[RZc] Roozemond R.C., van der Geer P., and Bonavida B., NK-resistant tumor cells become susceptible to NK lysis upon fusion with reconstituted liposomes containing NK-sensitive membrane structures, in **Membrane-Mediated Cytotoxicity**, Bonavida B. and Coller R.J. eds., Liss (1987), 173–187.

[SAa] Sakharov D.V., Matveev M.Yu., and Domogatsky S., Binding of affinity ligand with a three-dimensional target: The role of diffusion limitations, *Biophysika*, **36** (1991), 49–54 (in Russian).

[SEa] Segel L.A., On the validity of the steady state assumption of enzyme kinetics, *Bull. of Math. Biol.*, **50** (1988), 579–593.

[SHa] Sharon N., Surface carbohydrates and surface lectins are recognition determinants in phagocytosis, *Immunology Today*, **5** (1984), 143–147.

[SNa] Seung L.P., Seung S.K., and Schereiber H., Antigenic cancer cells that escape immune destruction are stimulated by the host cells, *Cancer Res.*, **55** (1995), 5094–5100.

[SOa] Solono-Munoz G., McGinley P.B., Woolfson R., and Bardsley W.G., Deviations from Michaelis-Menten kinetics, *Biochem. J.*, **193** (1981), 339–352.

[SUa] Shau H. and Golub H., Modulation of natural killer-mediated lysis by red blood cells, *Cellular Immunology*, **116** (1988), 60–72.

[TEa] Thiele D.L. and Lipsky E., The role of cell surface recognition structures in the initiation of MHC-unrestricted "promiscuous" killing by T cells, *Immunology Today*, **10** (1989), 375–381.

[THa] Thoma J.A., Thoma G.J., and Clark W., The efficiency linearity of the radiochromium release assay for cell-mediated cytotoxicity, *Cellular Immunology*, **40** (1978), 404–418.

[TIa] Timonen T., Patarroyo M., and Gahmberg C.G., CDIIa-c/CD18 and GP84(LB-2) adhesion molecules on human large granular lymphocytes and their participation in natural killing, *J. Immunology*, **141** (1988), 1041–1046.

[TRa] Thorn R.M. and Henny C.S., Enumeration of specific cytotoxic T cells, *Nature*, **262** (1976), 75–77.

[TRb] Thorn R.M. and Henny C.S., Kinetic analysis of target cell distinction by effector T cells. I. Delineation of parameters related to the frequency, *J. Immunology*, **117** (1976), 2213–2219.

[TRc] Thorn R.M. and Henny C.S., Kinetic analysis of target cells distinction by effector T cells. II. Changes in killer cell avidity as function of time and dose, *J. Immunology*, **119** (1977), 1973–1978.

[TUa] Tutt A., Greenman J., Stevenson G.T., and Glennie M.J., Bispecific $F(ab^{\gamma})_3$ antibody derivatives for redirecting unprimed cytotoxic T cells, *Eur. J. Immunology*, **21** (1991), 1351–1358.

[ULa] Ullberg M. and Jondal M., Recycling and target binding capacity of human natural killer cells, *J. Exp. Med.*, **153** (1981), 615–628.

[VAa] Vasiljeva L.B. and Butuzov V.F., **Asymptotic Analysis**, Nauka (1973) (in Russian).

[VIa] Vitolo D., Vujanovic N.L., Rabinowich H., Schlesinger M., Herberman R.B., and Whiteside T.L., Rapid Il-2-induced adherence of human natural killer cells: Expression of mRNA for cytokines and IL-2 receptors in adherent NK cells, *J. Immunology*, **151** (1993), 1926–1937.

[VOa] Van Oers M.H.J., De Goede R.E.Y., and Zeijlemaker W.P., Antibody dependent cytotoxicity: An analysis of effector cell-target cell interactions, *J. Immunology*, **121** (1978), 499–504.

[WEa] Weinstein J.N. and Van Osdol W., Early intervention in cancer using monoclonal antibodies and other biological ligands: Micropharmacology and the "binding site barrier", *Cancer Res.*, **52** (1992), 2747–2751.

[YOa] Yokoyama W.M. and Seaman W.E., The Ly-49 and NKR-1 gene families encoding lectin-like receptors on natural killer cells: The NK gene complex, *Annual Rev. Immunology*, **11** (1993), 613–635.

[ZEa] Zeijlemaker W.P., van Oers R.H., deCoede R.E., and Schellekens P.T., Cytotoxic activity of human lymphocytes: Quantitative analysis of T cell and K cell cytotoxicity, revealing enzyme-like kinetics, *J. Immunology*, **119** (1977), 1507–1514.

[ZUa] Zugary D., Bernardi J., and Jeannesson P., Studies on the mechanism of T-cell lethal hits and target cell lysis in multicellular conjugates, *J. Immunology*, **123** (1979), 1604–1609.

7

Tumor Heterogeneity and Growth Control

S. MICHELSON

Roche Bioscience
Research Support and Information Services
Palo Alto, CA, USA

AND
J.T. LEITH

Brown University
Radiation Biology Laboratories
Providence, RI, USA

ABSTRACT. Tumor growth control is described especially as it pertains to tumor heterogeneity. Four facets heterogeneity are reviewed; statistical or distributional heterogeneity, epigenetic or environmental heterogeneity, emergence of intrinsic or clonal heterogeneity, and the development of clonal subpopulations in a heterogeneous micro-environment. A model of tumor growth and its control is developed. Growth control is defined for a heterogeneous tumor composed of a cycling, proliferative compartment and a non-cycling, quiescent one. The paradigm for this form of heterogeneity is hypoxia in a solid tumor. It is used to establish a linkage between the carrying capacity of a tumor-bearing host for its tumor burden. The model is then applied to three disparate tumor growth phenomena. Each study is accompanied by an exploration of what we know (the experimental and clinical literature describing the phenomenon), what we think we know (a summary of the underlying growth processes we surmise accounts for the phenomenon), what we wish we know (areas which are still unexplored in the laboratory or clinic), and a description of the experiment and its analysis (a means of gathering and analyzing the missing information to complete a picture of the phenomenon in question).

7.1 Introduction

We believe that science, real science, is achieved when hypothesis, synthesis, and experimentation are harmonized within a coherent union. We think that science requires the design, implementation, and execution of good experiments within the context of a firm theoretical structure. We have always believed that data is not information. Rather, they are random snapshots of complex processes, inherently noisy and incomplete. Therefore, we believe that data require a context for interpretation, and experimentation, without a firm basis in a theoretical context, is merely collecting data from scattered venues with no central theme to build around. We believe that developing theoretical models without a firm grasp of the experiment, its implications, and its limits is *kinderspiel*. The elegance of theory, while intellectually exciting, is of no purpose if it fails to predict observation.

These are fairly strong comments, some may even call them declarations of faith. But we think they are, for the most part, valid. The questions we are asking in this article are: How do tumors grow? How do they react to their adverse environment? How do they control their own growth and manipulate those environments to their own advantage?

To more fully understand tumor growth we must identify the key players in the control process, and determine whether our theoretical models can predict complex tumor growth phenomena based upon observed data. The models we have developed help us move to the next level by suggesting areas in which our knowledge is lacking. They do it either by succeeding and identifying a signal that should exist for the model to work properly, or by failing and suggesting some assumption, analysis, or idea in the model which is too simplistic to describe the complex dynamics we are observing.

7.2 The Goal

We think that the goal of any theoretical program should be to gain a fundamental understanding of the phenomenon under investigation. In particular, in this article we are trying to determine which underlying control mechanisms are responsible for the complex phenomena observed in tumor growth. **Specifically, we believe that there is a dynamic signal processing mechanism in place, and that tumor growth is fundamentally enmeshed in its control sequences.** Our goal is to define the tumor growth environment as completely as possible, and suggest a reasonable control structure for these growth processes. From this basis, we will try to predict the kinds of behavior a tumor can exhibit while evolving in vivo. In parallel, we are advancing our experimental program to identify the key molecules (processing elements) in the control structure: where they are located and what they are doing in the tumor, the local stroma, and the systemic host. In other words, we want to know who sends what to whom and what do they do with it once they have got it.

7.3 The Plan

Given these goals, we must decide how best to go about achieving them. In general, we plan to:

1) Determine, **from first principles**, the basic mathematical and logical sequences a growth control process must go through to establish tumor growth. These theoretical sequences carry with them biological consequences, a "Gold Standard" against which we must test our model predictions.
2) Establish a "database" of tumor growth phenomena to act as an information bank of "Gold Standards" for developing our theoretical models.
3) Model as many of these phenomena as possible using the latest incarnation of our models, stretching them as far as possible, so that we may gain as much insight into the biology as we can.
4) Determine where we are missing information, and assess what bits of knowledge we need to complete our understanding of the phenomenon. To do this, we must work closely on an experimental design team to design and analyze the data from the next series of experiments.
5) Finally, we must determine where our models fail. It is foolish to believe that any theoretical structure is 100% correct all the time.

Along with determining which experiment needs to be done next, we must also determine how to best improve our model. MODELS SHOULD EVOLVE TOO!

7.4 The Foundation and Tools

Experimental data, derived from controlled laboratory experiments, and anecdotal observations, derived from clinical experience, must drive the theory towards a "first principles" explanation of the phenomena under study. The tools we use may be elegant, but in this system, if they do not describe, at least partially and in some reasonable way, the underlying processes controlling tumor growth, they are useless.

To do this, to build our models based on first principles, we exploit a tumor growth "database" which we have collated from our own laboratory experience and from information gleaned from the experimental and clinical literatures. Tumors evolve as complicated, heterogeneous micro-environments, and the mathematical tools needed to describe these complex structures require that we understand, as fully as possible, what "tumor heterogeneity" is. We must know what makes up the intricate society we call a tumor and the micro-ecology in which it grows. We must know how the tumor communicates with its host, both locally and systemically. And we must know how this kind of dynamic and heterogeneous micro-ecology asserts itself upon the growth dynamics of the tumor.

To that end, we will review the kinds of heterogeneity one can expect to observe in vivo, and the mathematical tools that have been developed to describe them. The review is divided into four subsections:

1) Distributional heterogeneity and models of the cell cycle;
2) Epigenetic heterogeneity and environmental factors in the development of a heterogeneous milieu;
3) Intrinsic heterogeneity and the emergence of cellular subpopulations;
4) Intrinsic heterogeneity and the interactions of competing subpopulations.

After our review, we will describe the latest incarnation of our own models, and in the later sections of this article, we will use them to model three different tumor growth phenomena.

7.4.1 Distributional heterogeneity and models of the cell cycle

In an exponentially growing tumor population, the observed cell cycle time is not a constant fixed across the entire population, but an average, derived statistically from a sampled distribution of life lengths. We use the term distributional heterogeneity to describe this sort of statistical phenomenon. In the late 1950s and throughout the 1960s a number of mathematical models (too numerous to list here!) were developed to account for cell cycle heterogeneities. The primary tool employed in these models was the stochastic age-dependent branching process. Individuals in a population aged with time, and, as a function of their age, gave birth to similar individuals to replenish and expand the population. The primary predictive measures of these kinds of models were the first and second statistical moments of the population size as a function of time.

The first mathematical formulations of this type of model applied to growing cellular populations were developed by Von Foerster [VOn] and Truco [TRa,b]. From their models, they predicted the mean size of the population at any time, as a function of the initial age distribution of the population, the age-dependent cellular birth rate, and the elapsed observation time. They showed that to maintain a population in steady state, as in an erythropoietic stem cell system, an intrinsic loss factor had to be included in the model so that cells were removed from the system as quickly as they were born. Whether the loss was due to differentiation, death, or migration, it had to be accounted for to maintain a steady state. As an extension of the theory, Rubinow [RUa,b] replaced cell age by a new variable, "cell maturity", which he hoped was a more "biologically reasonable" measure than mere chronological age. His efforts met with limited success.

All these early models describe a steady state in self-replenishing and pluripotent stem cell compartments. The loss rates and birth rates are in balance. But it is not hard to generalize these models to tumor growth by modeling a system that is out of balance.

The cell cycle is only one of a number of variables that are continuously distributed over a cellular population (e.g., cell volume, molecular concentrations, etc.). Each of these, known as a continuous structure variable, represents a facet of distributional heterogeneity. Tucker [TUc] has reviewed this class of mathematical models, and duplicating her efforts here would be a tedious exercise for the reader. However, it is sufficient to this discussion to note that these models all describe, in one manner or another, an underlying statistical distribution, and that these dynamics, within an "exponentially growing population" (a theoretical structure at best!) significantly overlap with the epigenetic and intrinsic heterogeneities described below.

A different type of approach was taken for modeling the emergence and development of these statistical distributions. A case in point is cell cycle asynchrony. Simply stated the question is "Why do tumors, which begin as a single malignantly transformed cell, develop into a population of **asynchronously** dividing progeny?". If each phase of the cell cycle were pre-programmed, as on a computer, the life lengths of all progeny would be identical. The assumption that no random errors/variations occur within the cell cycle dooms a population to synchronous growth. Clearly, this is not the case. Therefore, a new series of mathematical models had to be developed to account for this.

These new models described cellular growth as a stochastic process. They assumed that the life lengths of any tumor cell population are statistically distributed about a well defined mean over a well defined distribution. The models went on to assume that while cell maturation is a pre-defined phenomenon (i.e., cells get older as time goes by), the rate of maturation is a random variable, known only by the distribution it keeps.

The earliest models described the entire cell cycle as a single random state with life lengths distributed as in a gamma function [HAr]. Using this model, Harris developed a branching process to demonstrate that age and life length distributions (i.e., heterogeneities) can quickly arise in a population derived from a single cell [HAr]. Bronk, et al., [BRo] generalized this technique to account for random transit times across the four phases of the cell cycle. From these models, Bronk and colleagues were able to derive estimates for statistics such as "decay of synchrony", the distribution parameters for the age distributions, cell cycle label inhomogeneities, etc.

7.4.2 Epigenetic heterogeneity and environmental factors in the development of a heterogeneous milieu

Mathematical models which describe logistic growth as observed in most biological populations (including tumors in vivo) were developed as early as Gompertz and Verhulst. What this theory tells us is that initially, populations grow in proportion with their size, i.e., some proportion or segment of the population is continuously giving birth to new members. However, as the total population grows, that proportion declines, until at some point (maybe after "infinite time"), the rate of total population growth goes to zero. **This does not mean that the population is in stasis**. Rather, it means that the population birth rate and death rate are balanced. Until recently, these models only represented tumor growth in a phenomenological way, and were irrelevant to the discussion of heterogeneity. However, newer models describing logistic growth in terms of proliferating and non-proliferating subpopulations have recently been developed, requiring a new look at the problem.

Recall that the early logistic models say that the proportion of cells contributing to overall population growth decreases as the total population increases. Verhulst assumed that this decline was due explicitly to competition for dwindling resources. Gompertz, on the other hand, assumed a more phenomenological explanation, suggesting that the rate of overall population growth decreases dynamically with time. In either case, a simple analysis of tumor growth will suffice as an explanation of the logic:

Assume that a growing tumor is a sphere, and that the resources needed for cell proliferation completely surround the sphere. (The geometry of the sphere is the easiest to work with, but the argument can be easily extended to other closed volumes). Since nutrients (including oxygen), must diffuse through the radial depth of the sphere to get to the core of the tumor, some cells become hypoxic, quiescent, or non-proliferating. Those that do proliferate reside on the surface in a shell which is some number of cell diameters deep. This shell can then be approximated by an annulus, growing with the sphere's own radius like an area (r^2). The volume, however, continues to grow as r^3. Therefore, the proportion of proliferating cells in the total population decreases with increasing radius.

This line of reasoning is the basis for the models developed by Gyllenberg and Webb [GYa], Kendal [KEn], and Wette, et al., [WEc,d]. The primary difference between these models is the specification of the transition rates from the proliferating to non-proliferating compartments. We will return to this intriguing facet of tumor heterogeneity in the discussion of our own models below (see Section 7.4.5).

As a variation on a theme, Adam and Maggelakis [ADa] developed a spherical tumor model containing four populations: proliferating, hypoxic, anoxic, and necrotic. The epigenetic factor in this model is oxygen tension. However, their model also provides for the distribution of negative growth factors throughout the tumor volume. Oxygen and nutrients diffuse into the tumor from an "infinite" exterior source, and growth inhibitor diffuses out to the proliferating shell from the necrotic core. Diffusion dynamics are based upon the thicknesses of the four shells, and growth dynamics are regulated by differential signal processing in the four subpopulations.

We could use these kinds of models to describe other epigenetic factors [ROc], [LEd]. If we were to ignore tumor geometry as the source of our control signals, we could adapt these kinds of models to ones which describe a self-sustaining stem cell population associated with a differentiation pathway (i.e., tumor progression, e.g. [DAy], [CIa]). Strictly speaking, this type of model should be included in our review of intrinsic heterogeneity below. However, due to its structural similarity with these models, we include it here. Simply stated, the model assumes that a stem cell population differentiates into non-dividing "end cells". If one replaces the term "hypoxic" with the term "differentiated" the basic models are structurally identical.

The transition between differentiation states may be modeled as a random event, defined as an "either ... or" branch point, executed at mitosis (i.e., a stochastic, multi-type branching process). During any small time step, Δt, each cell in the system may divide and choose a differentiation pathway, remain as they are (your best bet!), or die. The probabilities for these events should be derived from well defined underlying transition rate distributions. In particular, Ciampi [CIa] uses his model to estimate the dynamics of stem cell repopulation (a key target for any therapeutic regimen).

Note the similarity between these models describing the establishment of epigenetic heterogeneity and those of Von Foerster, Truco, and Bronk presented above to describe cell cycle heterogeneity. Models describing the maturation of cells and the development of separate subpopulations

must be complementary. Cell cycle progression, cell maturation, cellular differentiation, and cellular mutation are all based on the biochemistry of DNA reproduction. Any attempt to model one, inherently includes all the others.

7.4.3 Intrinsic heterogeneity and subpopulation emergence

Intrinsic heterogeneity is defined by the presence of two or more distinct populations residing coincidentally within a single tumor. One question the theoretician asks is "How did the second (and third, and fourth, ...) population emerge in the first place?" There is good evidence to suggest that tumor populations on the whole are genetically more unstable than those of normal cells [GEr], [NOw]. We believe that the emergence of a subpopulation requires that an "event" take place, one which gives rise to a new and entirely different clone of cells. The arising clone must then survive within a potentially hostile environment. Cellular mutation is a perfect example of this kind of dynamic. But so is differentiation. Therefore, given this restrictive definition of subpopulation emergence, all models describing this phenomenon should be stochastic.

Since intrinsic heterogeneity implies the categorization of the population into two or more identifiable subpopulations, one area of considerable clinical interest is the emergence of drug resistance in a tumor. Goldie and Coldman have proposed some of the most notable models in this area, basing their research upon a generic cellular mutation which yields intrinsic resistance to a single cytotoxic agent [GOa–c], [COa,b]. Their models have also been extended to describe pleiotropic cross-resistance. Based on these models, they predict that the frequency of cross-resistance should be the product of the individual underlying single mutation rates. Since tumor cells express an increased genetic instability as compared to non-transformed cells, and since subpopulations compete for resources within a dynamic micro-environment (see below), the frequency of cross-resistance may, in fact, be quite a bit higher than what a simple mutation model would predict (see Kuczek and Chan, [KUz]).

There are two conclusions one can draw from these early models. First, even if the genetic mutation rate is small (i.e. 1 mutation in 10^6 mitoses), tumors presenting at an early clinical stage (approximately 1 cm^3) have negligible chance of being homogeneously chemosensitive. Assuming the Goldie–Coldman scenario (i.e., that resistant cells are **totally** resistant), one must conclude that upon presentation, the chances of curing any moderately large tumor are negligible. Even if caught early, massive levels of a vast array of drugs would be needed to cure the cancer.

Second, the dynamics of subpopulation emergence must be entirely subsumed into their single parameter for the mutation rate, the so-called "viable mutation rate". The problem with this approach is that it ignores the dynamic early growth of the new subpopulation in a potentially hostile or competitive environment. Remember that these cells must compete with their neighbors for nutritional/growth resources. The dynamics of early population emergence are quite complex, and, since estimates of mutation rates can be made only from surviving clones, the true underlying mutation rate may be many times higher than the viable mutation rate.

Michelson and Slate [MIg] developed a hybrid model of subpopulation emergence for multidrug resistant subclones based upon a stochastic birth-death-migration process. In their model, during any small time step, Δt, cells either give rise to two daughters of the same type (just as in a branching process), die, change their type, or stay the way they are. What is unique about this model is that the transition rates between states are defined by the intracellular distribution of a cytotoxic drug within both sensitive and resistant cells. The probability that a cell is killed by the drug is defined in terms of the concentration of drug at the target site inside each type of cell. Drug resistance is then modeled more mechanistically as a failure of drug uptake, increased efflux of drug from the cytoplasm (classical MDR), modulation of target site sensitivities, and/or increased repair/clearance from the target site. As opposed to the Goldie–Coldman hypothesis, no cell is 100% resistant, but traverses a spectrum of resistance as a function of the pharmacokinetics of the drug concentration.

To get a handle on the viable mutation rate, a model of a tumor micro-ecology (i.e., how clones compete, over what, etc.) [MIa] was extended to its stochastic variant [MIh]. The particulars of that model are discussed in much greater detail below. However, results derived from the stochastic analogues suggest that upon emergence, subpopulation extinction may be a highly probable outcome. However, once a subpopulation has become competitively established, the dynamics of the tumor's overall growth become a complex function of the individual growth characteristics of each subpopulation, and their interspecific competition rates. This suggests that surviving initial selection/competition pressures is a highly probabilistic exercise, but that once a new clone survives, and only then, is a mutation viable and, hence, observable.

Of course, drug resistance is only one facet of tumor heterogeneity. Michelson ([MIi], [MIj]) has used this same type of stochastic process to study the development of heterogeneous tumor subpopulations during the early stages of tumor progression when the selective pressure is an active anti-tumor immune response. A general simulation system for these kinds of hybrid models has been developed, and can be modified to include any sort of selection that is specified in a mathematically reasonable way [MIk].

The stability of the micro-ecology is another observable measure of tumor heterogeneity. By stability, we mean a measure of the resilience of the entire system to suffer a small perturbation and still remain essentially unchanged. Goel, et al., [GOe] wrote a seminal paper on the statistical theory of interacting populations within a random environment. In their discussion of system stability (see Section 5, page 256), they studied a macro-ecology, especially with respect to species diversity and invasion. They concluded that, on average, the more species one has in an ecosystem, the less likely the entire system is to go unstable. They found that most of the variance observed in the system is due to the normal random fluctuations in nominal noise ranges observed in each subpopulation. This makes sense on the micro-ecological level too. If one were to consider subpopulation emergence as a form of species invasion, then assuming a clone survives the initial competitive steps of emergence, the tumor system, as a whole, is significantly strengthened by its own diversity. Experimental examples of this basic principle can be found throughout the literature (see especially [HEa,b] and [POa,b]).

7.4.4 Intrinsic heterogeneity and interacting populations

In the previous section, we briefly touched upon the micro-ecological aspects of interacting cellular populations and why these dynamics are an important factor in dealing with tumor cell diversity. In this section we focus on the dynamics observed in these kinds of mixed populations of tumor cells, why these dynamics are observed, and how we can understand them to better plan our experiments.

The basic premise of these types of models is that intrinsically different cells must compete with each other for limited resources. Net growth of each subpopulation is defined as normal logistic growth minus cell loss due to competition. Remember that the early models of Truco and Von Foerster required explicit loss terms to reasonably model the steady state in a self-renewing stem cell population. If each subpopulation competes "well enough", an equilibrium between them can be achieved (as observed in the DLD-1 adenocarcinoma of the colon [LEe] or in the mammary carcinomas described by Heppner, et al., [HEa]).

The earliest mathematical models describing this phenomenon were developed by Jansson and Revesz [JAn]. They modeled the dynamic redistribution of diploid and tetraploid cells within an Ehrlich ascites tumor. Their model is equivalent to those used by population ecologists to describe speciation and growth in a macro-ecology. Their basic equations are given as:

$$\begin{cases} \dfrac{dX}{dt} = r_1 X\left(1 - \dfrac{X}{K_1} - c_1 Y\right) \\ \dfrac{dY}{dt} = r_2 Y\left(1 - \dfrac{Y}{K_2} - c_2 X\right). \end{cases} \tag{7.1}$$

Assuming the parameters of the model are constants, one can define four potential equilibria: (1) the origin at which both populations become extinct, (2) & (3) $(K_1, 0)$ and $(0, K_2)$ wherein one competitor eliminates the other, and (4) a stable equilibrium point (X^*, Y^*), i.e., a point at which a heterogeneous tumor exists. The criteria for selecting which of these four equilibria prevails are determined in terms of the two carrying capacities (the K's) and competition rates (the c's). Suffice it to say, that if each subpopulation competes equally well against the other, a stable mixed tumor is established. It is at this equilibrium point that tumor heterogeneity is observed.

Michelson, et al., [MIa] extended the Jansson and Revesz model to include a term for subpopulation emergence (see Eq. (7.2), below). The point of this extension was to include an emergence dynamic which allows one subpopulation to arise from the other. Our initial analyses used a constant mutation rate similar in scope to the Goldie–Coldman viable mutation rate. We showed that with this simple modification only three equilibria were obtainable since the emerging population could no longer be excluded by competition. The reason is that when random variation is ignored, as long as the parent cell population continues to grow, there is always a positive probability that a new cell will emerge. We did show, however, that under certain circumstances, we could drive the heterogeneous equilibrium point as close to the emergence axis as desired. It was this limitation (inherent in all deterministic models) that drove us to extend our models to their stochastic analogues as described above [MIh].

Given a tumor micro-ecology, what are the effects exerted upon the tumor by the host environment? Consider the classic case of the tumor bed effect (TBE). Therapeutic radiation damages the tumor bed as well as the tumor, resulting in increased hypoxia, poor stromal circulation, and deficient resources (nutrients, oxygen, etc.). The result is that the competition levels for scarce resources will increase, perhaps beyond some critical point, leading to the exclusion of a marginal competitor (CE III dynamics in our model [MIl]). Leith, et al., [LEf] were able to demonstrate this phenomenon experimentally in artificial heterogeneous xenografts of the DLD-1 tumor. The effects they observed were due to more than just the selective elimination of a radiosensitive cell population. Rather, the complete dynamic of the microecology came into play, and typical equilibria were disrupted by the TBE.

A similar study was carried out by Leith, et al., [LEg] with Mitomycin C as a selective agent in the DLD-1 colon tumor model. The effects of the drug are exerted differentially upon the two subpopulations within the DLD-1, but also affect the ability of the host to support the tumor. They showed that after treatment with Mitomycin C, the typical tumor grew to logistic levels of only 20% to 30% of those observed in control tumors. Assuming constant coefficients, these asymptotic effects cannot be explained exclusively by a "herd thinning" phenomenon. Since, in the constant coefficients case, the heterogeneous equilibrium is globally stable, the tumor should return to exactly the same state it was in independent of the displacement it experiences. However, Mitomycin C appears to affect the host's ability to support a regrowing tumor mass; the drug disrupts the hosts's ability to supply blood, oxygen, nutrients and/or growth factors to the local milieu. This results in destruction of the host environment, differential regrowth, and new competitive equilibria. The interesting point is that these dynamics can only be explained by the model when the carrying capacities are forced to vary with the treatment [MIk].

The model was extended to describe subpopulation induction. For the purposes of this discussion only, we distinguish between induction and emergence biologically: By emergence we mean the development of a new subpopulation due to a (random) mutational event. By induction we mean the dose dependent recruitment of a resistant subpopulation from a previously sensitive parent line.

The best example of this type of dynamic is the genetic upregulation of DHFR in the presence of Methotrexate [SCa,b]. While DHFR expression is not necessarily **induced** by Methotrexate treatment, its appearance in response to treatment is **functionally** (i.e., mathematically) equivalent to induction.

Gyori, et al., [GYo] extended Michelson's original model to include a time-dependent induction function. The shape of the function was designed to mimic the pharmacokinetics of a selective cytotoxic inducing agent *in vivo*. What Gyori and colleagues showed was that in the face of no environmental insults (as observed in the Mitomycin C case), the emerging population would, if the two populations were sufficiently competitive, establish an equilibrium as predefined by the micro-ecology. However, once environmental effects are taken into account, no simple quantitative predictions are possible.

One should note that these models have all included host effects as simple phenomenological measures of the host carrying capacity. This level of description is recognizably naive. Gatenby [GAt] has described carcinogenesis in terms of tumor-host micro-ecologies, ascribing a competitive advantage to the emerging tumor cells. Additionally, Michelson and Leith [MIc,d] have developed a class of models which includes tumor-host signal processing, via receptor-bound growth factors, as a modifier of growth regulation. These models are the focus of the remainder of this article. However, it is important to note the obvious: that tumor cells grow heterogeneously within a host. They grow in a micro-ecology, competing with each other and the host cells which surround them. They establish an adaptive system for survival, manipulating their environment as best they can. For us to understand tumor growth and its regulation, we must understand it within this theoretical context.

7.4.5 Our models of tumor growth

Given the complex nature of a tumor's micro-ecology, we have developed a series of models which, we think, address the interactive nature of the subpopulations making it up.

Assume a tumor is made up of two different kinds of cells, X and Y. Then the micro-ecology in which it is growing can be modeled by:

$$\begin{cases} \dfrac{dX}{dt} = r_1 X\left(1 - \dfrac{X}{K_1} - c_1 Y\right) - mX \\ \dfrac{dY}{dt} = r_2 Y\left(1 - \dfrac{Y}{K_2} - c_2 X\right) + mX\,, \end{cases} \tag{7.2}$$

where the r's are the Malthusian growth parameters of the individual populations, the K's are the carrying capacities for the individual populations, the c's are the interspecific competition rates (and could represent negative growth factor signaling), and m is the transition rate from the X-type to the Y-type. If Y is a non-cycling population (e.g., differentiated cells in wound healing, hypoxic cells in a tumor, etc.), then, r_2 becomes zero and, dropping subscripts, the model becomes:

$$\begin{cases} \dfrac{dX}{dt} = rX\left(1 - \dfrac{X}{K} - cY\right) - mX \\ \dfrac{dY}{dt} = mX\,. \end{cases} \tag{7.3}$$

What happens when the coefficients are held constant? We have shown [MId,e] that when the tumor grows faster than its transition rate and when there is no negative feedback from the quiescent population (the Y's), i.e., when $m < r$ and $c = 0$, then the proliferating part of the tumor (the X's) will grow to a fixed size, K, and the quiescent population will grow infinitely and linearly.

If we were to consider tumor hypoxia in a solid tumor as the paradigm of quiescence, then X would represent the proliferating tumor cells and Y would represent the hypoxic/anoxic tumor population. The Y cells emerge, i.e., the cells become hypoxic, because they are denied access to oxygen. Surprisingly then, it is not the growth of an infinite tumor which is so bothersome to us. Rather, it is the fact that in a solid tumor the oxic cells should be on, or at least near the surface, while the hypoxic cells constitute the interior of the solid tumor volume. In this case then, our model predicts that an infinite volume should be covered with a finite number of cells. This is patently absurd! Therefore, we had to develop a more sophisticated approach, one which includes tumor-host signaling, and feedback between the proliferating-hypoxic transfer rate, m, and the carrying capacity of the host, K.

The basic structure of the control sequences is presented in Figure 7.1. It shows the tumor as a pair of populations geometrically distributed as a sphere. The tumor, local, and systemic host signal processors are depicted as a triad of controllers. The communications lines are established by local and systemic soluble protein factors.

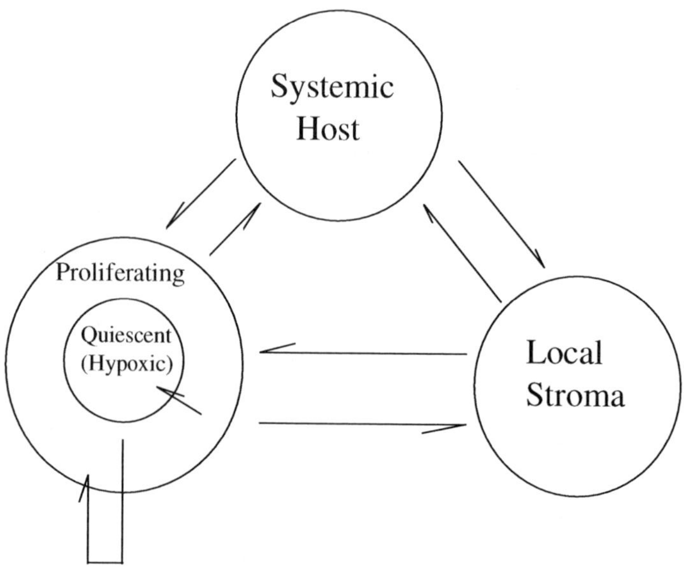

Figure 7.1 — The triad system of growth factor signal processing.

Given these control structures we have developed a mechanism based on the geometry of the tumor and the ability of the host to supply blood and nutrients to the tumor site to link transition from the proliferating rim to the hypoxic center, m, and the carrying capacity, K.

Let the X population represent the proliferating rim of a solid tumor, and let the Y population represents the portion of cells which are hypoxic and non-cycling. Define the emergence rate, m, as a function of both the geometry of the tumor and the diffusion rate of oxygen through the solid tumor mass. If we assume that the solid tumor grows spherically, which, for solid tumors, is not too far from the truth, and if we assume that tumor-derived adaptational signals result in local angiogenesis, then we can describe the total growth environment of the tumor as follows:

A tumor of volume V_{Total} can be considered as a shell of proliferating cells covering a ball of hypoxic (or anoxic or necrotic) cells of volume V_H. The depth of the proliferating rim, D, should be defined as a measure of blood vessel involution (a response of the local host to angiogenic signals sent from the proliferating cells and aimed at the local stroma) and the diffusability of oxygen. Therefore, the rate at which cells leave the proliferating rim and become hypoxic is a function of their radial distance to the nearest blood supply.

Define the survivorship function, $S(t)$, as the probability a cell remains oxic until time t, and the instantaneous risk the cell becomes hypoxic in the next dt time step as the function $f(t)$. Then the hazard function, $h(t)$, is defined as:

$$h(t) = \frac{f(t)}{S(t)} = -\frac{1}{S(t)}\frac{dS}{dt}(t)\,. \tag{7.4}$$

The hypoxic fraction, HF, is the ratio of the hypoxic volume (V_H) to the total volume (V_{Total}). Therefore, a reasonable estimate of the survivorship function is $(1 - HF)$. If the tumor has radius R^*, and the depth of the proliferating rim is D, then the HF is given by:

$$HF = \frac{V_H}{V_{\text{Total}}} = \frac{\frac{4}{3}\pi(R^* - D)^3}{\frac{4}{3}\pi R^{*3}} = \frac{(R^* - D)^3}{R^{*3}}\,. \tag{7.5}$$

Note that as R^* goes to infinity, HF goes to 1 unless D goes to infinity at least as fast, i.e., unless the total tumor remains proliferative. In a solid tumor that is highly unlikely. Then,

$$S(t) = 1 - HF = \frac{R^{*3} - (R^* - D)^3}{R^{*3}}\,, \tag{7.6}$$

and the hazard function becomes

$$h(t) = -\frac{S'(t)}{S(t)} = \frac{3\left[\frac{R^* - D}{R^*}\right]^2\left[\frac{(R^*D' - R^{*\prime}D)}{R^{*2}}\right]}{1 - \left[\frac{R^* - D}{R^*}\right]^3}\,, \tag{7.7}$$

where $'$ represents the time-dependent derivatives of R^* and D. Our transition rate parameter in Eq. (7.2), m, should be proportional to this hazard rate if the assumptions underlying this "Spherical Paradigm" are reasonable.

If D is constant, then $h(t)$ is given by

$$h(t) = \frac{3(R^* - D)^2 R^{*'} D}{R^* \left[R^{*3} - (R^* - D)^3\right]} . \tag{7.8}$$

For fixed K, if D is constant, as X goes to K, $R^{*'}$ goes to zero, $h(t)$ goes to zero, and an equilibrium is achieved. If D is time-dependent, then unless D grows as fast as the total tumor, when X goes to K, D' also goes to zero, and again an equilibrium is achieved.

If K is a function of adaptational signaling and if it goes to infinity with t, then R^* goes to infinity with t, and $h(t)$ goes to infinity, i.e., in an infinitely large, ideally spherical tumor, the population in the proliferating rim grows infinitely large, but becomes so minute in comparison to the rest of the tumor volume that the probability of becoming hypoxic in any dt time step is very nearly 1. This kind of heterogeneity can account for the logistic growth described earlier by Gyllenberg and Webb [GYa] since the proportion of cells proliferating is going to zero even though the total population grows infinitely.

A complete analysis of tumor growth in the presence of dynamic feedback between the hazard rate $h(t)$ and X, Y, and K is described in a previous work [MIe] and outlined in Section 7.5.1 below. The development of tumor dormancy, regression, and recurrence intimately depends on this interrelationship.

7.5 The Structure

In this section we will use the tools described above to develop our theory and to model three types of tumor growth. In each example, we will list what we know (experimental and clinical evidence), what we think we know (what the models and the theory suggest should be happening), and what we wish we knew (where the holes in our understanding are). We will also outline the kinds of statistical analyses and tools we have brought to bear on these data.

7.5.1 Paradigm #1: Tumor dormancy

We define tumor dormancy as a volumetric steady state, wherein the overall tumor growth rate is essentially nil, and yet the tumor remains a dynamic and viable entity. Given this general definition, a number of underlying biological phenomena may result in tumor dormancy: immunomodulation, anatomical sequestration and fibrosis, or development of a totally quiescent population. However, for the purposes of our discussion, we will focus on the subset of tumor dormancy that results when a dynamic equilibrium is established between the proliferating and quiescent subpopulations and the host. Regression represents a net loss of tumor cells, i.e., a negative growth rate, and, for the purposes of this article only, we define tumor recurrence as the re-emergence of a tumor from a dormant and possibly unobservable state, such as from an occult micro-metastasis. Recurrence requires the re-establishment of a positive growth rate. In mathematical terms, the derivative of the time-dependent volume curve for a dormant population is zero, for a regressing tumor it is negative, and for a recurring tumor it is positive.

To understand equilibrium, one can begin with normal tissue wound healing. Why do normal tissues stop growing while untreated tumors do not? The effects can not be accounted for by merely reducing r to zero in Eq. (7.3). That is equivalent to saying the proliferating cells are quiescent, an oxymoron. Rather, the proliferating compartment must either achieve steady state growth or vanish. If the proliferating compartment vanishes, one is left with a tissue composed completely of quiescent cells. For normally differentiated tissue, this is probably acceptable. For a tumor it probably is not.

What we know:

There are many reports of tumor dormancy and anecdotal evidence for its existence dating back to the 1950's. For example, tumor cells injected into the footpads of rats could remain dormant for months, yet be forced into regrowth by the surgical removal of the contralateral paw. In 1959, Fisher and Fisher [FIa–c] were able to show in rats, that of liver tumors that remained dormant for at least 5 months, 100% could be induced to recur after repeated laparotomies, even without resection of the liver. And perhaps most speculatively, surgeons have noted that resection of a primary tumor usually results in the immediate induction of occult micro-metastases.

Many experimental models of dormancy, regression, and recurrence have been described. Wijsman, et al., [WIj] have shown that in the EMR-86 rat mammary carcinoma maintenance of the tumor requires continuous systemic prolactin signals. Upon removal of an estrogen implant (a trigger for the prolactin signal) both epithelial and stromal cell populations regress, resulting in significantly smaller tumors. These tumors exhibit cell growth on the periphery while a cirrhotic stromal center emerges. Cell cycle studies suggest that the rim of the tumor is composed of cycling cells, and yet net growth of the nodule is essentially zero (i.e., an equilibrium, representing dormancy, is established).

Panis, et al., [PAn] injected DHDK12 colon carcinoma cell aggregates into the portal vein of rats, to see:

1) if they could establish dormant, occult tumor nodules;

2) if they could force these latent tumors into regrowth.

Tumor cells were injected intraportally, and eight weeks later a laparotomy was performed. Twenty-two of sixty-five rats had observable tumor nodules in the liver. The remainder ("tumor-free" rats) were randomized to two groups, one of which received a partial hepatectomy the other a sham laparotomy. The incidence of liver tumors in the two groups were then compared. In the control group, 20% of the animals developed secondary liver nodules, while in the hepatectomized group, 62% of the animals showed new observable nodules.

Panis suggests that these differences may be due to growth factor signaling, and he cites evidence for systemic release of growth factors after partial hepatectomy (also see [FIa–c], [NAm]). Leith, et al., [LEb] have shown that partial hepatectomy increases the growth potential of xenografted DLD-2 colon carcinomas, and that these effects can be blocked by systemic administration of suramin, a non-specific growth factor blocker.

What we think we know:

Stoll [STo] believes that suppression of oncogene expression and up- or down-regulation of growth factors and their receptors may precipitate spontaneous regression or dormancy. He also believes that tumor derived growth factors may be turned on and off via cascades of signals, processed sequentially through the local stroma or within the tumor itself. Mathematically, regression requires the derivative of the tumor volume curve be negative. If one defines the mass of the tumor as the sum of the proliferating and quiescent compartments, then if a loss function is applied to the proliferating compartment it would have to be fairly significant to result in these dynamics. dX/dt would have to be negative and greater in magnitude than mX. The argument is as follows:

Suppose tumor growth is described as in Eq. (7.3). Then the total tumor volume, Z, is just the sum of X and Y. If we were to induce a loss from the proliferating compartment alone, i.e., if we added a term like $-pX$ to the first equation, then the X population would be forced to zero and dX/dt would go to zero from above unless p is fairly large. But as X goes to zero, dY/dt also goes to zero, except that dY/dt is always positive, i.e., it is equal to mX.

Therefore, dZ/dt would go to zero from above unless $p > m$. If $p < m$, then at no time would dZ/dt be less than zero. In either case, the Y population grows asymptotically to some critical mass, say Y^*. This is biologically equivalent to establishing a totally quiescent population in a growing tumor. Michelson and Leith modeled this dynamic as a form of tissue differentiation in wound healing [MId–f], where the parameter m was an "on-off" function acting as a systemic differentiation signal. The results were exactly as predicted.

What we wish we knew:

In a recent paper [MIe], we proposed that dormancy can be of only one of two forms:

- TYPE I – all cells are quiescent (i.e., Y's in our model);
- TYPE II – there is a dynamic equilibrium established between proliferative and quiescent cells.

If we believe a tumor expresses TYPE I Dormancy, then recurrence depends upon a recruitment signal, and Eq. (7.3) is incomplete. A new model must be developed which must look something like:

$$\begin{cases} \dfrac{dX}{dt} = rX\left(1 - \dfrac{X}{K} - cY\right) - mX + nY \\ \dfrac{dY}{dt} = mX - nY\,, \end{cases} \tag{7.9}$$

where $n(\bullet)$ and $m(\bullet)$ are signal-based switches that account for recruitment and transition.

If we believe a tumor expresses TYPE II Dormancy, then the results outlined above by Panis with DHDK12 recurrence suggest that a local wound healing event may result in systemic signals that the tumor-stroma microenvironment "intercepts", forcing the tumor into a new growth phase. The fact that normally growing tumors exhibit increased volumes as the result of these signals, suggests that the intercepted message is being processed at the level of the parameter K. In our models [MIe], we have termed this phenomenon the "Coat-tail effect".

Panis quotes studies in humans that suggest that two different tumor cell populations make up the liver nodules he observed ([BRa]). One of the populations is proliferating, while the other is quiescent. If this is the case, and if the tumors do remain dormant for extended periods (e.g., 5 months), then the questions become, Are these tumors, in fact, expressing TYPE II dormancy, i.e., are they at equilibrium, and if so, can altering K, possibly by wound healing events, disrupt that equilibrium? Does disruption of K in the "Spherical Paradigm" alter the K-m feedback controller enough to account for these regrowth characteristics? On a more biological level, what signal ligands are involved, how are they received, what is done with them, etc.?

These are some of the things we wish we knew. There is, at present, only circumstantial evidence to help us answer these questions, and we propose the signal processing triad be used as a theoretical context for designing the next generation of experiments to tease apart some of these results.

The experiment and its analysis

When analyzing these data in our own experiments and when evaluating the literature, we have used the tumor volume as our primary endpoint to describe the growth, dormancy, regression, and recurrence. This growth phenomenon is a macro-variable, usually measured on the gross scale of milligrams of tissue or cubic millimeters of volume. Simple statistical designs (one-way designs, block designs, etc.) and analyses (t-tests, one-way ANOVAs, correlation studies, etc.) let us answer the questions: Which tumor is bigger than which? Which is growing and which is not? and then help us estimate final total volumes, growth rates, etc.

The real challenge for the designer and analyst is to analyze these data and derive from them reasonable estimates of the microparameters in his or her experiment. In a utopian world, estimating the parameters of Eq. (7.3) would require a series of nonlinear regressions on data derived under strictly controlled circumstances. Sometimes, however, the technology to do this is just not there. Therefore, we need to be able to derive gross estimates of some of these parameters from in vitro studies and artificial studies in vivo (i.e., in systems altered to control at least some of the variables involved). For example, we can estimate the Malthusian growth rates of tumor cells in culture by measuring the doubling time and mitotic indices of plated tumor cells. These measures are made in the absence of all host and local signal processing. We can add growth factor enhancers and blockers to the culture media to mimic growth in vivo, or we can alter the oxygen tension of the growth environment to mimic hypoxia. Estimates for the concentration and affinity of certain growth factors for their receptors and whether these receptors are even present on the tumor cells can be made using standard radioligand binding studies. The actual estimates are calculated using other nonlinear regression procedures. In vivo estimates of the plasma levels for particular growth factors can be derived from test animals throughout the observation period of our experiment to derive estimates for the dynamic pharmacokinetics of these endogenous molecules.

Once derived, these estimates can be used in our model, so that from simulation studies, gross ranges for all the other unknown parameters in our system can be derived. Additionally, a measure of inter-parameter correlation can be determined to yield some insight into the interdependence of these parameters. This bit of information helps us understand, **on a biological level**, whether there is an underlying relationship between any two parameters in our model. If significant interdependence is present, then the two dynamics which they represent may be related either by a common underlying signal or in some cause-effect manner.

7.5.2 Paradigm #2: Interlocking growth control

Tumor growth is intimately involved with other growth processes ongoing in the host. Data from as early as 1959 suggest that metastatic growth in the liver is dramatically enhanced when animals are subjected to partial hepatectomy [FIa–c]. And even earlier, Paschkis, et al., [PAs] showed that after tumor implant, animals receiving a partial hepatectomy subsequently exhibited enhanced liver growth when compared to non-implant controls. Others ([FId], [ASa], [LOi], and [NAm]) have shown that in the presence of partial hepatectomy, tumor growth is enhanced whether the tumor cells are injected intraportally (local to the liver) or subcutaneously (remote from the liver).

All these results suggest that some form of "crosstalk" is going on between the growing tumor and the regenerating liver. The fact that both subcutaneous tumor implants and intraportal injections exhibit these changes suggests that at least some component of the crosstalk is systemic.

What we know:

In a partial hepatectomy, approximately two-thirds of the liver is resected. The hepatectomized livers usually regrow, and will restore most of the lost volume. Partial hepatectomy produces significant increases in the plasma levels of a number of potential signals: hepatocyte growth factor [FUj], insulin-like growth factor binding protein-1 [GAh], transforming growth factors -α and -β [MEa], and acidic fibroblast growth factor [KAn]. At least some of these have been shown to be associated with rapid changes in gene expression [MOh]. Both insulin-like growth factor and transforming growth factor-α have been shown to stimulate proliferation of human lung and gastrointestinal tumor cells in vitro [DUr]. In our own laboratory, we have observed stimulation of human A431 epidermoid tumors in vivo by epidermal growth factor, a peptide which binds to receptors for transforming growth factor-α and b-FGF [LEa,c]. Taken as a whole, these results are consistent with the increased growth rates observed in the xenografted human colon tumors.

We have tried to understand the systemic growth control exerted by partial hepatectomy by performing the following experiment [LEb]: Animals received either a partial hepatectomy or sham operation, while tumor cells, human adenocarcinoma cells of the colon, were growing subcutaneously in the flanks. The volume, mitotic indices, and hypoxic fractions of the implants were measured. We found that the mice receiving partial hepatectomies exhibited increased tumor volume and mitotic indices. Additionally, these tumors exhibited decreased hypoxic fractions, suggesting improved neovascularization.

What we think we know:

The model we developed to study this particular phenomenon [MIf] posed a pair of interlocked growth control triads (schematically represented in Figure 7.2) as a mechanism which facilitates tumor-to-liver crosstalk. Our theoretical results suggest that the more intertwined the signal processing pathways become, the larger the tumor and liver appear to grow.

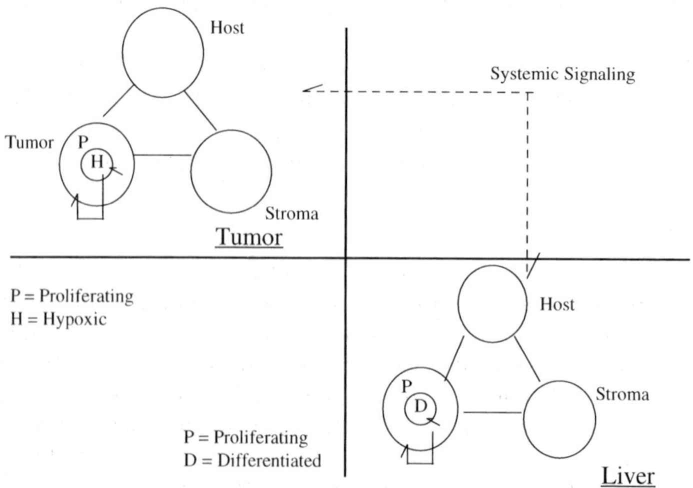

Figure 7.2 — Schematic diagram of the proposed interlocking mechanisms in tumor growth control and liver regeneration. Each tissue is controlled individually by its own triad. The triads communicate between each other through systemic signals. The growing tissues each are heterogeneous with a proliferating and quiescent compartment (hypoxic in the tumor, differentiated in the liver).

We have shown that secondary feedforward pathways (e.g., autocrine stimulation of the liver yielding greater growth signals to the tumor) can influence tumor growth. As a case in point, the largest tumors we observed were growing in a network in which a tumor cross stimulates an autocrinely regenerating liver. When put into the context of our theory, this makes sense. The liver stimulates its own growth, expanding its own proliferating compartment, resulting in greater systemic mitogenic signaling and increased mitotic indices in the tumor.

However, we also showed that a poorly controlled network can induce inefficiencies in the growth dynamics. A regenerating liver which routes its growth controlling signals through a tumor and back again will grow to a greater volume than one which receives no signals at all. But it will not grow as large as one which is autocrinely stimulated. Interestingly, as in the case of the tumor, the largest liver regrowth was observed when an autocrinely stimulated liver and tumor use mitogenic signals to converse.

Timing appears to be a crucial factor in this control network. We found that the transience of the proliferating liver compartment during regeneration (due to differentiation signaling) makes an adaptational signal for the liver (i.e., a tumor based signal that changes the host's carrying capacity for the liver) inconsequential. In our studies, the liver would have already redifferentiated long before any tumor-induced changes in carrying capacity for the liver could be exerted.

A similar result was observed when we simulated liver-based adaptational or neoangiogenic modifying signals acting on slow growing tumors. However, in faster growing tumors, our models were able to detect marked changes in growth when an adaptational signal emerging from the liver induced permanent changes in the tumor bed.

These results lead us to the conclusion that there are "early" and "late" stage effects exerted throughout the control network. Mitogenesis, whether autocrine or endocrine, would act on early stage growth acceleration. The ratio of the loss rate

$$(rX^2/K)_{\text{Tumor}}$$

to the pure growth rate, $(rX)_{\text{Tumor}}$, is minimal when the proliferating compartment is well supported, i.e.

$$X_{\text{Tumor}} \ll K_{\text{Tumor}} \,.$$

However, as the tumor grows, i.e. as this ratio approaches 1, the effects become more pronounced. If the host's carrying capacity for the tumor, K_{Tumor}, is under dynamic and adaptive control, as K_{Tumor} increases, this ratio shrinks, and overall tumor growth is enhanced. Clearly this effect is maximized at the later stages of tumor growth.

Finally, the hypoxic fractions in our simulation studies did not decrease. A result which stands in stark contrast to the experimental results observed by Leith, et al., [LEb]. This could be due to two factors:

1) The sphere is too simplistic as a model for the tumor geometry, and new tumor growth is asymmetric and irregular, spreading along subcutaneous surfaces and thus avoiding hypoxia; and/or

2) There are effects exerted on the depth and make up of the proliferating rim by the growth factor signals.

In the ideal sphere (or any other **fixed**, concave, closed structure like it), the only way to decrease the hypoxic fraction is to make the blood vessel involutions deeper and/or the oxygen diffusion gradients greater. While this explanation cannot be ruled out, it seems unlikely to us since it requires the induction of new signal processing machinery in the tumor-stroma control diad and at the oxic-hypoxic interface.

Rather than suggesting the induction of new receptors and/or signal processing elements in the tumor or at the hypoxic-oxic interface, we believe that accelerated tumor growth is due to new adaptational signals, especially those resulting in neoangiogenesis, which are by their very nature, asymmetric. The physical constraints of the tumor environment (e.g. subcutaneous implant sites), the geometric heterogeneity of the signals and their diffusion kinetics, and the differential responses inherent in all complex tissue systems should result in divergence from ideal sphericity.

Harkening back to early calculus, it was shown that given a fixed volume, the minimum surface area needed to cover that volume is the sphere. If the depth of the proliferating rim is small compared to the total tumor radius, then the oxic growth fraction, i.e., the proliferating rim, is probably acting more like a surface area growing on the tumor ball than as a volume growing on its own. The more the tumor diverges from sphericity, the more it becomes either asymmetric or irregular, the less efficiently the volume is covered, i.e., the greater the ratio of the surface area to total volume becomes. Since the surface is represented by the oxic, proliferating cells, the smaller the hypoxic fraction must be.

What we wish we knew:

To interpret our theoretical results correctly, we must place them into a reasonable biological context by linking our observations with plausible biological entities (e.g., receptors and growth factors). Clearly, there is good experimental evidence that growth in normal and neoplastic tissue systems is reciprocal. Though a spectrum of growth factors probably plays a role in the control mechanism, one intriguing candidate molecule which activates host cell growth during liver regeneration is hepatocyte growth factor HGF, see [MAt], [FAu]. HGF has been studied extensively in partially hepatectomized animals, and it has been associated with signal processing in lung, kidney and spleen epithelia [MAt]. It has also been shown to have mitogenic and motogenic effects on endothelial cells [RUb], effects which could be involved in neoangiogenesis. In other words, HGF does not act on the tumor directly (after all why should an adenocarcinoma of the colon have receptors for HGF?). Rather, it modifies the ongoing conversation between the tumor and its local stroma, i.e., it modifies the functional form of K_{Tumor}.

However, many other growth factors which possess angiogenic properties are also increased after partial hepatectomy (i.e., HGF, TGF-α, a-FGF, etc.). Therefore, increased tumor growth rates and decreases in tumor hypoxia may result from the additive interaction of some or all of these factors in the signal processing control structures of the tumor-stroma diad, see [MAt], [RUb].

Given this theory and these biological constraints what we really want to know is, What signals are actually emerging from the regenerating liver? Is HGF sufficient? Why would a tumor have receptors for HGF? Does the stromal epithelium have receptors for this signal? If so, how is it processed? Is there really a late phase and early phase response due to the transience of the liver signal and is there permanent alteration of the tumor's local support stroma? If so, how sensitive are these timing issues to the relative sizes of r_{Tumor} and K_{Tumor}? Can we design an experiment in which we alter the dynamics of the tumor-liver growth system by using different tumor cell lines with different growth characteristics or receptor spectra, i.e., can we test for particular types of signaling so as to separate the "early" and "late" stage components?

The experiment and its analysis

As in the dormancy study, we have used tumor volume as one of our primary end-points. However, in this study we also measured the hypoxic fractions of the implants, their mitotic indices, and liver regeneration. As before, these are macro-variables. Their units are percents, milligrams of tissue, or cubic millimeters. Initially, one would think that a simple two-by-two factorial design should be used to run this kind of experiment. The two factors would be Implant (YES or NO) and Partial Hepatectomy (YES or NO). However, simple statistical analysis (two-way ANOVAs) was precluded since all data related to any tumor would be missing in the case where no implant was made. Therefore, separate t-tests had to be developed to answer our questions against the appropriate controls. For example, to measure the effect of hepatectomy on tumor growth, a t-test compared the group receiving the implant and the hepatectomy to that receiving the implant and a sham laparotomy. Note, that great care had to be taken to avoid inflated false positives due to multiple comparisons within the experiment.

Our real challenge is to design and analyze data derived from an experiment which could provide reasonable estimates of the microparameters of our model. The technology to do this is presently unavailable. Measuring plasma levels of each of the growth factors and determining the receptor status for each in the tumor is a time-consuming and expensive process. The same must be done for the local stroma. And to complicate matters further, some measure of the modifying effects on the tumor-stroma conversation must also be estimated. We used tumor-based parameters (from data similar to those derived for the dormancy studies) and guesses from knowledgeable experts on liver regrowth to derive gross estimates of some of the other parameters in the model. These provided some insight into the kinds of dynamic we could expect in vivo. One idea for designing a new experiment to try and clarify these issues is to develop a multivariate vector of responses for each growth factor — it's expression and secretion rates — over a spectrum of tumor cell lines. Then we can try and run this same experiment with those tumors that appear to be in the "extremes" of our multivariate space. The point would be to see how sensitive each is to the purported systemic signals originating in the regenerating liver.

All the tools we brought to bear on the tumor dormancy data — simulation, nonlinear regression, and correlation — can be applied here. Each tool provides us with an insight into the biological processes underlying the gross phenomenon we call tumor growth. But again, we contend that designing an experiment in the absence of these theoretical structures makes identification and interpretation of these particularly important data more difficult and prone to error.

7.5.3 Paradigm #3: Concomitant resistance

"Concomitant resistance" is actually a misnomer. For many years it was believed to be an immunologically based phenomenon. It occurs when the growth of a second tumor implant (usually designated as the secondary) is inhibited by the presence of the first implant (usually designated the primary).

It was originally assumed that this type of inhibition was due to nutrient deprivation (Ehrlich, 1906, [EHr], the earliest guess). The reasoning went as follows: A growing tumor draws on all the nutrient resources of the host, indiscriminately starving normal tissues and other tumor implants as it grows. Later, secreted anti-mitogens were suspected as the causal agents [GOr]. And later still, there was speculation that the inhibitory response on the secondary was due to transplantation trauma [PRa].

In Paradigm #2 we were able to relate the growth of a tumor implant to that of a regenerating liver after partial hepatectomy. Accelerated growth was observed in both tissues when compared to appropriate controls. But when both tissues are tumor implants, as in the case of concomitant resistance, the growth of one of them is inhibited. Why would that be? What growth factors/inhibitors in the body are most likely to be causing this "aberrant" effect, and how are they represented as acting in our models?

What we know:

Primary tumor implants are artificial constructs of complex evolutionary processes. Tumors emerge within the host from one malignantly transformed cell. That cell will almost immediately initiate an ongoing conversation with the host to insure survival and eventual growth. The viability of the nascent tumor is usually mediated by growth factors and adaptational signals evolving at the tumor site. Secondary implants are another artificial construct, which are meant as experimental models of metastatic growth. The interactions between the two implants, then, is only suggestive of the dynamics one should observe between a true primary tumor and its metastatic satellites. However, given these limitations, we can still gain some insights from the double implant experiment. It is known, for example, that if the first implant is well established and thriving, growth in the secondary implant will usually be inhibited. These results have been observed with both immunogenic and non-immunogenic tumors and when the implants are made into nude mice [RUg], [GOR], [DYe]. However, if the secondary is an unusually fast or aggressive tumor, the first implant may, in fact, cease growing, and enter a dormant or steady state [RUg]. Most importantly, it appears that resection of the primary after the secondary has achieved volumetric stasis induces recurrence at the remote site.

Ruggiero and colleagues [RUh] found that the serum from mice bearing either immunogenic or non-immunogenic tumor implants exhibited growth inhibitory activity in vitro. This suggests that there is a systemic, anti-mitogenic signal which acts remotely and directly on the proliferating cells of the secondary. The assumption, of course, is that the source of this signal is the primary. O'Reilly and colleagues [ORe], on the other hand, have recently identified a molecule which appears to interrupt the conversation between metastases and their local support stroma. Again, the assumption here is that the source of the signal is the primary. But now the target is the local stroma surrounding the new growth site, and the suppression of growth is achieved indirectly.

What we think we know:

Given the artificiality of the experimental implant model, it is fair to say that concomitant resistance is an especially artificial construct. It is meant to describe the growth of occult, static, micro-metastases in the presence of a primary tumor, and explain the clinical observation that post-surgical trauma can recruit nascent metastases into recurrence. It is characterized by the systemic inhibition of one tumor implant by another. The questions we ask are what is the nature of this dynamic control, and can we theoretically characterize the kinds of inhibition employed?

Michelson and Leith [MIn] studied these dynamics using a pair of interlocking triad model systems like that in Eq. (7.3). Tumor-to-tumor interaction was described in either of two ways. The first model assumed that inter-tissue communication depends upon an interaction between the two tumor sites (i.e., the effects exerted by each tumor upon the other are proportional to the product of the two populations). The second model assumed that any inhibitory effects exerted by one tumor upon the other are strictly proportional to the size of the sending population. The models representing these two cases are given as follows:

$$\begin{cases} \dfrac{dX_1}{dt} = r_1X_1\left(1 - \dfrac{X_1}{K_1} - c_1Y_1 - \mu_1X_2\right) - m_1X_1 \\ \dfrac{dY_1}{dt} = m_1X_1 \\ \dfrac{dX_2}{dt} = r_2X_2\left(1 - \dfrac{X_2}{K_2} - c_2Y_2 - \mu_2X_1\right) - m_2X_2 \\ \dfrac{dY_2}{dt} = m_2X_2\,, \end{cases} \tag{7.10}$$

and

$$\begin{cases} \dfrac{dX_1}{dt} = r_1X_1\left(1 - \dfrac{X_1}{K_1} - c_1Y_1\right) - \mu_1X_2 - m_1X_1 \\ \dfrac{dY_1}{dt} = m_1X_1 \\ \dfrac{dX_2}{dt} = r_2X_2\left(1 - \dfrac{X_2}{K_2} - c_2Y_2\right) - \mu_2X_1 - m_2X_2 \\ \dfrac{dY_2}{dt} = m_2X_2\,, \end{cases} \tag{7.11}$$

where X_i and Y_i represent the proliferating and quiescent compartments of each of the two tumor implants, and the r's, K's, c's, and m's are defined as in Eq. (7.3). Tumor-to-tumor interaction is represented by the μ's. Classically, these terms would represent competition for limited resources (as would have been suggested by Ehrlich in 1906), but in our models they represent negative or inhibitory growth signals.

In our study of concomitant resistance, we looked closely at the various steady states defined by each of these model systems. We tried to determine what relationships, if any, existed between the two dynamic subsystems to establish a steady state, since, in its most theoretical sense, concomitant resistance is actually a phenomenon in which the secondary implant is at steady state.

We showed that concomitant resistance can be either real or apparent, and that if the models' coefficients were held constant, i.e., no dynamic signal processing is allowed in the tumors' micro-environments, then the only way to achieve concomitant resistance is by forcing one of the two tumor implants into a total quiescence (Type I Dormancy). If that is true, then the push required to force that tumor back into regrowth when the competitive partner is removed, must be an auxiliary systemic signal which recruits quiescent cells back into proliferation (as outlined above in Eq. (7.9)). Assuming this signal actually exists, then we must assume that there exists some sort of receiver at the tumor site for it to act upon. If true, these are important implications to our ultimate understanding of normal tumor growth, tumor dormancy, and, especially, tumor recurrence after resection of a primary tumor.

When we allowed the transition rate from the proliferating to quiescent compartments to vary (the parameter m as described in Paradigm #1), then either tumor could attain a dynamic equilibrium, and a state resembling concomitant resistance was achievable. If that is the true state of affairs, then tumor recurrence could be initiated by an increase in the parameter K. In other words, disruption of the steady state could be due to enhanced support for the proliferating cells. Increased mitogenesis is not sufficient. The enhancing signal can result from direct induction of new blood vessels, perhaps due to systemic wound healing signals, or by the removal of an antagonist molecule like angiostatin [ORe] which blocks adaptational signals emerging from the secondary and aimed at the stromal vasculature. To further this discussion only, we term the first mechanism as an "explicit disruption" and the second as an "implicit disruption" of the steady state.

Both mechanisms are intriguing. If we assume that the enhanced signal processing is due to an explicit process, then we must assume that there is a basal signal extant at the implant site, and that a systemic enhancer signal is released at the resection site (i.e., the wounding process) which acts directly on the epithelial vasculature. A possible candidate molecule for this kind of process is VEGF. If we assume that regrowth is an implicit phenomenon, then we must assume that there is a basal signal emerging from the secondary and aimed at its local support stroma which is being blocked by a systemic antagonist, and that removal of the antagonist results in the resumption of normal angiogenesis. A candidate molecule for this pathway is angiostatin.

We also showed that "apparent" concomitant resistance can emerge if the two implants are growing at disparate overall rates. "True" concomitant resistance, a growth dynamic observed when one implant is at complete volumetric stasis, can only accrue if the tumor is in a dynamic equilibrium (Type II Dormancy as in the Spherical Paradigm outlined above in Eqs. (7.7) and (7.8)), or if one of the implants is entirely quiescent (Type I Dormancy). If we constrain our models to the constant coefficients case, we have shown that the second explanation is the only possible alternative.

What we wish we knew:

Prehn [PRb] suggests that concomitant resistance can be fully explained by the geometry of the growing tumor and the access proliferating tumor cells have to circulating growth inhibitors. The logic is as follows: Large tumors are poorly vascularized, thus restricting the circulating inhibitors from gaining access to the bulk of the tumor. A smaller implant like the secondary would thus provide these anti-mitogens greater access over its entire volume. Prehn goes on to suggest that simple removal of the anti-mitogenic signal is equivalent to induction by a positive one. We question that assumption. But if he is correct, then a non-constant recruitment term must be added to our model, as a "switch" to be thrown upon excision. The recruitment signal would have to force quiescent cells back into cycle for the mitogenic signal to be processed. The biology of this type of signal has yet to be fully specified.

The mathematics of recruitment have been addressed by Webb, [WEb], and Gyllenberg and Webb [GYb]. The model they developed is similar to that in Eq. (7.9). They showed that for the linear case, there exist regions in the period-intensity phase space which define stability, extinction, or instability. The nonlinear extension of their theory assumes that the transition rates between the two cell types (the $m(\bullet)$ and $n(\bullet)$ in Eq. (7.9)) are functions of the total tumor size. These studies define even more complex regions in the phase space. If the secondary implant is actually totally quiescent, more extensive functional forms of the recruitment signal are probably required to account for concomitant resistance.

However, given the theory as we have constructed it, a dynamic equilibrium between the proliferating and quiescent compartments is a viable alternative. With this theory as a guide, we can re-examine Prehn's [PRb] solution to the concomitant resistance "paradox". Prehn suggests that the signal emerging from the primary implant is purely anti-mitogenic, i.e., it forces normally proliferating cells into quiescence. The reason that the larger tumor is not affected by inhibitory signals is that access to the signal by the proliferating cells of the larger tumor is impaired by the decreased flow of blood in the mass. Our problem with this argument is as follows:

If the larger implant is freed from the effects of the inhibitory signal because it has such poor vascularization and blood flow, then why is it well-oxygenated enough for the proliferating cells to grow? And even if the vascularization of the mass is sufficient for maintaining an active proliferating compartment, why are the cells which secrete the signal not being affected themselves?

We know that negative autocrine signal processing occurs with TGF-β in some cells lines [ROb]. Why should this system be any different? What Prehn must reconcile is the fact that poor vascularization, while it will may block intratumoral access to any purported inhibitor, must inherently also deny proliferating cells access to nutrients, oxygen, waste clearance, etc.

Of course alternative hypotheses are possible. One could suggest that the receptors of the primary tumor are down-regulated, making it immune to its own inhibitory signals. Or one could conjecture that there are subpopulations within the proliferating cells of the primary that are immune to these inhibitory growth signal. But one is then left with the need to explain why these same forces are not extant in the secondary implant, why excision of the primary induces the secondary into regrowth, and why a faster growing secondary overtakes the primary.

We think that the simple geometric argument is insufficient to explain these complex growth phenomena. The only way to achieve stasis is either when an implant is totally quiescent or when it achieves a dynamic equilibrium. We have shown that when there exists a link between the carrying capacity of the host for the proliferating compartment of the tumor and the transfer rate from proliferation into the quiescence (modeled as oxygen diffusion across a solid mass in the "Spherical Paradigm") we can achieve that dynamic equilibrium. Though the tumor is volumetrically at stasis, there is an active proliferating compartment at steady state. We have also shown [MIe] that one can describe dormancy and recurrence as a function of the stability of this linkage. If, as we suggest, there is a disruption of this link, either due to explicit signals (e.g., systemic wound healing) or implicit ones (e.g., systemic reduction of an angiogenic antagonist), an implant at dynamic equilibrium can easily be recruited back into recurrent growth.

The linkage we have defined depends upon the carrying capacity and the transfer rate into quiescence (K and m). Changing the carrying capacity in our model assumes that there is a signal which is processed locally by the tumor stroma, and results in the induction of greater blood flow, nutrient access, etc. If the signal is explicit, its source is systemic and its trigger is probably the wounding due to resection. If it is implicit, a systemic antagonist is removed from blocking a local adaptational signal. Whether mitogenic signals are also involved is still a question.

7.6 Conclusions

To paraphrase Einstein, a model should be the simplest one possible that explains our data, but one which is no simpler. Historically, the mathematical modeling of tumor growth and its control began with a number of early and simple models applied to gross measures of population growth (estimated cell numbers in culture, numbers of surviving colonies upon plating, and tumor volume in vivo). As technology advanced, as our knowledge about tumor growth expanded, the simple models had to give way to more sophisticated theory. The review of these tools in Section 7.4 above is meant as a brief overview of this evolution. And as the story of tumor growth continued to unfold, it became clear that the original assumptions about a tumor being a homogeneous mass of cells growing in a fairly fixed environment were too simplistic to represent reality. The theory needed to develop again. The result was that there is now an overlap of the models which were meant to describe tumor growth control with those meant to describe tumor heterogeneity. To that end we presented the models we have been developing in Section 7.4.5.

But the development of the theory prompted the need for even more sophisticated and advanced experiments; experiments designed to identify key growth factors, their receptors, and the interactions they sustain. From these experiments we have been able to accumulate a "knowledge base" of tumor growth phenomena, each with its own limitations, but, when taken in toto, providing a fairly reasonable portrait of this complex process. The need to understand these phenomena in depth, to model them, and to identify areas in which vital information may still be missing is fundamental to the evolution of our models. To that end, we presented three paradigms of complex tumor growth. We chose these examples because, though they are all linked to the same underlying theoretical structures, they represent very dissimilar kinds of tumor growth.

Our models suggest that certain signals must exist for us to see these disparate types of tumor growth. We may ruminate on where they might originate and where they are aimed. But our results remain only theoretical speculations until we are able to identify in our laboratories the molecules, receptors, and second messengers the theory represents. To do this, we must be able to design specific experiments and analyze our data based upon the theoretical context of our models. To that end, we have suggested a variety of experimental design and statistical analysis techniques which we have employed in our own studies.

7.7 References

[ADa] Adam J.A. and Maggelakis S.A., Diffusion regulated growth characteristics of the spherical prevascular carcinoma, *Bull. Math. Biol.*, **52** (1990), 549–582.

[ASa] Asaga T., Suzuki K., Umeda M., Sugimasa Y., Takemiya S., and Okamoto T., The enhancement of tumor growth after partial hepatectomy and the effect of sera obtained from hepatectomized rats on tumor cell growth, *Japanese J. Surg.*, **21** (1991), 669–675.

[BRa] Brattain M.G., Fine W.D., Khaled F.M., Thompson J., and Brattain D.E., Heterogeneity of malignant cells from a human colonic carcinoma, *Cancer Res.*, **41** (1981), 1751–1756.

[BRo] Bronk B.V., Dienes G.J., and Paskin A., The stochastic theory of cell proliferation, *Biophys. J.*, **8** (1968), 1353–1398.

[CIa] Ciampi, Kates A.L., Buick R., Kruikov Y., and Till J.E., Multi-type Galton–Watson process as a model for proliferating human tumour cell populations derived from stem cells: Estimation of the stem cell self-renewal probabilities in human ovarian carcinomas, *Cell Tissue Kinet.*, **19** (1986), 129–140.

[COa] Coldman A.J. and Goldie J.H., A model for the resistance of tumor cells to cancer chemotherapeutic agents, *Math. Biosci.*, **65** (1983), 291–307.

[COb] Coldman A.J., Goldie J.H., and Ng V., The effects of cellular differentiation on the development of permanent drug resistance, *Math. Biosci.*, **74** (1985), 177–198.

[DAy] Day R.S., A branching process model for heterogeneous cell populations, *Math. Biosci.*, **78** (1986), 73–90.

[DUr] Durrant L.G., Watson S.A., Hall A., and Morris D.L., Co-stimulation of gastrointestinal tumor cell growth by gastrin, transforming growth factor-α and insulin-like growth factor-1, *Br. J. Cancer*, **63** (1991), 67–70.

[DYe] Dye E.S., Role of concomitant antitumor immunity in restraining tumor metastases, in **Mechanisms of Host Resistance to Infectious Agents, Tumors, and Allografts**, Steinman R.M. and North R.J. eds., Rockefeeler University Press (1986), 197–411.

[EHr] Ehrlich P., Experimentelle Coarcinomatuien an Mausen, *Arb. Koniglichen Inst. Exp. Ther. Frankfurt*, **1** (1906), 65–103.

[FAu] Fausto N., Growth factors in liver development, regeneration, and carcinogenesis, *Progress in Growth Factor Research*, **3** (1991), 219–234.

[FId] Fidler I.J., Orthotopic implantation of human colon carcinoma into nude mice provides a valuable model for the biology and therapy of metastasis, *Cancer and Metastat. Rev.*, **10** (1991), 229–243.

[FIa] Fisher B. and Fisher E.R., Experimental studies of factors influencing hepatic metastases I. The effect of the number of tumor cells injected and the time of growth, *Cancer*, **12** (1959), 926–928.

[FIb] Fisher B. and Fisher E.R., Experimental studies of factors influencing hepatic metastases II. Effect of partial hepatectomy, *Cancer*, **11** (1959), 929–932.

[FIc] Fisher B. and Fisher E.R., Experimental studies of factors influencing hepatic metastases III. Effect of surgical trauma with special reference to liver injury, *Ann. Surg.*, **150** (1959), 731–744.

[FUj] Fujiwara K., Nagoshi S., Ohno A., Hirata K., Ohta Y., Mochida S., Tomiya T., Higashio K., and Kurokawa K., Stimulation of liver growth by exogenous human hepatocyte growth factor in normal and partial hepatectomized rats, *Hepatology*, **18** (1993), 1443–1449.

[GAh] Gahary A., Minuk G.Y., Lao J., Gauthier T., and Murphy L.J., Effects of partial hepatectomy on hepatic insulin-like growth factor binding protein-1 expression, *Hepatology*, **15** (1992), 1125–1131.

[GAt] Gatenby R.A., Population ecology issues in tumor growth, *Cancer Res.*, **51** (1991), 2542–2547.

[GEr] German J., **Chromosomal Mutation and Neoplasia**, Alan R. Liss (1983).

[GOa] Goldie J.H. and Coldman A.J., A mathematical model for relating the drug sensitivity of tumors to their spontaneous mutation rate, *Cancer Treat. Rep.*, **63** (1979), 1727–1733

[GOb] Goldie J.H. and Coldman A.J., The genetic origin of drug resistance in neoplasms: Implications for systemic therapy, *Cancer Treat. Rep.*, **67** (1984), 923–931.

[GOc] Goldie J.H., Coldman A.J., and Gudauskas G.A., Rationale for the use of alternating non-cross-resistant chemotherapy, *Cancer Treat. Rep.*, **66** (1982), 439–449.

[GOe] Goel N.S., Maitra S.C., and Montroll E.W., On the Volterra and other nonlinear models of interacting populations, *Rev. Modern Physics*, **43** (1971), 231–276.

[GOr] Gorelik E., Concomitant tumor immunity and resistance to a second tumor challenge, *Adv. Cancer Res.*, **39** (1983), 71–120.

[GYa] Gyllenberg M. and Webb G.F., Quiescence as an explanation of Gompertzian tumor growth, Vanderbilt University Technical Report MAT-A264 (1989).

[GYb] Gyllenberg M. and Webb G.F., A nonlinear structured population model of tumor growth with quiescence, *J. Math. Biol.*, **28** (1990), 671–694.

[GYo] Gyori I., Michelson S., and Leith J.T., Time-dependent subpopulation induction in heterogeneous tumors, *Bull. Math. Biol.*, **50** (1988), 681–696.

[HAr] Harris T.E., **In The Kinetics of Cell Proliferation**, Stohlman F. ed., Grune and Stratton (1959).

[HEa] Heppner G.H., Tumor heterogeneity, *Cancer Res.*, **44** (1984), 2259–2265.

[HEb] Heppner G.H., Miller B.E., and Miller F.R., Tumor subpopulation interactions in neoplasms, *Biochim. Biophys. Acta*, **695** (1983), 215–226.

[JAn] Jansson B. and Revesz L., Analysis of the growth of tumor cell populations, *Math. Biosci.*, **19** (1975), 131–154.

[KAn] Kan M., Huan J., Mansson P., Yamsumitsu H., Carr B., and McKeehan W., Heparin-binding growth factor type II (acidic fibroblast growth factor): A potential biphasic autocrine and paracrine regulator of hepatocyte regeneration, *Proc. Natl. Acad. Sci.*, **86** (1989), 7432–7436.

[KEn] Kendal W.S., Gompertzian growth as a consequence of tumor heterogeneity, *Math. Biosci.*, **73** (1985), 103–107.

[KUz] Kuzcek T. and Chan T.C.K., Mathematical modeling for tumor resistance, *JNCI*, **80** (1988), 146–147.

[LEa] Leith J.T., Harrigan P., Padfield G., and Michelson S., Modification of growth rates and hypoxic fractions of xenografted A431 tumors by sialoadenectomy or exogenously supplied epidermal growth factor, *Cancer Res.*, **51** (1991), 4111–4113.

[LEb] Leith J.T., Padfield G., and Michelson S., Effects of partial hepatectomy on the growth characteristics and hypoxic fractions of xenografted DLD-2 human colon cancers, *Rad. Res.*, **132** (1992), 263–268.

[LEc] Leith J.T., Papa G., Quaranto L., and Michelson S., Modification of the volumetric growth responses and steady state hypoxic fractions of xenografted DLD-2 human colon carcinomas by administration of basic fibroblast growth factor or suramin, *Br. J. Cancer*, **66** (1992), 345–348.

[LEd] Leith J.T. and Michelson S., Tumor radiocurability: Relationship to intrinsic tumor heterogeneity and the tumor bed effect, *Inv. and Metast.*, **10** (1990), 329–351.

[LEe] Leith J.T., Michelson S., Faulkner L.E., and Bliven S., Growth properties of artificial heterogeneous human colon tumors, *Cancer Res.*, **47** (1987), 1045–1051.

[LEf] Leith J.T., Faulkner L.E., Bliven S.F., and Michelson S., Tumor bed expression in xenografted artificial heterogeneous colon tumors, *Int. J. Radiat. Oncol. Biol. Phys.*, **15** (1988), 151–158.

[LEg] Leith J.T., Faulkner L.E., Bliven S.F., and Michelson S., Compositional stability of artificial heterogeneous tumors in vivo: Use of

Mitomycin C as a cytotoxic probe, *Cancer Res.*, **48** (1988), 2669–2673.

[LOi] Loizidou M.C., Lawerence R.J., Holt S., Carty N.J., Cooper A.J., Alexander P., and Taylor I., Facilitation by partial hepatectomy of tumor growth within the rat liver following intraportal injection of syngeneic tumor cells, *Clin. and Exp. Metastasis*, **9** (1991), 335–349.

[MAa] Marusic M., Bajzer Z., Freyer J.P., and Vuk-Pavlovic S., Analysis of growth of multicellular tumour spheroids by mathematical models, *Cell Prolif.*, **27** (1994), 73–94.

[MAb] Marusic M. and Vuk-Pavlovic S., Prediction power of mathematical models for tumor growth, *J. Biol. Sys.*, **1** (1993), 69–78.

[MAt] Matsumoto K. and Nakamura T., Hepatocyte growth factor: molecular structure, roles in liver regeneration, and other biological factors, *Crit. Revs. in Oncogenesis*, **3** (1992), 27–54.

[MEa] Mead J.E. and Fausto N., Transforming growth factor alpha may be a physiological regulator of liver regeneration by means of an autocrine mechanism, *Proc. Natl. Acad. Sci.*, **86** (1989), 1558–1562.

[MIa] Michelson S., Miller B.E., Glicksman A.S., and Leith J.T., Tumor microecology and competitive interactions, *J. Theor. Biol.*, **128** (1987), 233–246.

[MIb] Michelson S. and Leith J.T., Autocrine and paracrine growth factors in tumor growth, *Bull. Math. Biol.*, **53** (1991), 639–656.

[MIc] Michelson S. and Leith J.T., The autocrine-paracrine-endocrine triad of tumor growth control, in **Proceedings of Third International Conference on Communications and Control**, Victoria, B.C., Oct. 16–18 1991, Mohler R.H. and Wells W. eds., Vol. 2 (1992), 481–490.

[MId] Michelson S. and Leith J.T., Growth factors and growth control of heterogeneous cell populations, *Bull. Math. Biol.*, **55** (1992), 993–1011.

[MIe] Michelson S. and Leith J.T., Dormancy, regression, and recurrence: Towards a unifying theory of tumor growth control, *J. Theor. Biol.*, **169** (1994), 327–338.

[MIf] Michelson S. and Leith J.T., Interlocking triads of growth control in tumors, *Bull. Math. Biol.*, **57** (1995), 345–366.

[MIg] Michelson S., Tran H., Ito K., and Leith J.T., Stochastic models for subpopulation emergence in heterogeneous tumors, *Bull. Math. Biol.*, **51** (1989), 731–747.

[MIh] Michelson S., Comparison of stochastic models for tumor escape, in **Immunology and Epidemiology**, Hoffman G.W. and Hraba

T. eds., Lecture Notes in Biomathematics, Vol. 65, Springer-Verlag (1986).

[MIj] Michelson S., Immune surveillance: Towards a tumor specific model, in **Theoretical Immunology**, Part II, Perelson A. ed., Addison-Wesley (1988), 37–56.

[MIk] Michelson S., A system for Monte Carlo simulation of heterogeneous tumor cell populations, in **Mathematical Models in Medicine: Diseases and Epidemics**, *Adv. Math. and Computers in Med.*, **20** (1990), 139–148.

[MIl] Michelson S. and Leith J.T., Environmental stress induced by the tumor bed effect leads to subpopulation exclusion within heterogeneous neoplasms: Modeling studies, *Radiation Res.*, **115** (1988), 533–542.

[MIm] Michelson S. and Leith J.T., Effects of differential cell kill on the dynamic composition of heterogeneous tumors, in **Mathematical Models in Medicine: Diseases and Epidemics**, *Adv. Math. and Computers in Med.*, **20** (1990), 149–160.

[MIn] Michelson S. and Leith J.T., A theoretical explanation of "Concomitant Resistance", *Bull. Math. Biol.*, **57** (1995), 733–747.

[MOh] Mohn K.L., Melby A.E., Tewari D.S., Laz T.M., and Taub R., The gene encoding rat insulin-like growth factor binding protein-1 is rapidly and highly increased in regenerating liver, *Molec. Cell Biol.*, **11** (1991). 1393–1401.

[NAm] Namieno T., Takeichi N., Hata Y., Uchinao J., and Kobayashi H., Kinetic changes of liver regeneration and hepatocellular carcinoma cells after partial hepatectomy in rats, *Gastroenterologia Japonica*, **26** (1991), 29–36.

[NOw] Nowell P.C., Mechanisms of tumor progression, *Cancer Res.*, **44** (1986), 3801–3805.

[ORe] O'Reilly M.S., Holmgren L., Shing Y., Chen C., Rosenthal R.A., Moses M., Lane W.S., Chao Y., Sage E.H., and Folkman J., Angiostatin: A novel angiogenesis inhibitor that mediates the suppression of metastases by a Lewis Lung carcinoma, *Cell*, **79** (1994), 315–328.

[PAn] Panis Y., Ribeiro J., Chretien Y., and Nordlinger B., Dormant liver metastases: An experimental study, *Br. J. Surg.*, **79** (1992), 221–223.

[PAs] Paschkis K.E., Cantarow A., Stasney J., and Hobbs J.H., Tumor growth in partially hepatectomized rats, *Cancer Res.*, **15** (1955), 579–582.

[POa] Poste G., Doll J., and Fidler I.J., Interactions among clonal subpopulations affect stability of the metastatic phenotype in polyclonal populations of the B16 melanoma cell, *PNAS*, **78** (1981), 6226–6230.

[POb] Poste G., Greig R., Tzeng J., Koestler T., and Corwin S., Interactions between tumor cell subpopulations in malignant tumors, in **Cancer and Metastases: Biological and Therapeutic Aspects**, Nicolson G.L. and Milas L. eds., Raven Press (1984).

[PRa] Prehn R.T., The inhibition of tumor growth by tumor mass, *Cancer Res.*, **51** (1991), 2–4.

[PRb] Prehn R.T., Two competing influences that may explain concomitant tumor resistance, *Cancer Res.*, **53** (1993), 3266–3269.

[ROb] Roberts A.B., Anzano M.A., Wakefield L.M., Roche N.S., Stern D.F., and Sporn M.B., Type beta transforming growth factor: A bifunctional regulator of cellular growth, *PNAS*, **82** (1985), 119–123.

[ROc] Rockwell S., Effect of host age on the transplantation, growth, and radiation response of EMT6 tumors, *Cancer Res.*, **41** (1981), 527.

[RUb] Rubin J.S., Chan A.M., Bottaro D.P., Burgess W.H., Taylor W.G., Cech A.C., Hirschfeld D.W., Wong J., Miki T., Finch P.W., and Aaronson S.A., A broad-spectrum human lung fibroblast-derived mitogen is a variant of hepatocyte growth factor, *Proc. Natl. Acad. Sci.*, **88** (1991), 415–419.

[RUc] Rubinow S.I., A maturity-time representation for cell populations, *Biophysical J.*, **8** (1968), 1055–1073.

[RUd] Rubinow S.I., A simple model of a steady state differentiating cell system, *J. Cell Biol.*, **43** (1969), 32–39.

[RUg] Ruggerio R.A, Buatuoabad O.D., Bonfil R.D., Meiss R.P., and Pasqualini C.D., "Concomitant immunity" in murine tumors of non-detectable immunogenicity, *Br. J. Cancer*, **51** (1985), 37–48.

[RUh] Ruggerio R.A, Buatuoabad O.D., Cramer P., Bonfil R.D., and Pasqualini C.D., Correlation between seric antitumor activity and concomitant resistance in mice bearing nonimmunogenic tumors, *Cancer Res.*, **50** (1990), 7159–7165.

[SCa] Schimke R.T., Gene amplification, drug resistance, and cancer, *Cancer Res.*, **44** (1984), 1735–1742.

[SCb] Schimke R.T., Gene amplification in cultured cells, *J. Biol. Chem.*, **44** (1988), 1735–1742.

[STo] Stoll B.A., Spontaneous regression of cancer: New insights, *Biotherapy*, **4** (1992), 23–30.

[TRa] Truco E., Mathematical models for cellular systems: The Von Foerster equation. Part I, *Bull. of Math. Biophys.*, **27** (1965), 283–303.

[TRb] Truco E., Mathematical models for cellular systems: The Von Foerster equation. Part II, *Bull. of Math. Biophys.*, **27** (1965), 449–471.

[TUc] Tucker S.L., Cell population models with continuous structure variables, in **Cancer Modeling**, Brown B.W. and Thompson J.R. eds., Marcel Decker (1987).

[VOn] Von Foerster H., Some remarks on changing populations, in **The Kinetics of Cellular Proliferation**, Stohlman F. ed., Grune and Stratton (1959).

[WEb] Webb G.F., A nonlinear cell population model of periodic chemotherapy treatment, *WSSIAA*, **1** (1992), 569–583.

[WEc] Wette R., Katz I.N., and Rodin E.Y., Stochastic processes for solid tumor kinetics I. Surface regulated growth, *Math. Biosci.*, **19** (1974), 231–255.

[WEd] Wette R., Katz I.N., and Rodin E.Y., Stochastic processes for solid tumor kinetics II. Diffusion regulated growth, *Math. Biosci.*, **19** (1974), 311–338.

[WIj] Wijsman J.H., Cornelisse C.J., Keijzer R., van de Velde C.J.H., and van Dierendonck J.H., A prolactin-dependent, metastasizing rat mammary carcinoma as a model for endocrine related tumour dormancy, *Br. J. Cancer*, **64** (1991), 463–468.

8

Biological Glossary

F. CAVALLO AND K. BOGGIO

University of Torino
Dipartimento di Scienze Cliniche e Biologiche
Orbassano, Italy

ABSTRACT. The aim of this biological glossary is to help mathematically oriented, but biologically disoriented readers.

8.1 Glossary

Adenocarcinoma: a malignant tumor of epithelial cells in a glandular pattern.

aFGF: acidic fibroblast growth factor, a member of the family of fibroblast (q.v.) growth factors that promotes the growth of epithelial cells, has angiogenic potential (see "angiogenesis"), and can be produced by tumor cells.

AIDS: acronym for "acquired immunodeficiency syndrome", a disease caused by infection by the human immunodeficiency (HIV) virus. It becomes clinically evident when most of the patient's CD4+ (q.v.) T lymphocytes are lost, with the result that opportunistic pathogens are able to establish life-threatening diseases.

Anastomosis: a natural or surgically created, direct or indirect junction between two blood vessels or other tubular structures.

Anatomical sequestration: immunological isolation caused by from physical barriers to antigens (q.v.) and lymphocytes and resulting in the non-rejection of foreign tissue. Sites isolated in this way are called "immunologically privileged sites".

Angiogenesis: development of blood vessels stimulated by endothelial cell growth factors. Many tumors produce angiogenic factors essential for provision of the energy they require to survive.

Angiostatin: a factor that inhibits angiogenesis by preventing the proliferation of epithelial cells. This inhibition can impede the growth of tumors.

Anoxia: a state of no oxygen that creates major tissue distress (see also "hypoxia").

Antibodies (or immunoglobulins): proteins in body fluids that specifically bind the determinant (or epitope, q.v.) of an antigen (q.v.). Antibodies bind and neutralize pathogens or prepare them for uptake and destruction by phagocytes. Their overall structure is similar. Every antibody, however, has a single external antigen binding site, i.e. a particular conformation that allows it to bind its specific antigen.

Antigen: any substance (usually foreign) that induces the formation of an antibody (q.v.), by which it is then bound, or by a T-lymphocyte receptor (q.v.). The name is derived from anti(body) and the suffix "gen" (producing).

Antiserum (pl. antisera): the fluid of clotted blood from an immune individual. Antisera contain heterogeneous collections of antibodies that bind the antigen used for immunization. This heterogeneity makes each antiserum unique.

Autocrine: an adjective referring to growth factors or hormones that influence the metabolism and behavior of the cell that produces them.

Autoimmunity: a condition in which substances naturally present in the body are treated as antigens, resulting in an abnormal immune response and damage to the body's own tissues on the part of antibodies (known as autoantibodies) produced against these "self-antigens".

Avascular growth phase: the initial growth phase of a tumor, prior to its vascularisation. The few tumor cells already present are fed by fluids from the surrounding tissues.

B cells, (B lymphocytes): one of the two major classes of lymphocytes. Their antigen receptor (q.v.) is a cell-surface immunoglobulin molecule. Upon activation by antigen, B cells differentiate into plasma cells producing antibody of the same specificity as their initial receptor.

Benign: referring to a tumor containing cells that closely resemble normal cells. Benign tumors stay where they are. They do not grow into (infiltrate) nor destroy their surroundings, and do not spread to other parts of the body (see "malignant" and "metastasis").

Cancer: defective gene regulation of cell proliferation resulting in the uncontrolled multiplication of one or more clones (q.v.). The defect usually arises in a single cell, which then gives rise to a clone of actively proliferating daughter cells. These form a mass, i.e. a tumor, which grows locally at first and may eventually spread to distant sites by metastasis (q.v.). See also "neoplasia".

Capillary sprouts: the first signs of angiogenesis (q.v).

CD3: a polypeptide complex composed of five chains (γ, δ, ε, ζ, and η) and associated with the T-cell receptor and functions in signal transduction.

CD4: a lymphocytes molecule found on the T lymphocytes (usually T helper cells) that recognize antigenic peptides associated with a class II glycoprotein of the major histocompatibility complex (q.v).

CD8: a lymphocytes molecule found on the T lymphocytes (usually T cytotoxic cells) that recognize antigenic peptides associated with a class I glycoprotein of the major histocompatibility complex (q.v).

Cell cycle: the ordered sequence of events whereby a cell reproduces itself by duplicating its contents and dividing into two. See also "mitotic".

Cell differentiation: the process by which a cell acquires a clearly specialized function or character. It usually involves changes in gene expression.

Cell maturation: the stage following division and prior to differentiation during which the organelles of a cell, i.e. its specialized components, grow and make it ready to perform the operations peculiar to its type.

Chemochines: small cytokines (q.v) involved in the migration and activation of cells, especially macrophages (q.v) and lymphocytes. They play a central part in inflammatory responses.

Chemotactic stimulus: any substance that induces chemotaxis (q.v).

Chemotaxis: motile response of a cell or organism that carries it towards (positive chemotaxis) or away from (negative chemotaxis) a chemical substance.

Chemotherapy: the use of drugs that inhibit cell proliferation in the treatment of (usually malignant) diseases or infections.

Christopher Robin: see "Winnie the Pooh".

Clone: a population of identical cells or DNA molecules descended from a single progenitor.

Collagen: a triple-helical protein that forms fibrils of great tensile strength; a major component of the extracellular matrix (q.v.) and connective tissues.

Collagenase: an enzyme that catalyses the cleavage of peptide bonds into triple-helical collagen (q.v).

Concomitant resistance: resistance to a second tumor challenge conferred by a growing tumor.

Cytokines: numerous low-molecular-weight proteins that regulate the intensity and duration of the immune response by exerting a variety of effects on lymphocytes and other immune cells. They act on specific cytokine receptors (q.v.) on the cells they affect. Cytokines made by lymphocytes are often called lymphokines. Cytokines are also called interleukins (q.v.).

Cytoplasm: viscous contents of a cell contained within the plasma membrane outside its nucleus. The part of the cytoplasm not contained in any cell component is called the cytosol.

Cytotoxic: detrimental or destructive to cells.

Cytotoxic T lymphocyte (CTL): a killer lymphocyte that recognizes the target peptide presented by the glycoproteins of the major histocompatibility complex (q.v.) and thus mediates the lysis of other cells. A few CTL are CD4+ (q.v.), most are CD8+ (q.v.).

Desmosome: specialized cell-cell junction, usually formed between two epithelial cells, consisting of dense plates of protein into which intermediate filaments in the two adjoining cells insert themselves.

Diploid: containing two sets of homologous chromosomes and hence two copies (alleles) of each gene or locus (q.v.). Somatic (or body) cells, i.e. cells other than the male and female sex cells (spermatozoon and ovum), contain the diploid number of chromosomes (2n) characteristic of a species.

Dormancy: a period in which an incipient tumor remains in a steady state.

Effector cell: any cell capable of mediating an immune function without the need for further differentiation.

Endocrine: adjective used of a hormone produced by a gland or cell and secreted into the bloodstream to act on distant cells or tissues.

Endothelial cells: flat cells that line blood vessels and regulate exchanges between the bloodstream and surrounding tissues. They usually rest on a basal lamina.

Enzymes: proteins that catalyze a specific chemical reaction.

Epitope: a site on an antigen (q.v.) that is recognized and bound by a particular antibody or a T-cell receptor (q.v.). Also called an antigenic determinant.

Exophytic masses (outgrowths): a noninvasive neoplasm (q.v.) projecting from an epithelium.

Extracellular matrix (ECM): complex network of polysaccharides (e.g. glycosaminoglycans or cellulose) and proteins (e.g. collagen q.v.) secreted by cells. Serves as a structural element in tissues and also influences their development and physiology.

Fibroblast: common cell type found in connective tissue. Secretes an extracellular matrix (q.v.) rich in collagen (q.v.) and other macromolecules. Migrates and proliferates readily in damaged tissues and in tissue cultures.

Fibrosis: an abnormal amount of fibrous tissue in an organ due to proliferation of interstitial connective tissue stimulated by a previous or ongoing disease process.

Ganglioside: any glycolipid containing one or more N-acetylneuraminic acid (sialic acid) residues. Found in the plasma membrane of eukaryotic cells and especially abundant in neurons; confers a net negative charge on most animal cells.

Growth factor: an extracellular polypeptide molecule that binds to a cell-surface receptor (q.v.) and triggers a signal-transduction pathway that leads to cell proliferation or cell differentiation (q.v.).

Hamster: one of several species (especially Cricetus cricetus) of rodents of the Cricetidae family used as laboratory animals, especially for vitamin assays and selected disease studies.

Haptotaxis: orientation movement in response to a stimulus provided by contact with a solid body.

Histocompatibility: term used in immunology to describe the genetic system that codes cell surface differences leading to the rejection of tissue and organ grafts. This results from immunological recognition of histocompatibility (H) antigens. See also "major histocompatibility complex".

Hyaluronidases: enzymes that randomly cleave β-N-acetyl-hexosamine glycosidic bonds in hyaluronic acid, chondroitin, and chondroitin sulfates.

Hypoxia: oxygen deficiency (see also "anoxia").

Immunomodulation: therapeutic alteration of the activity of the immune system with drugs or biological components (i.e. Bacteria, cytokines etc.) to either boost a useful response (immunostimulation) or suppress a counter-productive response (immunosuppression), as in some autoimmune diseases (see "autoimmunity") or to prevent the rejection of transplants.

Immunotherapy: treatment with immunostimulants (active immunotherapy) or re-infusion of the patient's own antibodies or immune system cells after stimulation in vitro (passive immunotherapy).

Inhibitors: natural or synthetic substances capable of stopping or slowing down a particular biological process.

Interferons (IFN): circulating glycoproteins that induce an antiviral state in other cells and regulate the immune response. IFN-γ is mainly produced by T cells (q.v.) and is responsible for several forms of immunomodulation (q.v.).

Interleukins (IL): generic term for cytokines (q.v.) produced by leukocytes (white cells). They primarily affect the growth and differentiation of hematopoietic (literally "blood making") and immune-system cells.

Ligand: any molecule recognized by a receptor (q.v.).

Locus (pl. loci): the place occupied by one or more genes on a specific chromosome.

Lumen: cavity enclosed by an epithelial sheet (in a tissue) or by a membrane (in a cell). Usually refers to the space inside a tube (artery, vein, intestine etc.).

Macrophages: large, migratory mononuclear cells found in most organs. Of great importance in the defense of the body because they engulf other cells (phagocytosis), process and present antigens (q.v.) to T cells (q.v.),secrete cytokines (q.v.) and take part in antibody (q.v.)-dependent cytotoxicity.

Malignant: denoting any neoplasm (q.v.) known to have the property of invading and destroying its surroundings and spreading to other parts of the body by metastasis (q.v.). See also "benign".

Melanocytes: cells that produce melanin, the pigment that gives a brown to black color to the skin and hair.

Melanoma: a neoplasm (q.v.) derived from cells capable of forming melanin.

Metabolism: the sum of the chemical changes that occur in living cells.

Metabolites: generic term used for any of the intermediate, end or waste products of metabolism (q.v.).

Metastasis: the transfer of tumor cells from a primary malignant (q.v.) tumor to a secondary site.

Methotrexate: a dihydrofolate analog. Inhibitor (q.v.) of eukaryotic dihydrofolate reductase. Used in chemotherapy (q.v.).

Major histocompatibility complex (MHC): a complex of genes encoding cell-surface molecules required for antigen presentation to T lymphocytes (q.v.) and rapid graft rejection. Its molecular products are classified as class I, class II and class III glycoproteins.

Mitomycin C: inhibitor (q.v.) of DNA synthesis and nuclear division. See also "mitotic".

Mitotic: adjective referring to mitosis, i.e. the normal division of the nucleus during the cell cycle (q.v.) that results in the condensation of DNA into visible chromosomes.

Molecular biology: study of the structure and functions of the molecules that form living organisms.

Necrosis: morphologic changes associated with the death of cells or groups of cells due to chemical or physical injury. It results in extensive debris that must be removed by phagocytosis (see "macrophages").

Neoplasia: uncontrolled cell proliferation; formation of a neoplasm (q.v.).

Neoplasm: a synonym for cancer (q.v.) or malignant (q.v.) tumor.

Neovascularization: formation of new vessels in response to a stimulus, such as the secretion of angiogenic factors. See "angiogenesis".

Paracrine: adjective referring to the production by a cell of a cytokine (q.v.) or growth factor (q.v.) that acts by binding to the receptors (q.v.) near target cells. See also "endocrine".

Parenchymal cells: the epithelial cells of a gland that perform its specific function (secretion).

Phenotype: the observable character conferred on a cell or organism by the expression of particular genes.

Prevascular growth: same as "avascular growth phase" (q.v.).

Proliferating rim: rim rich in cells during proliferation.

Promotor: DNA sequence to which RNA polymerase binds to begin transcription, i.e. the transfer of genetic information.

Protease: descriptive term for the proteolytic enzymes (q.v.).

Protein: the major macromolecular constituent of cells. A linear polymer of amino acids linked together by peptide bonds in a specific sequence.

Proteinases: enzymes, such as trypsin, that hydrolyze protein (q.v.) by means of internal cleavages.

Proteolytic enzymes: enzymes that catalyze the hydrolysis of the internal or external amino acids of the peptide chains that form a protein (q.v.).

Radiation therapy (radiotherapy): the use of X-rays, gamma rays, protons, ions and other forms of radiation to treat tumors and diseases.

Receptor: cell-surface molecule that binds a specific extracellular signaling molecule (ligand, q.v.) and initiates a response in the cell.

Regulatory elements: parts of a gene that regulate its expression.

Replication (cellular): mitotic (q.v.) expansion of a cell populations.

Signal-transduction pathway: a series of intracellular events triggered by binding of a signaling molecule to a receptor (q.v.) that convert an extracellular signal into a cellular response.

Spheroid (multicellular): spherical clump of cells cultivated in vitro as a useful model for the study of solid tumors.

Stem cell: a totipotent cell whose daughter cells can differentiate into other types.

Superantigens: molecules that stimulate a large subset of T cells (q.v.) by binding to class II glycoproteins of the major histocompatibility complex (q.v.).

T cell receptor (TCR): antigen-binding-molecule expressed on the surface of T cells and associated with CD3 (q.v.). It is a disulfide-linked heterodimer of the highly variable α and β chains. An alternative receptor made up of variable γ and δ chains is expressed with CD3 on a subset of T cells. This receptor specifically interacts with peptides bound to class I or class II glycoproteins of the major histocompatibility complex (q.v.).

T cells (T lymphocytes): any of several subsets of lymphocytes defined by their development in the thymus and by heterodimeric receptors (q.v.) associated with the CD3 (q.v.) proteins. See also "B cells".

T-helper (Th) lymphocyte: generally a CD4+ class II MHC-restricted T cell (q.v.) that plays a central role in both humoral and cell-mediated (delayed-type) immunity by secreting numerous cytokines (q.v.). In vitro, subset Th1 secretes interleukin-2 and interferon-γ (see "interleukin" and "interferon"), subset Th2 secretes interleukin-4, interleukin-5, interleukin-6, and interleukin-10. This difference also reflects different biological functions: Th1 is responsible for classic cell-mediated function and activation of cytotoxic T lymphocytes (q.v.), whereas Th2 is more effective as a helper for B lymphocyte (q.v.) activation.

Tetraploid: adjective referring to a cell having four full sets of homologous chromosomes and hence four copies of each gene or locus (q.v.). After the S phase of the cell cycle (q.v.), when DNA replication occurs, and before cell division, somatic cells (see "diploid") are tetraploid.

Tumor: see "Cancer".

Tumor biology: study of the biological characteristics of tumors.

Tumor heterogeneity: dissimilarity of the characteristics of a single tumor's cells.

Vaccination: intentional administration of a harmless or less harmful form of a pathogen to induce a specific immune response that protects the individual against later exposure to the same pathogen. Vaccination can also be performed by injecting foreign molecules.

Vascular growth phase: an advanced stage in the growth of a tumor, when its survival depends on the oxygen and nourishment provided by its newly formed blood vessels. See also "avascular growth phase".

Winnie-the-Pooh: a teddy bear extremely fond of honey, and the leading character (along with Christopher Robin, the author's son, and his other toy animals) in a series of adventures in two children's classics published by the English writer A.A. Milne in 1926 and 1928.

Xenograft: a graft transplanted from a donor of one species to a host of another species.